HAS

1999

Hospital

Accreditation

Standards

Joint Commission Mission

The mission of the Joint Commission on Accreditation of Healthcare Organizations is to improve the quality of care provided to the public through the provision of health care accreditation and related services that support performance improvement in health care organizations.

© 1999 by the Joint Commission on Accreditation of Healthcare Organizations

All rights reserved. No part of this publication may be reproduced in any form or by any means without written permission from the publisher.

Printed in the U.S.A.

Requests for permission to make copies of any part of this work should be mailed to:
Permissions Editor
Department of Publications
Joint Commission on Accreditation of Healthcare Organizations
One Renaissance Boulevard
Oakbrook Terrace, Illinois 60181

ISBN: 0-86688-625-7
ISSN: 1522-1083

For more information about the Joint Commission, please visit our Web site at http://www.jcaho.org

Contents

Introduction 1

The Accreditation Cycle: Official Accreditation Policies and Procedures 7

Accreditation Participation Requirements 41

Standards and Intents

Section I: Patient-Focused Functions
Patients Rights and Organization Ethics (RI) 47
Assessment of Patients (PE) 61
Care of Patients (TX) 77
Education (PF) 113
Continuum of Care (CC) 121

Section II: Organization-Focused Functions
Improving Organization Performance (PI) 129
Leadership (LD) 143
Management of the Environment of Care (EC) 163
Management of Human Resources (HR) 187
Management of Information (IM) 193
Surveillance, Prevention, and Control of Infection (IC) 215

Section III: Structures with Functions
Governance (GO) 219
Management (MA) 225
Medical Staff (MS) 229
Nursing (NR) 275

Glossary 281

Index 309

Introduction

The *1999 Hospital Accreditation Standards* (*HAS*) contains the standards, intent statements, accreditation policies and procedures, and the glossary from the *Comprehensive Accreditation Manuals for Hospitals: The Official Handbook* (*CAMH*). This introduction is designed to provide you with information on the following topics:
- New materials for this edition; and
- Accreditation process initiatives: continuous accreditation, the Orion Project, and the use of performance measures in the accreditation process. The following sections introduce important developments relevant to hospital accreditation. For the purpose of readability and ease of use, this introduction is organized in a question-and-answer format.

If, after reading the *HAS*, you have questions about this book or the accreditation process, please contact the Joint Commission. Table 1, pages 2 and 3, includes a list of resources for your convenience.

What's New in the *HAS*?

Changes to the *HAS* have been made in response to suggestions from customers and relate to important issues that clearly support quality patient care. In the past year, many chapters have been revised and improved to include additional information requested by customers. Table 2, page 4, summarizes the major revisions that occurred during 1998.

How Is Technology Enhancing the Accreditation Survey Process?

The Surveyor Laptop Technology Project.
In January 1996, the Joint Commission implemented surveyor laptop technology into the survey process. Surveyors now use laptop computers to enter their survey findings on site. The laptop computers are equipped with specially designed decision-support software. The software is designed to
- improve the validity and reliability of the survey results;
- enable surveyors to provide the hospital with a preliminary report on site at the end of the survey; and
- reduce turnaround time on the hospital's final accreditation report.

Each member of the survey team gathers and inputs data into the laptop computer. The special software guides the gathering of data, integrates team members' findings, scores the standards, aggregates scores, and compiles a draft survey report. Since the software completes the scoring, the reliability and validity of the accreditation process are significantly improved.

Preliminary Reports. Among the advantages of the surveyor laptop technology is the production of a draft accreditation decision report for review before the survey team leaves the hospital. This preliminary report is provided to the hospital's chief executive officer and used during the survey team's presentation of the survey findings at the Leadership Exit Conference. These reports are preliminary; the final *Official Accreditation Decision Report* may differ from the preliminary report. A final accreditation decision is made following review of the survey findings at the Joint Commission's central office. This process is designed to minimize and, in most cases, eliminate the differences between the preliminary and final reports.

The Joint Commission cautions hospitals that want to make their preliminary reports public that the preliminary report is *not* a final decision. Hospitals are encouraged to use the preliminary report

Table 1. Whom Do I Call?

The following is a list of information resources at the Joint Commission. You can contact the appropriate person by phone, mail, or fax.

By phone: The Joint Commission's **main** telephone number is **630/792-5000**. If you are telephoning, you can also contact the appropriate department directly for the specific issues listed below. The Joint Commission's business hours are 8:30 AM to 5:00 PM central standard time, Monday through Friday. Customer service representatives are available from 8:00 AM to 5:00 PM central standard time Monday through Friday. The **Customer Service** telephone number is **630/792-5800**.

By mail: Mail materials to the Joint Commission at the following address:
Joint Commission on Accreditation of Healthcare Organizations
One Renaissance Boulevard
Oakbrook Terrace, IL 60181

By fax: The Joint Commission's main fax number is **630/792-5005**.

Call the Hospital Accreditation Operations
East 630/792-5872 (CT, DC, DE, KY, MA, MD, ME, NC, NH, NJ, NY, RI, SC, VA, VT, WV)
South 630/792-5019 (AL, AR, FL, GA, LA, MS, PR, TN, TX)
West 630/792-5014 (AK, AZ, CA, CO, HI, ID, KS, MT, NE, ND, NM, NV, OK, OR, SD, UT, WA, WY)
Midwest 630/792-5021 (IA, IL, IN, MI, MN, MO, OH, PA, WI)
if you have a question about
- application for survey for hospitals;
- scheduling of surveys;
- survey agenda or survey process;
- status of your survey report;
- content of your survey report;
- written progress reports (WPRs);
- focused surveys; and
- surveys of home organizations.

Call the Department of Standards at 630/792-5900 if you have a question about
- interpretation of hospital standards and
- development of hospital standards.

Call Customer Service at 630/792-5800 if you have a question about
- general information about Joint Commission products, services, mission, or history;
- your organization's accreditation status or history;
- obtaining a free Joint Commission Publications or Education catalog;
- orders for Joint Commission publications and registration for education seminars; and
- performance reports.

Call the Pricing Unit at 630/792-5115 if you have a question about
- survey fee information.

Table 1. Whom Do I Call? (continued)

Call the Department of Publications at 630/792-5498 if you have a question about
- Joint Commission publications.

Call the Department of Education at 630/792-5398 if you have a question about
- custom education programs.

Call the Department of Communications at 630/792-5631 if you have a question about
- publicizing your accreditation.

Call the ORYX Information Line at 630/792-5085 if you have a question about
- the requirements for the ORYX initiative, the scoring of the requirements, or the effect on the survey process;
- performance measurement systems;
- the technicalities of data submission; or
- ORYX PLUS.

Call the Sentinel Event Hotline at 630/792-3700 if you have a question about
- providing information about a Joint Commission accredited organization;
- the Joint Commission sentinel event policy; and
- self-reporting a sentinel event.

Call the Speakers' Bureau at 630/792-4633 if you have a question about
- arranging for a Joint Commission expert to address your organization's staff on issues of concern.

Information About Other Joint Commission Accreditation Programs

Ambulatory care accreditation	630/792-5732
Behavioral health care accreditation	630/792-5788
Health care networks accreditation	630/792-5295
Home care accreditation	630/792-5754
Laboratory accreditation	630/792-5771 or 630/792-5778
Long term care accreditation	630/792-5721 or 630/792-5791
Long term care pharmacy accreditation	630/792-5752

for quality improvement purposes only. However, if a hospital chooses to publicize its preliminary report, it should emphasize that the findings are preliminary.

The Joint Commission will not be able to comment to members of the news media or community on the findings and decision reflected in the preliminary report. The accreditation decision and report are official only after the final accreditation decision report is sent to the hospital.

Web site. The Joint Commission's award-winning Web site is a valuable resource for hospitals. It provides

- up-to-date information about Joint Commission initiatives, including the Sentinel Event policy, Accreditation Watch, and ORYX;
- a complete collection of ORYX listed performance measurement systems and candidate measurement systems with links to their Web sites;
- information about accreditation programs;

1999 Hospital Accreditation Standards

Table 2. Summary of Major Revisions During 1998

Chapter	Content Summary
Introduction	■ Explanation of Quality Check™ ■ Summary of 1998 revisions
The Accreditation Cycle	■ Revised survey postponement policy ■ Revised public information policy ■ Revised sentinel event policy, root cause analysis information, and Accreditation Watch information *(handwritten: Risk)* ■ New Integrated Survey Process description ■ Integrated Survey Process expanded to include all psychiatric hospitals and behavioral health care components of small hospitals ■ Revised public release of compliant information policy
Accreditation Participation Requirements	■ Clarified requirement 7
Patient Rights and Organization Ethics (RI)	■ Revised RI.1.3.5 and intent statement ■ Revised RI.2 standard and intent statement
Care of Patients (TX)	■ Deleted TX.7.1.3.1 through TX.7.1.3.1.3 ■ Renumbered TX.7.1.3.2 through TX.7.1.3.3 ■ New TX.7.5, TX.7.5.1, TX.7.5.2, TX.7.5.3, TX.7.5.3.1, TX.7.5.3.2, TX.7.5.4, and TX.7.5.5 standards and intent statements
Improving Organization Performance (PI)	■ Revised PI chapter standards and intent statements
Leadership (LD)	■ New LD.4.3.4 standard and intent statement ■ Corrected leaders definition
Management of the Environment of Care (EC)	■ Revised intent statements for EC.1.3, EC.1.4, EC.1.5, EC.1.6, EC.1.7, EC.1.8, EC.1.9, EC.2.6, EC.2.12, EC.4, and EC.4.2 ■ Revised EC.1.7 standard ■ Revised EC.2.10, EC.3.2, EC.4.1, EC.4.3, and EC.4.4 standards and intent statements ■ Deleted EC.4.1.1, EC.4.1.2, EC.4.2.1, EC.4.2.2, EC.4.3.1, EC.4.3.2, EC.4.3.2.1, EC.4.4.1, and EC.4.4.2

continued on next page

Table 2. Summary of Major Revisions During 1998 (continued)

Chapter	Content Summary
Medical Staff (MS)	■ New notes for MS.5.4.3.1 through MS.5.4.3.2 intent statement ■ Corrected leaders definition
Nursing (NR)	■ Revised intent statement for NR.1
Glossary	■ Revised definitions, including the corrected leaders definition

© Joint Commission 1998.

- an electronic version of the *National Library of Healthcare Indicators*, a collection of 225 performance measure indicators judged to have face-validity; and
- other news and information.

A complete directory of Joint Commission accredited organizations is also available on the Web site. This new directory, Quality Check,™ includes the following information for each accredited health care organization:

- organization name, address, telephone number, and Web site address with e-mail contact, if available;
- accreditation decision based on the most recent full survey and accreditation date;
- current accreditation status and accreditation status effective date; and
- an easy-to-use, printable performance report (1996, 1997, 1998, and future reports).

The Joint Commission's Web site address is http://www.jcaho.org.

What Is Continuous Accreditation? Why Should My Hospital Be Interested in It?

Continuous accreditation refers to the process by which a hospital continuously evaluates and improves its processes to maintain performance that constantly meets or exceeds accreditation requirements. The Joint Commission is committed to helping hospitals move toward continuous accreditation.

For some hospitals accredited by the Joint Commission, the accreditation process involves a three-year performance measurement and improvement cycle driven by the timing of the triennial survey. In the 12 months prior to the survey, the hospital may devote considerable resources to getting ready for the survey. Performance improvement efforts may be undertaken and results measured in order to meet survey requirements. Upon completion of the survey, the hospital may return to "business as usual" and may reduce its focus on performance improvement efforts.

By participating in continuous accreditation efforts, hospitals monitor and improve their performance on a year-round, year-in-and-year-out basis. At any point in their triennial accreditation cycle, hospitals know how they are doing, are aware of performance areas, and know whether performance improvement efforts are achieving the desired results. Continuous improvement efforts help hospitals maintain the highest possible quality of patient care and services. In addition, hospitals can use their resources more wisely, avoiding the high cost of "gearing up" for a Joint Commission survey.

Hospitals interested in continuous accreditation efforts can perform continuous self-assessment using the accreditation standards in this book. The *CAMH* provides a tool for ongoing self-evaluation against nationally recognized standards. Hospitals may wish to focus on one or two chapters each month to review their processes and evaluate their progress with performance improvement initiatives. This kind of continuous self-assessment helps hospitals prepare for their Joint Commission survey by maintaining readiness through an ongoing self-assessment process.

What Is the Continuous Survey Readiness Project?

The Continuous Survey Readiness (CSR) project, formerly known as Orion, is an initiative designed to create a continuous accreditation process on a regional level, test accreditation models, and test an alternative process for reporting survey findings to hospitals. It also provides a platform to test customer-recommended changes to the accreditation process. Customers have indicated that they would like the accreditation process to be "close to home" and less resource intensive. They also want continuous Joint Commission support for their services and improvement initiatives and to be involved in decisions made about the accreditation process. CSR is currently being tested in Pennsylvania, Arizona, Tennessee, and Georgia.

How Will the Use of Performance Measures Be Integrated in the Accreditation Process?

The Joint Commission's current triennial, on-site survey process is evolving to include performance measurement data to continually assure the public and other interested stakeholders that continuous attention is being given to the care provided by health care organizations.

Following the data submission by the performance measurement system to the Joint Commission, Joint Commission staff will use criteria to review data trends and determine if contact with the health care organization is indicated (for example, a phone call, a request for a written progress report, or an on-site survey). Such reviews will begin once enough data points are available, presumably by the end of 1999. Particular attention will be given to the way in which the health care organization uses the data to analyze processes and improve care. In addition, a summary of organization performance data will be provided to surveyors for use during the regular on-site triennial survey.

The Accreditation Cycle: Official Accreditation Policies and Procedures

Chapter Overview

This chapter provides information relevant to all hospitals interested in Joint Commission accreditation, whether they are applying for the first time or on a renewal basis. The chapter describes the Joint Commission's official accreditation policies and procedures. They apply to all hospitals either currently accredited by, or seeking accreditation by, the Joint Commission.

The chapter includes information relevant to hospitals

- *at all times* (general information), including accreditation eligibility; survey scope, options, and fees; and information, and public information policies;
- *before the survey,* including an overview of the survey process, survey application and scheduling, the survey team and agenda, notifying the public about a Joint Commission survey, and conducting public information interviews;
- *during the survey,* including how the Joint Commission handles patient care or safety concerns, on-site survey activities, the use of laptop technology during the survey, and preliminary accreditation reports;
- *following the survey,* including accreditation decisions, survey report revision requests, and decision appeals; and
- *before the next survey,* including monitoring between surveys, the duration of accreditation awards, the accreditation renewal process, notification of organization changes between surveys, and unscheduled and unannounced surveys.

The chapter is organized into major sections reflecting these categories. You will be able to locate the policies and procedures applicable to your hospital according to where your hospital is in the accreditation process or cycle. A hospital must follow the policies and procedures described in this chapter in order to participate and continue to participate in the accreditation process. A hospital that fails to follow the policies and procedures described in this chapter may be considered to have withdrawn from the accreditation process.

Note: *The "Accreditation Participation Requirements" chapter (pages 41 through 46) includes specific requirements for accreditation participation. Requirements 1 through 3 and 7 through 10 are existing policies within this "Accreditation Cycle" chapter and are currently effective for accreditation purposes. Cross-references to the accreditation participation requirements can be found in the applicable sections of this chapter.*

General Information

This section provides information relevant to a hospital either applying for Joint Commission accreditation or seeking continued accreditation. Since this material is revised on a regular basis, all hospitals are encouraged to review it.

Hospitals Eligible for Survey

General Eligibility Requirements. Any hospital may apply for a Joint Commission accreditation survey under the standards in this book* if the following requirements are met:
- The hospital is in the United States or its territories or, if outside the United States, is operated by the United States government, under a charter of the United States Congress, or for other hospitals outside of the United States that meet the following criteria:
  - ❑ The nature of the health care practices in the applicant hospital is compatible with the intents of Joint Commission standards;
  - ❑ With the use of available translators, as necessary, the surveyors can effectively communicate with substantially all of the hospital's management and clinical personnel and at least half of the hospital's patients, and can understand medical records and documents that relate to the hospital's performance; or
  - ❑ United States citizens make up at least 10% of the hospital's patient population
      OR
    A United States government agency contracts with the hospital to provide services to United States citizens
      OR
    United States citizens preferentially use the hospital in that country.
- The hospital assesses and improves the quality of its services. This process includes a review of care by clinicians, when appropriate.
- The hospital identifies the services it provides, indicating which services it provides directly, under contract, or through some other arrangement.
- The hospital provides services addressed by the Joint Commission's standards.

Purpose of a Survey

A Joint Commission accreditation survey provides an assessment of a hospital's compliance with standards and their intent statements developed by the Joint Commission. The Joint Commission evaluates a hospital's compliance based on
- verbal information provided to the Joint Commission;
- on-site observations by Joint Commission surveyors; and
- documents provided by the hospital.

The survey is key to accreditation. The Joint Commission's accreditation process seeks to help organizations identify and correct problems and improve the quality of care and services provided. In addition to evaluating compliance with standards and their intent statements, significant time is spent in consultation and education.

Scope of Accreditation Surveys

General Survey Categories. The Joint Commission surveys and accredits health care organizations using standards from one or more of the following manuals:
- *Comprehensive Accreditation Manual for Ambulatory Care*;
- *Comprehensive Accreditation Manual for Behavioral Health Care*;
- *Comprehensive Accreditation Manual for Health Care Networks*;
- *Comprehensive Accreditation Manual for Home Care*;
- *Comprehensive Accreditation Manual for Hospitals: The Official Handbook*;

---

* The Joint Commission will work with the hospital to determine which standards from other accreditation programs are applicable.

- *Comprehensive Accreditation Manual for Long Term Care* (includes standards for dementia special care units and subacute care programs);
- *Comprehensive Accreditation Manual for Long Term Care Pharmacies*;
- *Comprehensive Accreditation Manual for Pathology and Clinical Laboratory Services*;
- *Accreditation Manual for Preferred Provider Organizations*; and
- *Comprehensive Accreditation Manual for Managed Behavioral Health Care.*

Tailored Surveys. The Joint Commission tailors its survey to reflect the services offered by the organization. The Joint Commission creates a tailored survey for an organization providing services covered by standards in more than one of the accreditation manuals listed above. The tailored survey will be based on the services provided by the hospital as reported in its Application for Survey. The Joint Commission provides the organization with a copy of each of the manuals to be used in the survey before it is conducted. The Joint Commission determines which manuals are applicable based on information provided in the Application for Survey.

Integrated Survey Process. In January 1998, the Joint Commission launched the Integrated Survey Process (ISP) for small hospitals with an average daily census of less than 40 that have long term care and/or home care services. The ISP reduces duplication by offering a single survey with a single team of surveyors and replaces the tailored survey process, which requires additional surveyors for additional components evaluated in small hospitals. The new process includes evaluating performance in those functions that are common across the hospital's components once for the entire organization. Through the ISP, small hospitals with one additional component (long term care or home care services) will be surveyed by two surveyors for three days. Small hospitals with both of these components will be surveyed by two surveyors for four days. Beginning in January 1999, the ISP will be extended to include behavioral health care components (partial hospitalization and residential services) in small hospitals and all psychiatric hospitals regardless of size. The ISP will be expanded to include additional settings in the future.

Single Accreditation Awards. The Joint Commission survey, assuming satisfactory compliance, provides one accreditation award for all of the organization's services, programs, and related organizations. Included in each organization's survey and accreditation decision are all services, programs, and related organizations that are
- organizationally and functionally integrated or
- publicly represented as a part of the organization.

Organizational and functional integration refer to the degree to which the service, program, or related entity is owned and operated by the applicant organization. A service, program, or related entity is any organized health care delivery site that is eligible for survey. These include, among others, physician practices owned or operated by hospitals, rural clinics, laboratories, and hospices, as well as other organizations traditionally accredited by the Joint Commission.

Organizational integration exists when the applicant organization's governing body, either directly or ultimately, controls budgetary and resource allocation decisions for both the applicant organization *and* the service, program, or related entity included in the survey. Organizational integration also exists when separate corporate entities share more than 50% of the same governing body membership.

Functional integration exists when the entity meets three of the following criteria, including criterion 1 or 2:
1. The applicant organization and the service, program, or related entity
    - use the same process for determining membership of licensed independent practitioners in practitioner panels or medical or professional staff or
    - have a common organized medical or professional staff.

2. The applicant organization's human resources function hires and assigns staff at the service, program, or related entity and has the authority to
   - terminate staff at the entity,
   - transfer staff between the applicant organization and the entity, and
   - conduct performance appraisals of the staff who work in the entity.
3. With few exceptions, the applicant organization's policies and procedures are applicable to the service, program, or related entity.
4. The applicant organization manages significant operations of the service, program, or related entity; that is, the service, program, or related entity has little or no management authority or autonomy independent of the applicant organization.
5. The service, program, or related entity's patient records are integrated in the applicant organization's patient record system.
6. The applicant organization applies its performance improvement program to the entity and has authority to implement actions intended to improve performance at the service, program, or related entity.
7. The applicant organization bills for services provided by the service, program, or related entity under the name of the applicant organization.

The Joint Commission assesses an organization's public representation of its services by examining letterhead, brochures, telephone book listings, and other advertising media. Commonality of names may also be relevant.

The Joint Commission evaluates all health care services provided by the organization for which the Joint Commission has standards and makes one accreditation decision and survey report. An organization must be prepared to provide evidence of its compliance with each applicable standard. To gain accreditation, an organization must demonstrate *overall* compliance with the standards and their intent statements, not necessarily compliance with *each* standard and its intent statement.

Contracted Services. The Joint Commission evaluates the hospital's assessment of the quality of services provided under contractual arrangements. The Joint Commission reserves the right to evaluate, as part of its survey, services provided by another organization or provider.

However, the Joint Commission will not ordinarily do so if the contracted organization is separately accredited by the Joint Commission. It may, however, survey performance issues between the contracted organization and the applicant organization, regardless of the accreditation status of the contracted organization. The Joint Commission also surveys services provided on site under contract.

Multihospital Option

The Joint Commission offers multihospital systems that own or lease at least two hospitals the option of a modified survey process. This option has three components:
- A corporate orientation;
- A consecutive survey of participating organizations with the same survey team leader; and
- A corporate summation.

A system may choose to have either a corporate orientation, a corporate summation, or both. The orientation session provides an opportunity for corporate staff to orient the survey team to the structure and practices of the system. The survey team will also survey centralized corporate services, documentation, and policies and procedures applicable to Joint Commission standards. The corporate summation provides an overall analysis of the system's strengths and weaknesses. It also provides consultation and education related to accreditation survey findings across the system. There is a separate fee for the corporate orientation and corporate summation.

Continuity in the composition of the survey team will be maintained by the survey team leader. The remaining members of the survey team will rotate every third or fourth survey, depending on the location of the hospitals being surveyed. The survey team leader will compile the information necessary to support the corporate summation.

A rotating surveyor is selected to survey a hospital within a system based on the region in which the hospital is located and to which the surveyor is assigned. Therefore, although the team leader may cross geographic regions and survey outside of his or her assigned region, rotating surveyors will be selected to survey system hospitals only within their assigned region.

Through the multihospital option, the Joint Commission accredits the individual health care organizations that are part of a multihospital system, not the system itself. Therefore, each hospital within a system will receive its own accreditation decision and report. The findings and decision for one hospital within a system will have no bearing on those of another hospital within the system.

Early Survey Policy

A hospital wishing to be accredited by the Joint Commission may choose one of two Early Survey Policy Options described here. Under Option 1 and Option 2, hospitals are required to undergo two surveys. However, the nature of the surveys and the potential outcomes differ. The first survey under Option 2 is a full accreditation survey, rather than the more limited first survey under Option 1. The Joint Commission has been notified by the Health Care Financing Administration (HCFA) that Option 2 will also meet the needs of hospitals seeking Medicare certification. It is the hospital's responsibility to confirm with HCFA the use of this option for the purposes of Medicare certification. The Public Information Policy (pages 20 through 23) applies to both Option 1 and Option 2 described below.

The side bar on page 13 highlights Early Survey Options 1 and 2 and describes the potential outcomes of each survey.

Option 1 (Provisional Accreditation)
A. *Eligibility.* This option is available to any hospital that is currently not accredited *except* a hospital that has been denied accreditation because it provided falsified information within the past year. Hospitals must declare during the application process that they wish to be surveyed under this option.
B. *The First Survey.* When a hospital chooses Option 1, the Joint Commission will conduct two on-site surveys. It can conduct the first survey as early as two months before the hospital begins operating, provided it meets the following criteria:
   - It is licensed or has a provisional license, according to applicable law and regulation;
   - The building in which the services will be offered or from which the services will be coordinated is identified, constructed, and equipped to support such services;
   - It has identified its chief executive officer or administrator; its director of clinical or medical affairs; its nurse executive, if applicable; and its director of clinical services; and
   - It has identified the date it will begin operations.

   Generally, the first survey uses a limited set of standards and assesses only the hospital's physical facilities, policies and procedures, plans, and related structural considerations.
C. *Provisional Accreditation.* The Joint Commission grants provisional accreditation to a hospital in overall compliance with the standards and their intent statements assessed in the first survey under Option 1. A hospital *not* in overall compliance must reapply and begin the accreditation process again. A hospital that meets the decision rules for conditional accreditation will also be granted provisional accreditation status.

   The provisional accreditation decision will include assignment of a "special type I recommendation" indicating the requirement for survey against the full set of applicable standards, including all track record requirements. Other type I recommendations may also be assigned based on survey findings from the first survey.

For a hospital operating when the survey is conducted, the effective date for its provisional accreditation status is the day after the survey was conducted. For a hospital not in operation, the effective date is the day after it begins operating. If the hospital is not in operation at the time of survey, the hospital must confirm in writing the date it begins operating.

Provisional accreditation status remains until the hospital has completed a second, full survey or the Joint Commission has withdrawn the Provisional Accreditation. The Joint Commission may withdraw provisional accreditation
- when a hospital that was not providing services at the time of the first survey does not begin services when expected;
- if a hospital does not meet the survey eligibility criteria (see page 8); or
- if a hospital fails to accept the date of the second survey.

In these cases, the hospital must begin the accreditation process again.

D. *The Second Survey.* The second survey is a full accreditation survey. The Joint Commission conducts this survey
- approximately six months after the first survey; and
- at least four months after the hospital has begun operating.

The hospital's accreditation status, based on survey results, will change to
- accreditation with commendation;
- accreditation;
- accreditation with type I recommendations;
- conditional accreditation;
- preliminary nonaccreditation; or
- not accredited.

The effective date of the accreditation decision is the day after the second survey.

A type I recommendation(s) addresses insufficient or unsatisfactory compliance with standards and their intent statements in a specific performance area. A hospital receiving any such recommendations is required to resolve them within specified time frames to remain accredited. The hospital's three-year accreditation cycle begins the day after the second survey was conducted, unless the Joint Commission reached a decision not to accredit.

Option 2

A. *Eligibility.* Option 2 is available only to a hospital that has
- never been surveyed by the Joint Commission;
- been in actual operation for at least one month;
- cared for at least ten patients by the time of the first survey with at least one patient in active treatment at the time of survey.

B. *The First Survey.* When a hospital chooses Option 2, the Joint Commission will conduct an initial full accreditation survey. If the hospital demonstrates satisfactory compliance with standards and their intent statements in the first survey, it will be granted Accreditation with type I recommendations, including a "special type I recommendation" for insufficient track record of compliance. This accreditation decision reflects the preliminary nature of the assessed performance. At a minimum, the recommendations will relate to limited or absent track records of performance in the functional areas where these are required. The effective date of the accreditation decision is the day after the *first* survey.

Early Survey Policy Options

Option 1

First survey
Can be conducted up to two months before operations begin. Survey of a limited set of standards addressing physical plant, policies and procedures, plans, and related structural considerations for patient care.

Successful outcome:
Provisional accreditation.

Second survey
Full survey conducted approximately six months after the first survey.

Possible outcomes:
Change in Provisional Accreditation status to Accreditation with Commendation, Accreditation with or without Type I Recommendations, Conditional Accreditation, or Preliminary Nonaccreditation. The effective date of the accreditation decision is the day after the *second* survey.

Option 2

First survey
Must be in operation at least one month and has demonstrated a defined minimum level of patient care service with at least one patient in active treatment at the time of survey.

Possible outcomes:
Accreditation with Type I Recommendations, including a "Special Type I Recommendation" for insufficient track record of compliance; Conditional Accreditation; or Preliminary Nonaccreditation.

Second survey
Conducted four months after the first survey. Survey addresses track record requirements not evaluated during the initial survey and may address standards compliance issues identified in the first survey. Based on the findings of either survey, follow-up activities such as focused surveys and written progress reports might be required.

Possible outcomes:
Accreditation with or without Type I Recommendations, Conditional Accreditation, or Preliminary Nonaccreditation. The effective date of the accreditation decision is the day after the *first* survey.

C. *The Second Survey.* The hospital will undergo a follow-up survey in four months to address track record requirements that could not be assessed during the first survey due to the limited time of operation. The full scope of applicable standards will be reviewed with particular attention being paid to the issue of sustained performance since the first survey. Other follow-up activities such as focused surveys and written progress reports may be required on the basis of survey findings from either of the two surveys.

Initial Surveys

Hospitals that are not currently accredited and that are seeking accreditation are eligible for an Initial Survey. The full scope of applicable standards will be reviewed during the survey. The scoring of the standards will be based on a 4-month track record of compliance, rather than the 12-month track record of compliance required for triennial surveys.

Sentinel Events

A sentinel event is an unexpected occurrence involving death or serious physical or psychological injury, or the risk thereof. Serious injury specifically includes loss of limb or function. The phrase, "or the risk thereof," includes any process variation for which a recurrence would carry a significant chance of a serious adverse outcome.

Such events are called "sentinel" because they signal the need for immediate investigation and response. Accredited organizations are expected to identify and respond appropriately to *all* sentinel events occurring in the organization or associated with services that the organization provides or provides for. Appropriate response includes a thorough and credible root cause analysis, implementation of improvements to reduce risk, and monitoring of the effectiveness of those improvements. An organization that completes an acceptable root cause analysis in response to a sentinel event will *not* be placed on Accreditation Watch.*

Organizations' activities in response to sentinel events will be routinely assessed as part of all triennial and random unannounced surveys.

Reporting of Sentinel Events to the Joint Commission

Organizations are encouraged to report a sentinel event to the Joint Commission if the event has resulted in an unanticipated death or major permanent loss of function not related to the natural course of the patient's illness or underlying condition,[†‡] or the event is one of the following (even if the outcome was not death or major permanent loss of function):

- Suicide of a patient in a setting where the patient receives around-the-clock care (such as a hospital, residential treatment center, crisis stabilization center);
- Infant abduction or discharge to the wrong family;
- Rape;[§]
- Hemolytic transfusion reaction involving administration of blood or blood products having major blood group incompatibilities; or
- Surgery on the wrong patient or wrong body part.**

---

* **Accreditation Watch** An attribute of an organization's Joint Commission accreditation status. A health care organization is placed on Accreditation Watch when a sentinel event has occurred and a thorough and credible root cause analysis of the sentinel event has not been completed within a specified time frame. Although Accreditation Watch status is not an official accreditation category, it can be publicly disclosed by the Joint Commission.

† "Major permanent loss of function" means sensory, motor, physiologic, or intellectual impairment not present on admission requiring continued treatment or life-style change. When "major permanent loss of function" cannot be immediately determined, reporting is not expected until either the patient is discharged with continued major loss of function, or two weeks have elapsed with persistent major loss of function, whichever occurs first.

‡ A distinction is made between an adverse outcome that is related to the natural course of the patient's illness or underlying condition (not reportable) and a death or major permanent loss of function that is associated with the treatment, or lack of treatment, of that condition (reportable).

§ The determination of "rape" is to be based on the health care organization's definition, consistent with applicable law and regulation. Reporting of an allegation of rape is not expected. The five-day time frame for reporting begins when a determination is made that a rape has occurred. Reporting of a rape is not expected where such reporting is prohibited by law.

** All events of surgery on the wrong patient or wrong body part are reportable, regardless of the magnitude of the procedure.

An organization that reports a sentinel event to the Joint Commission within five business days of its occurrence (or its discovery by the organization) and submits to the Joint Commission an acceptable root cause analysis (as described below) within 45 days of reporting the event, will *not* be placed on Accreditation Watch.

If the Joint Commission receives an inquiry about the accreditation status of the organization during the 45-day analysis period, the organization's accreditation status will be reported in the usual manner without reference to the sentinel event. If the inquirer specifically references the sentinel event, the Joint Commission will acknowledge that it is aware of the event and is working with the organization through the *sentinel event review process*.

An organization which experiences a sentinel event that does not meet the criteria for review under the Sentinel Event Policy is expected to complete a root cause analysis. However, the root cause analysis need not be made available to the Joint Commission.

Figure 1, page 16, is a flowchart depicting the sentinel event process and Table 1, pages 17 through 20, details the steps taken during this process by both the Joint Commission and the organization experiencing a sentinel event.

Information Accuracy and Truthfulness Policy

Information provided at any time during the accreditation cycle by the hospital and used by the Joint Commission for accreditation purposes must be accurate and truthful.* Such information may
- be provided verbally;
- be obtained through direct observation by Joint Commission surveyors;
- be derived from documents supplied by the hospital to the Joint Commission; or
- involve data transmitted electronically to the Joint Commission.

The Joint Commission requires each hospital seeking accreditation to engage in the accreditation process in good faith. The Joint Commission may deny or remove accreditation from any hospital failing to participate in good faith by falsifying information presented in the accreditation process, among other possible acts.

The Joint Commission's information policy includes the following:
1. A hospital must never provide the Joint Commission with falsified information during the accreditation process. The Joint Commission construes any efforts to do so as a violation of the hospital's obligation to engage in the accreditation process in good faith.
2. Falsification is defined for this policy as the fabrication, in whole or in part, of any information provided by an applicant or accredited hospital to the Joint Commission. This includes, but is not limited to, any redrafting, reformatting, or content deletion of documents.
3. The hospital may submit additional material that summarizes or otherwise explains original information submitted to the Joint Commission. These materials must be properly identified, dated, and accompanied by the original documents.
4. Annually, each hospital must submit to the Joint Commission a signed certification attesting to the accuracy and truthfulness of all information provided, or to be provided, throughout the accreditation cycle. Such certification should be signed by the chief executive officer, the chairperson of the governing body, and the chief of the medical staff (or leader of the professional staff).
5. The Joint Commission does not release the hospital's accreditation award or survey report until it has received the hospital's properly signed certification for the current year.

---

* See Requirement 9 on page 45 in the Accreditation Participation Requirements chapter.

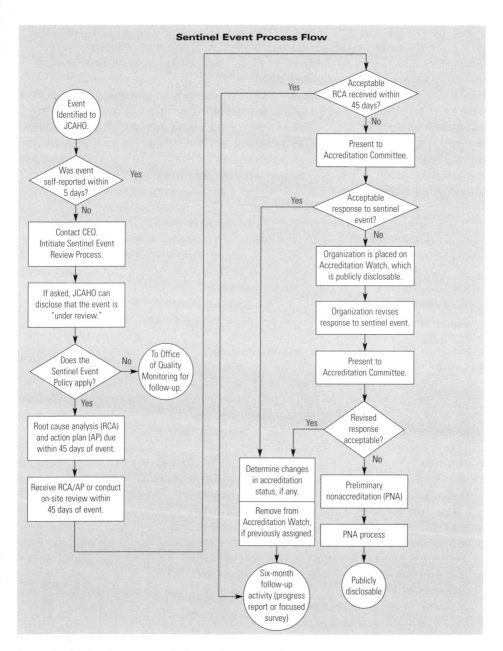

Figure 1. *This flowchart represents the Sentinel Event process.*

6. The Joint Commission conducts an evaluation when it has cause to believe that an accredited hospital may have provided falsified information. Except as otherwise authorized by the president of the Joint Commission, the evaluation includes an unannounced on-site survey.

This survey uses special protocols designed to address the alleged information falsification. It assesses the degree of actual hospital compliance with the standards and their intent statements that are the subject of the allegation, if appropriate.

The Accreditation Cycle: Official Accreditation Policies and Procedures

Table 1. The Sentinel Event Procedures

Voluntary Self-Reporting of Sentinel Events to the Joint Commission
- If an organization wishes to self-report an occurrence in the subset of sentinel events that are subject to review by the Joint Commission, the organization will be required to complete a self-reporting form. To be considered a "self-reported sentinel event," this form must be received by the Joint Commission no later than five business days following the event, or the organization's becoming aware of the event.
- The organization will be required to
  - prepare an acceptable root cause analysis and action plan within 45 calendar days of the self-report, and
  - submit those documents to the Joint Commission, or otherwise provide for Joint Commission evaluation of its response to the sentinel event under an approved protocol, within 45 calendar days of the self-report.

Sentinel Events That Are Not Self-Reported
- If the Joint Commission becomes aware of a sentinel event subject to review under the Sentinel Event Policy that was not self-reported by the organization, the Chief Executive Officer of the organization is contacted, and a preliminary assessment of the sentinel event is made.
- The organization will be required to
  - prepare an acceptable root cause analysis and action plan within 45 calendar days of the event, or of its becoming aware of the event, and
  - submit those documents to the Joint Commission, or otherwise provide for Joint Commission evaluation of its response to the sentinel event under an approved protocol, within 45 calendar days of the event, or of its becoming aware of the event.

On-site Review of a Sentinel Event
- An on-site review of a sentinel event will usually not be conducted unless it is determined that there is a potential ongoing threat to patient health or safety or potentially significant non-compliance with major Joint Commission standards. If an on-site ("for-cause") review is conducted, the organization will be billed an appropriate amount to cover the costs of conducting such a survey.

Disclosable Information
- If, during the 45-day analysis period, the Joint Commission receives an inquiry about the accreditation status of an organization that has experienced a sentinel event, the organization's accreditation status will be reported in the usual manner without making reference to the sentinel event.
- If the inquirer specifically references the sentinel event, the Joint Commission will acknowledge that it is aware of the event and is working with the organization through the *sentinel event review process.*

Initiation of Accreditation Watch
- If an organization has experienced a sentinel event but fails to submit or otherwise make available an acceptable root cause analysis and action plan, or otherwise provide for Joint Commission evaluation of its response to the sentinel event under an

continued on next page

Table 1. The Sentinel Event Procedures (continued)

approved protocol, within 45 days of the event, or of its becoming aware of the event, a recommendation will be made to the Accreditation Committee to place the organization on Accreditation Watch. If the Accreditation Committee places the organization on Accreditation Watch, the organization will then be permitted an additional 15 days to submit an acceptable root cause analysis and action plan, or otherwise provide for Joint Commission evaluation of its response to the sentinel event under an approved protocol.
- The Accreditation Watch status will be publicly disclosed, and the organization will be offered assistance in performing a root-cause analysis of the event.
- In all cases of organization refusal to permit review of information regarding a sentinel event in accordance with the Sentinel Event Policy and its approved protocols, the initial response by the Joint Commission is assignment of Accreditation Watch. Continued refusal may result in loss of accreditation.

The Organization's Response
Any organization that experiences a sentinel event subject to the Sentinel Event Policy must:
- Execute a root cause analysis that
  - focuses primarily on systems and processes, not individual performance;
  - progresses from special causes in clinical processes to common causes in organizational processes; and
  - identifies potential improvement in processes or systems that would tend to decrease the likelihood of such events in the future, or determines, after analysis, that no such improvement opportunities exist.
- Develop an action plan that
  - is based on the root cause analysis; and
  - as appropriate, identifies changes to be made in systems and processes—either through redesign or development of new systems or processes—that would reduce the risk of such events occurring in the future.
- Implement (after initial testing, if appropriate) the system and process improvements identified in its action plan.
- Design and apply an appropriate approach for evaluating the effectiveness of the improvements.

Submission of Root Cause Analysis and Action Plan
- The organization that experiences a sentinel event subject to the Sentinel Event Policy is asked to submit two documents:
  - the complete root cause analysis, including its findings; and
  - the resulting action plan that describes the organization's risk reduction strategies and strategy for evaluating their effectiveness.
- The root cause analysis and action plan are *not* to include the patient's name or the names of care givers involved in the sentinel event.
- Alternatively, if the organization has concerns about increased risk of legal exposure as a result of sending the root cause analysis documents to the Joint Commission, three additional options for on-site review are available:

continued on next page

Table 1. The Sentinel Event Procedures (continued)

- ❑ An on-site visit by a specially trained surveyor to review the root cause analysis and action plan, at a charge sufficient to cover the direct costs of the visit.
- ❑ An on-site visit by a specially trained surveyor to conduct interviews and review relevant documentation to verify the appropriate response to the sentinel event, at a charge sufficient to cover the direct costs of the visit. For purposes of this review activity, "relevant documentation" includes, at a minimum, any documentation relevant to the organization's process for responding to sentinel events, and the action plan resulting from the analysis of the subject sentinel event (to serve as the basis for appropriate follow-up activity).
- ❑ Where the organization meets specified criteria respecting the risk of waiving legal protection for root cause analysis information shared with the Joint Commission, an on-site visit by a specially trained surveyor to conduct interviews and review relevant documentation to obtain information about:
  - the process the organization uses in responding to sentinel events, and
  - the relevant policies and procedures preceding and following the organization's review of the specific event, and the implementation thereof,
  sufficient to permit inferences about the adequacy of the organization's response to the sentinel event, at a charge sufficient to cover the direct costs of the visit.
- ■ A request for on-site option 1, 2, or 3 must be received by the Joint Commission at least 15 days prior to the due date for the root cause analysis and action plan.

The Joint Commission's Response
- ■ Staff assesses the acceptability of the organization's response to the sentinel event, including the thoroughness and credibility of any root cause analysis information reviewed and the organization's action plan, and brings a recommendation to the Accreditation Committee at its next meeting following the due date for the organization's response.
- ■ If the response is unacceptable, the organization is required to address the inadequacies and submit, or make available for review, a new root cause analysis and action plan, or otherwise provide for further Joint Commission evaluation of its response to the sentinel event, within 15 days of notification that the Accreditation Committee has found the response to be unacceptable.
- ■ Depending on the nature and extent of the inadequacies of the organization's initial response to the sentinel event, the Joint Commission will determine whether an on-site visit should be made to assist the organization in understanding how to conduct an appropriate root cause analysis and develop an action plan.
- ■ If on review, the organization's response is still not acceptable, or the organization fails to respond, staff will recommend to the Accreditation Committee that the organization be placed in Preliminary Nonaccreditation. If approved by the Accreditation Committee, this accreditation decision would be publicly disclosed, and the process for resolution of Preliminary Nonaccreditation would be initiated.
- ■ When the organization's response (initial or revised) is found to be acceptable, the Joint Commission issues an *Official Accreditation Decision Report* that:

continued on next page

Table 1. The Sentinel Event Procedures (continued)

- ❑ reflects the Accreditation Committee's determination to continue or modify the organization's current accreditation status and terminate the Accreditation Watch (if previously assigned); and
- ❑ assigns an appropriate follow-up activity, typically a written progress report or follow-up visit to be conducted within six months.

Follow-up Activities
- The follow-up activity will assess, based on applicable standards, the implementation of system and process improvements identified in the action plan, the means by which the organization will continue to assess the effectiveness of those efforts, and the resolution of any type I recommendations. The follow-up activity will be conducted when the organization believes it can demonstrate effective implementation, but no later than six months following receipt of the *Official Accreditation Decision Report.*
- A decision to maintain or change the organization's accreditation status as a result of the follow-up activity or to assign additional follow-up requirements will be based on existing decision rules unless otherwise determined by the Accreditation Committee.
- Each sentinel event evaluated under the Joint Commission's Sentinel Event Policy will be reviewed at the organization's next full accreditation survey. This review will focus on implementation of risk reduction strategies and the effectiveness of these actions.

Handling Sentinel Event-Related Documents
- Upon completing the review of any submitted root cause analysis and action plan and abstracting the required data elements for the Joint Commission's Sentinel Event Database, the original root cause analysis documents will be returned to the organization and any copies will be shredded. Handling of these sensitive documents is restricted to specially trained staff in accordance with procedures designed to protect the confidentiality of the documents. The action plan resulting from the analysis of the sentinel event will be retained to serve as the basis for the follow-up activity.
- Once the action plan has been implemented to the satisfaction of the Joint Commission, as determined through follow-up activities, the Joint Commission will return the action plan to the organization.

7. The Joint Commission immediately takes action to deny accreditation or remove the accreditation award from an accredited hospital whenever the Joint Commission is reasonably persuaded that the hospital has provided falsified information.
8. The Joint Commission notifies responsible federal and state government agencies of any hospital subject to such action.
9. If a hospital becomes not accredited because it provided falsified information, the Joint Commission prohibits it from participating in the accreditation process for a period of one year. The president of the Joint Commission, for good cause only, may waive all or a portion of this waiting period.

Public Information Policy

The Joint Commission is committed to making relevant and accurate information about surveyed health care organizations available to interested persons. Information regarding the performance of a health care organization not only assists providers in improving their services, but also helps educate consumers. It also may help consumers and purchasers make informed choices in selecting health care providers. At the same time, it is important that confidentiality be maintained for certain information to encourage candor in the accreditation process. This candor facilitates improvement of the quality of health care to the benefit of the public.

Performance Reports. Performance reports are designed to provide useful and understandable information about the performance of organizations accredited by the Joint Commission. The Joint Commission began releasing organization-specific performance reports in December 1994 for most types of health care organizations undergoing full surveys after January 1, 1994. Reports for laboratories subsequently became available for those labs surveyed after January 1, 1995. Reports for health care networks will become available once this accreditation program includes a statistically significant sample. Joint Commission performance reports for each accredited organization include the following information:
- The date of the most recent triennial survey;
- The accreditation decision based on the most recent triennial survey;
- An organization's current accreditation status, including any designation attached to that status, such as Accreditation Watch, and the date on which that designation became effective;
- The date of the most recent follow-up activity for the organization, if any;
- The organization's overall evaluation score, based on the triennial survey, and national comparison to scores for comparable organizations;
- The organization's score for each performance area evaluated and national comparisons to scores for comparable organizations;
- Performance areas with recommendations for improvement;
- Subsequent change(s) in accreditation status, if any;
- Subsequent resolution of recommendations for improvement and the date(s) of resolution for specific performance areas;
- Subsequent new performance area(s) having recommendations for improvement and the date(s) assigned;
- The organization's updated overall evaluation score and performance area scores; and
- Organizational and operational components included in the accreditation survey.

Each accredited organization is afforded the opportunity to prepare a commentary of up to two pages regarding its performance report. The commentary is to accompany any organization performance reports distributed by the Joint Commission.

Each performance report released by the Joint Commission is also to be accompanied by an explanatory document that supports the accurate interpretation of the report.

The Joint Commission also may provide access to performance reports through the Internet and may make available information contained in performance reports to other third-party providers of information.

Performance measurement data will be included in performance reports when those data become an integral part of the accreditation process. These data will be released provided that the following conditions are met:
- The data are accompanied by an explanation of their
  - source or derivation;
  - accuracy, reliability, and validity;
  - appropriate uses; and
  - limitations and potential misuses.
- No data will be published unless it contains at least 12 monthly data points.
- No data will be published until the organization has had an opportunity to comment on them.

Information That is Publicly Disclosed on Request. In addition to information provided in performance reports, the following information may be obtained by writing or calling the Joint Commission:
- The organization's accreditation history;
- Any special recognition conferred on the organization, such as the Ernest A. Codman Award or participation in ORYX PLUS;
- Survey fees paid by an accredited organization;
- The organization's scheduled survey date(s) once the organization has been notified of the dates;
- Confirmation of the occurrence of a sentinel event in an accredited organization and the Joint Commission's intent to evaluate this occurrence;
- Applicable standards used for an accreditation survey;
- For a tailored survey, the organizational component(s) contributing to a conditional accreditation or denial of accreditation decision;
- Whether there were any type I recommendations for which the Joint Commission had no, or insufficient, evidence of resolution when an organization withdrew from accreditation;
- The performance areas for which the Joint Commission had no, or insufficient, evidence of resolution of type I recommendations when an organization withdrew from accreditation; and
- Whether an on-site evaluation of an organization in which a sentinel event has occurred is to be or has been conducted.

Public Release of Complaint Information. The Joint Commission responds to complaints received about accredited organizations. Complaints may be forwarded by HCFA or other federal or state agencies having oversight responsibilities for health care organizations, or may be received directly from consumers, payers, or health care professionals. The Joint Commission addresses all complaints that pertain to quality of care issues within the scope of Joint Commission standards.

The Joint Commission releases the following information relating to complaints about accredited organizations upon request:
- The applicable standards areas involved in a Joint Commission complaint review;
- Since the last triennial survey, the
  - number of written complaints filed against an accredited organization,
  - number of complaints investigated by the Joint Commission, and
  - performance areas in which type I recommendations were issued as a result of complaint evaluation activities; and
- When an unannounced or unscheduled survey is based on information derived from a complaint or public sources, the nature of the complaint or information upon which the survey is based.

The Joint Commission also provides the following information to complainants regarding their complaints:
- The course of action to be taken regarding the complaint;
- Whether the Joint Commission has decided to take action regarding an organization's accreditation status following completion of the complaint investigation;
  - If the Joint Commission has decided to take no action, the complainant is to be so advised.
  - If the Joint Commission has taken action, the complainant is to be advised in conformance with the guidelines for release of complaint information as set forth above.

Release of Aggregate Performance Data. The Joint Commission reserves the right to publish or release aggregate performance data.

Confidential Information. The Joint Commission keeps confidential the following information received or developed during the accreditation process:
- Information relating to compliance with specific accreditation standards obtained from an organization before, during, or following the accreditation survey;

- The content of an organization's root cause analysis prepared in response to a sentinel event or in response to other circumstances specified by the Joint Commission;
- All other materials that may contribute to the accreditation decision (for example, survey report forms, medical records);
- Written staff analyses and Accreditation Committee minutes and agenda materials; and
- The *Official Accreditation Decision Report.*

This policy applies to all organizations with an accreditation history, except as provided below or by law, or as authorized by responsible organization officials.

Data Release to Government Agencies.* The Joint Commission provides federal, state, or local government agencies specific accreditation-related information under the following circumstances:

- When the Joint Commission identifies a serious situation in an organization that may jeopardize the safety of patients or the public; and
- When an organization, certified for participation in a federal or state program or licensed to operate on the basis of its accreditation, is assigned a Conditional Accreditation, Preliminary Nonaccreditation, or Not Accredited decision. The Joint Commission so advises the organization's chief executive officer and provides timely notice to local, state, and federal authorities having jurisdiction. The information provided to government agencies includes
  - ❏ the accreditation decision, including any designation attached to that status, such as Accreditation Watch;
  - ❏ all type I recommendations;
  - ❏ a statement, if any, provided by the organization regarding the validity of the Joint Commission survey finding; and
  - ❏ for conditionally accredited organizations, a copy of the approved plan of correction and the results of the plan of correction follow-up survey.

Joint Commission Right to Clarify. The Joint Commission reserves the right to clarify information, even if the information involved would otherwise be considered confidential, when an organization disseminates inaccurate information regarding its accreditation.

Performance Reports

The Performance Report provides summary information about a hospital's performance on current Joint Commission standards relating to quality of care and service. Performance Reports are created at the organization level and provide comparative accreditation information gathered from similar organizations surveyed nationwide. A Performance Report includes such information as

- the organization's accreditation decision;
- a listing of the areas having specific recommendations for improvement;
- performance area scores (with national comparative data); and
- an overall evaluation score (with national comparative data).

---

* Section 92, PL 96-499, of the Omnibus Budget Reconciliation Act of 1980, requires that Medicare providers include, in all their contracts for services costing $10,000 or more in any 12-month period, a clause allowing the Secretary of the U.S. Department of Health and Human Services (DHHS), the U.S. Comptroller General, or their representatives to examine the contract and the contractor's books and records. The Joint Commission herein stipulates that if its charges to any such organization amount to $10,000 or more in any 12-month period, the contract or any agreement on which such charges are based and any of the Joint Commission's books, documents, and records that may be necessary to verify the extent and nature of Joint Commission costs will be available to the Secretary of DHHS, the Comptroller General, or any of their duly authorized representatives for four years after the survey. The same conditions will apply to any subcontracts the Joint Commission has with related organizations if the payments under such contracts amount to $10,000 or more in any 12-month period.

Results of follow-up activities are also reported on the Performance Report, including current information regarding
- the organization's accreditation status;
- performance area scores;
- the remaining performance areas that have recommendations for improvement.

A Performance Report is created once an organization's accreditation decision is final. If an organization requests a revision to its *Official Accreditation Decision Report* or its survey report, the Joint Commission will not release the hospital's Performance Report until the revision is addressed.

On receipt, an organization has 30 days to submit a Two-Page Commentary on the Performance Report. The commentary is optional. The Joint Commission sends the Performance Report, an explanatory document, and the organization's commentary to individuals requesting the organization's Performance Report. The Joint Commission sends only the Performance Report and the explanatory document if an organization chooses not to prepare a commentary. The Performance Report is available to the public 30 days after its receipt by the organization.

Survey Fees

The Joint Commission determines survey fees annually as needed to maintain the cost of its operations. Surveyed hospitals are charged for all surveys with the exception of focused surveys and random unannounced surveys. The Joint Commission bases a hospital's survey fees on several factors, including the volume and type of services provided, and the survey's length and location. A hospital may request a longer survey, but a fee will be charged for the additional time. Such requests should be sent to the hospital's accreditation service specialist. Contact the Pricing Unit at the Joint Commission at 630/792-5115 for a fee schedule or more information on survey fees.

The Joint Commission sends an invoice when it schedules a hospital for survey. It asks the hospital to pay the fees according to specified terms. The Joint Commission charges a hospital the fee rate in effect at the time of survey. For an initial survey, a hospital must send a nonrefundable processing fee with the Application for Survey. The Joint Commission credits this payment toward the hospital's total fee.

The Joint Commission offers hospitals two payment options. A hospital can either
- pay the full survey fee when billed or
- spread the payments over a three and one-half-month period.

Under the second option, a hospital must pay one-half of the full survey fee at the time of billing (about six weeks before the survey date) and the balance no later than 60 days after the survey date.

A hospital *that did not pay* its survey fee in full prior to issuance of the accreditation decision and report must remit the outstanding balance within 60 days from receipt of the report. Failure to provide timely payment may result in the loss of accreditation. The Joint Commission notifies a hospital with significant standards compliance problems of either a conditional accreditation or a preliminary nonaccreditation decision as soon as possible, whether or not payment has been received.

Before the Survey

A hospital seeking to undergo the accreditation process for the first time will want to read this section. It provides information on the steps leading to a full accreditation survey. These include the application process, the assignment of an accreditation service specialist, survey scheduling, the assignment of a survey team, the development of a survey agenda, public notification of the survey, and the conduct of a public information interview.

The Accreditation Cycle: Official Accreditation Policies and Procedures

A hospital seeking to renew its accreditation may wish to review selected information, including the description of the application for resurvey process, policies regarding survey scheduling, postponements, and delays, the notification of the public about a forthcoming Joint Commission survey, and the conduct of a public information interview.

Application for Survey

A hospital begins the accreditation process by completing an Application for Survey. This document provides essential information about a hospital, including ownership, demographics, and types and volume of services provided.

The Application for Survey
- describes the hospital seeking accreditation;
- requires the hospital to provide the Joint Commission with all official records and reports of public or publicly recognized licensing (for example, a state license), examining, reviewing, or planning bodies;*
- authorizes the Joint Commission to obtain any records and reports not possessed by the hospital; and
- when accepted, establishes the terms of the relationship between the hospital and the Joint Commission.

A hospital may request an Application for Survey by writing to

Joint Commission on Accreditation of Healthcare Organizations
Packaging Unit
One Renaissance Boulevard
Oakbrook Terrace, IL 60181

or by calling 630/792-5519.

The Joint Commission sends an application for resurvey to accredited hospitals approximately six months before the due date of their next triennial survey. Hospitals that have not received an Application for Survey four months before their due date should call the Joint Commission at the number listed above. The Joint Commission will notify the hospital of the scheduled survey at least four weeks before the survey date.

Accuracy of the Application Information. The Joint Commission schedules surveys based on information provided in the hospital's Application for Survey. With the information provided, the Joint Commission determines the number of days required for a survey and the composition of the survey team.

Inaccurate information in the Application for Survey may necessitate an additional survey, which could delay the Joint Commission's accreditation decision and survey report. The hospital may also incur additional survey charges.

Handling Changes During the Application Process.[†] The hospital must notify the Joint Commission immediately if it undergoes a change that modifies the information reported in the Application for Survey. Information that must be reported includes
- a change in ownership;
- a change in location;
- a significant increase or decrease in the volume of services;
- the addition of a new type of health service; or
- the deletion of an existing health service or site of care.

---

* See Requirement 1 on page 42 in the Accreditation Participation Requirements chapter.

† See Requirement 2 on page 42 in the Accreditation Participation Requirements chapter.

The Joint Commission may schedule an additional survey for a later date if its surveyor or survey team arrives at the hospital and discovers that a change was not reported. The Joint Commission may also survey any unreported services addressed by its standards. The Joint Commission will make the final accreditation decision for the hospital only after surveying all services provided by the hospital for which the Joint Commission has standards. Information reported in the Application for Survey is bound by the Joint Commission's policy on information accuracy and truthfulness (see page 15).

Role of the Accreditation Service Specialist
The Joint Commission assigns an accreditation service specialist to each hospital scheduled for a triennial survey. This person serves as the primary contact between the hospital and the Joint Commission. He or she coordinates survey planning and covers policies, procedures, accreditation issues or services, and inquiries throughout the accreditation cycle. The accreditation service specialist also helps the hospital to customize its survey agenda to reflect its unique structure and characteristics. The accreditation services specialist makes the most efficient use of staff and surveyor time during the survey.

Survey Scheduling and Postponements
Schedules for Surveys. The Joint Commission schedules surveys systematically and efficiently to keep survey fees to a minimum. Therefore, hospitals are encouraged to accept scheduled survey dates. Resurveys are scheduled within 45 days before or after the hospital's triennial due date. A hospital's first full accreditation survey, an initial survey, must be scheduled within one year from the time the Joint Commission receives the hospital's application.

Special Requests. The Joint Commission tries to honor written requests specifying dates during which a hospital prefers not to be surveyed. The hospital should make the request with the completed Application for Survey, whenever possible. However, circumstances may prevent the Joint Commission from accommodating these requests.

Definition of Postponement. Under limited circumstances, the Joint Commission can provide for the postponement of surveys beyond the 45-day window. A postponement is a hospital's request to alter an already scheduled survey date or to alter the survey date before it is actually scheduled. A hospital should direct a request for a postponement to its accreditation service specialist.

Survey Postponement Policy. A request to postpone a survey may be granted if one or more of the following criteria are met:
- a natural disaster or other major unforeseen event has occurred that has totally or substantially disrupted operations;
- the organization is involved in a major strike, has ceased admitting patients, and is transferring patients to other facilities or organizations;
- patients and/or the organization are being moved to a new building on the day or days of the survey; or
- the Joint Commission has provided less than four weeks advance notice to the organization (by telephone or in writing) of the survey date(s).

Note: If a survey postponement is requested because of a natural disaster, strike, or movement to a new building, an on-site extension survey may be required if the organization is continuing to provide patient care services.

If one or more of the listed criteria are met, a survey may be postponed for up to six months from the anniversary or due date. If the postponement or delay is to be more than six months and the organization is accredited, an on-site extension survey will normally be conducted.

An organization undergoing its first Joint Commission survey will be required to specify on its application for survey the month in which it wishes to be surveyed. Following the scheduling of the survey, the organization would only be permitted to postpone its survey if it meets the above criteria.

Fees for Postponements. The Joint Commission may, at its option, approve a survey postponement for a hospital not meeting any of the criteria described above. In such cases, the hospital is charged a fee to defray costs and may be required to undergo an extension survey. The Joint Commission will charge the base fee for the survey of each program being postponed. The Joint Commission reserves the right, however, to deny any request for a postponement, regardless of the hospital's willingness to pay the special fee.

Timeliness of Application and Deposits. The Joint Commission requires a hospital to submit a new Application for Survey if the hospital does not accept a scheduled survey within one year. This ensures that the hospital's information is current.

A nonrefundable, nontransferable survey deposit is required for initial surveys only. The Joint Commission applies the deposit to the hospital's survey fee if a survey is conducted.

Forfeiture of Survey Deposit. A hospital scheduled for an initial survey will forfeit its survey deposit if its survey is not conducted within 12 months of submission of its application. The hospital must then reapply and submit a new survey deposit to begin the accreditation process again.

The Survey Agenda

The Joint Commission's accreditation service specialist works with the hospital to develop a tentative survey agenda based on survey task assignments required as part of the survey. A generic agenda template will be sent to all hospitals with a similar number of required survey days and similar survey teams. The draft of the tentative agenda is reviewed and revisions made, as appropriate.

The hospital and its accreditation service specialist collaboratively develop the final agenda used for the accreditation survey. A planning questionnaire is sent to the hospital approximately six months before the hospital's due date for survey to facilitate this process. The questionnaire solicits information about
- the hospital's patient care settings including inpatient, ambulatory/outpatient, special care, imaging, and anesthetizing units or locations, and
- optional survey activities the hospital may wish to have included in the survey.

The Joint Commission provides other materials to assist the hospital in identifying
- staff that should be involved in various survey activities, and
- documents that should be available to the surveyors during the on-site survey.

The final agenda reflects survey activities, and the staff and documents required during the survey.

Notifying the Public About a Joint Commission Survey

The Joint Commission evaluates all relevant information about a hospital's compliance with applicable standards. It therefore requires a surveyed hospital to inform the public of a scheduled full survey and invite them to provide the surveyor or survey team with relevant information.* The hospital must provide an opportunity for members of the public to participate in a public information interview during a full survey, including both surveys under Option 2 of the Early Survey Policy (see pages 11 through 13). A full survey refers to the survey of all components of a hospital under all applicable standards. The public includes, but is not limited to
- patients and their families;
- patient advocates and advocacy groups;

---

* See Requirement 7 on page 44 in the Accreditation Participation Requirements chapter.

- members of the community for whom services are provided; and
- personnel and staff.

Public Posting. The surveyed hospital is responsible for making the public information interview process widely known and effective as a source of compliance information in the accreditation process. The Joint Commission requires a hospital scheduled for full survey to post announcements of
- the survey date,
- the opportunity for a public information interview, and
- how to request an interview.

In the event that all hospital components are not surveyed at the same time, the posting requirement applies at the time the primary program is surveyed. For example, if an organization with hospital, long term care, and home care components is scheduled for a tailored survey in which the hospital is the primary program and each component's survey is scheduled for a different date, the notice of survey is to be posted consistent with the hospital's survey dates.

To maximize participation, postings must be made throughout the hospital, including components being surveyed at a different time, in the form provided by the Joint Commission. See Figure 2, page 29, for an example of a Public Notice form. This example may be used by the hospital, or the hospital may design its own Public Notice form that conveys the same information as this example. A hospital should post notices in staff eating areas, break rooms, on bulletin boards near major entrances, and in treatment or residential areas. In addition, the hospital must provide each staff person with a written announcement of the survey, if such postings are not likely to be seen by all staff.

Advance Notice. The Joint Commission requires a hospital scheduled for survey to post public notices at least 30 days before the scheduled date. A hospital receiving the scheduled date less than 30 days before the survey date should post public notices promptly. Notices must remain posted until the survey is completed.

Informing the Community. The hospital must take reasonable steps to inform its community of the opportunity for public information interviews during the full survey at least 30 days before the survey. Steps include
- informing all advocacy groups (such as organized patient groups and unions) that have substantively communicated with it in the previous 12 months;
- reaching other members of the community through means such as a public service announcement on radio or television, a classified advertisement in a local newspaper, or a notice in a community newsletter or other publication;* and
- informing individuals who inquire about the survey of the survey date(s) and opportunity to participate.

Compliance with the Public Information Interview Policy. The surveyor(s) reviews the hospital's compliance with the policy outlined above. The team indicates at the exit conference whether it believes the hospital has complied with the policy and reports on this to the Joint Commission. An initial failure to comply with the public information interview policy ordinarily results in a type I recommendation (see "Accreditation Decision" on page 34). As a result, the Joint Commission may also conduct a postsurvey public information interview, if requested.

In addition, the surveyor(s) conducting a postsurvey public information interview also conduct(s) whatever follow-up survey he or she (they) believes appropriate in view of the information obtained during the public information interview. A hospital's subsequent failure to comply with the Joint Commission's public information interview policy may result in loss or denial of its accreditation. A fee is associated with public information interviews conducted after the survey of a hospital that is not in compliance with the public information interview policy.

---

* This type of notification must be published or broadcast at least once.

> **PUBLIC NOTICE**
>
> The Joint Commission on Accreditation of Healthcare Organizations will conduct an accreditation survey of _____ on _____.
> (Insert the name of your organization)   (Insert your survey dates)
>
> The purpose of the survey will be to evaluate the organization's compliance with nationally established Joint Commission standards. The survey results will be used to determine whether, and the conditions under which accreditation should be awarded the organization.
>
> Joint Commission standards deal with organizational quality of care issues and the safety of the environment in which care is provided. Anyone believing that he or she has pertinent and valid information about such matters may request a public information interview with the Joint Commission's field representatives at the time of the survey. Information presented at the interview will be carefully evaluated for relevance to the accreditation process. Requests for a public information interview must be made in writing and should be sent to the Joint Commission no later than five working days before the survey begins. The request must also indicate the nature of the information to be provided at the interview. Such requests should be addressed to:
>
> **Division of Accreditation Operations**
> **Accreditation Service Specialist**
> **Joint Commission on Accreditation of Healthcare Organizations**
> **One Renaissance Boulevard**
> **Oakbrook Terrace, IL 60181**
>
> The Joint Commission will acknowledge such requests in writing or by telephone and will inform the organization of the request for any interview. The organization will, in turn, notify the interviewee of the date, time, and place of the meeting.
>
> This notice is posted in accordance with the Joint Commission's requirements and may not be removed before the survey is completed.
>
> **Date Posted:**_____

Figure 2. *A sample Public Notice form.*

Conduct of the Public Information Interview

Handling Requests.* Individuals requesting a public information interview are to forward their requests and the nature of the information they will provide in writing to the Joint Commission. The hospital must explain this process in its communications. To ensure participation, individuals are encouraged to forward written requests as soon as possible, and no later than five days before the scheduled survey.

---

* See Requirement 8 on page 45 in the Accreditation Participation Requirements chapter.

Sometimes an individual may make a written request for a public information interview directly to the hospital. When this occurs, the hospital must promptly forward it to the Joint Commission. A hospital receiving *oral requests* should instruct individuals to make the request in writing and mail them to the Joint Commission. The hospital should provide individuals needing assistance in doing this with the necessary support.

Scheduling Interviews. The hospital must provide potential public information interview participants with sufficient advance notice. The Joint Commission acknowledges all public information interview requests and provides the hospital with copies of the acknowledgments. Prior to the survey, the Joint Commission schedules a time-limited public information interview to be conducted during the survey. The hospital is responsible for notifying the individuals requesting public information interviews of the interview's exact date, time, and place. The hospital must try to alleviate any potential concerns about reprisals to individuals who participate in the interview process.

Interview Eligibility. Individuals whose written requests arrive late or who simply appear at the stated time, requesting the opportunity to be heard without a prior written request, are heard by a Joint Commission surveyor if time permits. Otherwise, the surveyor informs them that it is not possible to honor their requests and then offers them the opportunity to provide a subsequent written statement.

Individuals contacting the Joint Commission and stating an interest in supplying information anonymously are informed that they may provide written complaints through the Joint Commission's complaint process. The Joint Commission will maintain confidentiality, as requested.

The Interview Process. The Joint Commission's survey team conducts the public information interview. A representative of the surveyed hospital may attend, unless the individual requesting the public information interview asks that no representative from the hospital be present. The Joint Commission will honor such requests. The interview will be conducted on the hospital's premises, whether a representative from the hospital is present or not. The hospital is expected to provide reasonable accommodations for all public information interviews.

An interview consists of the orderly receipt of information, orally or in writing, within a set time limit. The interview is *not* a debate between a hospital's representative and an interviewee. Surveyors may, however, ask clarifying questions.

In addition, surveyors will not debate with or convey conclusions to any interviewee. Rather, the Joint Commission considers the information gathered by the survey team along with its findings and recommendations during the survey process.

During the Survey

This section includes information relevant to a hospital that has applied for an accreditation survey and is ready for the survey process. It provides an overview of the survey process itself, the survey team and its leadership, and surrounding issues. These include how the Joint Commission handles findings of patient care or safety concerns, preliminary reports and how they are prepared, and the conduct of a leadership exit conference.

The Survey Process in Brief

Overview. During an accreditation survey, the Joint Commission evaluates a hospital's performance of functions and processes aimed at continuously improving patient outcomes. The survey process focuses on assessing performance of important patient-centered and organization functions that support quality patient care. The process has moved away from evaluating specific departments and services. The survey team described below assesses a hospital based on the performance-focused standards included in this book. Surveys are designed to be individualized to each hospital, to be consistent, and to support the hospital's efforts to improve performance. Depending on the scope of the survey, hospitals receive a 2-, 3-, 4-, or 5-day survey, conducted on a triennial basis.

Survey Team Composition. Accreditation surveys usually are conducted by a survey team rather than an individual surveyor. The composition of a hospital's survey team is based on the information provided in its Application for Survey. In most instances, a hospital survey team is composed of three surveyors: an administrator, a nurse, and a physician. In smaller hospitals with an average daily census of less than 40 patients, the survey team is composed of two surveyors, usually, but not always, a nurse and a physician. All surveyors assess and provide consultation regarding all functions addressed by the standards.

In addition, depending on the hospital's service configuration, there may be a specialized surveyor addressing such areas as long term care, home care, behavioral health, or ambulatory care services. The findings of specialized surveyors are integrated into the hospital's accreditation decision and survey report.

Survey Team Leadership. One of the experienced surveyors on each hospital survey team is designated as the "team leader." The team leader is responsible for integration, coordination, and communication of on-site survey activities. In addition to direct participation as an active member of the survey team, the team leader serves as the primary point of on-site contact between the hospital and the Joint Commission. Among other responsibilities, the team leader leads the opening conference and the daily and exit briefings.

Opening Conference and Performance Improvement Overview. After the hospital has completed the presurvey steps described in pages 24 through 30, the first actual survey activity involves an opening conference. This conference lays the groundwork for the survey.

Following the opening conference, hospital staff orient the survey team to the hospital's approach to performance improvement. This is an opportunity for a hospital to showcase its program to measure, assess, and improve its performance of the important functions addressed by the standards.

Document Review. After completing the opening conference and the performance improvement overview, the surveyors begin the assessment process by reviewing key documents that focus on the hospital's performance. Documents include committee minutes, reports of performance-improvement activities, measurement data, and reports to medical staff and hospital committees and the governing body. Certain bylaws, planning documents, and other evidence of performance also will be included.

Interviews with Organization Leaders. Interviews with the hospital's leaders occur both early and at later stages in the survey process. Interviews address the collaboration of senior leaders in the performance improvement process and the roles played by administration, department directors, medical staff, and nursing leaders.

Visits to Patient Care Settings. Visits to patient care settings play a major role in the hospital survey process. Surveyors visit settings where patients' needs are assessed or where patients receive care. Settings include inpatient units, operating rooms, ambulatory/outpatient clinics, and anesthetizing, emergency, imaging, rehabilitation, and other locations.

During these visits, the survey team interacts with managers, direct care providers—including members of the medical staff, other hospital staff, and patients. The team also
- tours the setting to address environment of care, infection control, patient care, staff communication, and patient rights issues; and
- reviews open medical records with a multidisciplinary group of providers.

Team members integrate their findings to assess compliance levels.

Function Interviews. These interviews gather a multidisciplinary group of the hospital's staff who have important responsibilities related to a given function. They follow up on issues identified in the document review and reflect observations made by surveyors in visits to patient care settings.

Scoring Compliance Against Track Record Requirements. Accredited organizations are expected to remain in continuous compliance with the standards and their intent statements throughout the interval between surveys. However, for practical purposes in conducting the survey, surveyors will ordinarily limit their evaluation of the organization's track record of compliance. In addition to the performance expectations described in the scoring section of each functional chapter, and subject to exercise of appropriate discretion, hospitals ordinarily will be expected to show a track record of compliance for one year before a triennial survey. Surveyors may evaluate compliance over a shorter or longer time frame depending on circumstances encountered during the survey. For example, the required time frame for full compliance with applicable standards and intents for new services will not exceed the time the service has been in operation. In another example, certain activities that are conducted infrequently, such as biennial credentialing, may require evaluation over a longer interval to ensure an adequate sample size for valid assessment.

For a triennial survey, a hospital's track record generally will impact the scoring of standards according to the following matrix:

Score 1 12 months before survey
Score 2 9 to 11 months before survey
Score 3 6 to 8 months before survey
Score 4 5 months or less before survey
Score 5 No process in place

During initial or focused surveys, a hospital's track record generally will impact the scoring of standards according to the following matrix:

Score 1 4 months before survey
Score 2 3 months before survey
Score 3 2 months before survey
Score 4 1 month before survey
Score 5 Less than 1 month before survey

Feedback Sessions. Final scores about compliance are not reached until all patient care settings have been visited and all other assessment interviews and activities have been conducted. However, surveyors will communicate their observations at daily briefings and during a medical staff luncheon, as requested by the hospital.

Final On-Site Survey Activities. At the leadership exit conference, described on page 33, the survey team will present complete survey findings, a preliminary written report, and a potential accreditation decision.

Patient Care or Safety Concerns

The Joint Commission may consider for accreditation purposes a surveyor's finding that some aspect of a hospital's operation is having or may have a direct, adverse effect on patient health or safety. The Joint Commission may obtain expert consultation regarding these findings.

Surveyors will notify the hospital's chief executive officer and Joint Commission corporate office staff immediately if they identify any condition they believe poses an immediate threat to public or patient safety. The president of the Joint Commission, or if the president is unavailable, a designated vice president, can then issue an expedited preliminary nonaccreditation decision based on such notification. He or she will promptly inform the hospital's chief executive officer and appropriate governmental authorities of this decision. The Accreditation Committee of the Board of Commissioners will confirm or reverse the decision at its next meeting.

Laptop Technology and Preliminary Reports

Use of Laptop Technology. Each day, after the survey team performs the activities described on pages 30 through 32, team members enter survey data and documentation on laptop computers. These computers are equipped with specially designed decision-support software. The software guides the accurate entry of findings, integrates the findings of multiple surveyors, and calculates standard-level scores, thereby allowing surveyors, as a team, to review the information and make necessary adjustments.

Presentation of a Preliminary Report. The survey team reviews the results of integrated individual findings. Then, with the use of laptop-based decision support software, the team produces a preliminary report on-site. Preliminary reports include the accreditation decision grid, preliminary type I and supplemental recommendations (as applicable), the projected outcome or potential accreditation decision, and any follow-up requirements. The findings of specialized, add-on surveyors (see page 31) are integrated as a part of the preliminary report.

The team leader meets with the hospital's chief executive officer prior to the leadership exit conference (see below) and provides him or her with a copy of the preliminary report. The CEO determines whether or not the preliminary report is distributed at the leadership exit conference. The survey team uses preliminary report contents in making its leadership exit conference presentations.

Use of the Preliminary Report. Recognizing that many hospitals are eager to release the results of their accreditation survey immediately following the survey, it must be emphasized that this is a preliminary report, not a final decision. The final decision will be made following an appropriate review at the Joint Commission's central office. In some instances, a change will be made in the accreditation report. Therefore, hospitals are encouraged to not make any formal announcement as a result of a preliminary report.

In choosing to publicize the preliminary report, hospitals should state that the findings are preliminary. If the Joint Commission is contacted by members of the media or community we will not be able to confirm any accreditation decision because no such decision will have yet been made. Once the final report is sent to the hospital, the accreditation decision is officially public.

Leadership Exit Conference

Joint Commission surveyors confer with the hospital's chief executive officer and other leaders* as part of a leadership exit conference for each survey. The purpose of the conference is to
- review the preliminary report, if the CEO determines it will be made available;
- gain agreement between the team and the hospital regarding survey findings; and
- report to the hospital the potential accreditation decision based on the findings.

The survey team leader presides during the conference. The team leader and the other surveyors present their findings on any significant standards compliance issues. In addition, they discuss underlying causes of the compliance issues and recommend improvements. Each member of the team presents findings by function. The surveyors provide the hospital's representatives with an opportunity to clarify issues and respond to recommendations. The surveyors also confer on survey findings that may not be directly related to the standards, if requested.

Following the close of the leadership exit conference, the survey team will, as appropriate
- revise or include additional information from the conference in the team's report;
- identify, for the Joint Commission's central office staff, challenged findings that have not been resolved; and
- issue a new preliminary report, if needed.

---

* **leaders** The leaders described in the leadership function include at least the leaders of the governing body; the chief executive officer and other senior managers; department leaders; the elected and the appointed leaders of the medical staff and the clinical departments and other medical staff members in organizational administrative positions; and the nurse executive and other senior nursing leaders.

After the Survey

This section includes information relevant to a hospital that recently has participated in an accreditation survey. Material includes information on types of accreditation decisions, how to request revisions to the survey report, how to appeal "not accredited" decisions, and how to use and display an accreditation award.

Accreditation Decision

The Joint Commission provides the organization with an accreditation decision in its *Official Accreditation Decision Report*. This accreditation decision involves processing the surveyors' findings according to specific aggregation rules and decision rules established by the Accreditation Committee of the Board of Commissioners. The "Accreditation and Appeal Procedures" chapter outlines specific accreditation procedures.

There are seven possible accreditation decisions:
1. Accreditation with Commendation;
2. Accreditation;
3. Accreditation with Type I Recommendations;
4. Provisional Accreditation;
5. Conditional Accreditation;
6. Preliminary Nonaccreditation; and
7. Not Accredited.

Table 2 (pages 35 through 37) provides a description of each category and the conditions that lead to it.

A hospital's wish to withdraw from the accreditation process after undergoing survey and before a final decision has been made does not terminate the decision-making process. The Joint Commission will reach a final accreditation decision.

Requests for Revision to the *Official Accreditation Decision Report*

The hospital has 30 days from receipt of its *Official Accreditation Decision Report* to request, in writing, a revision of any portion of the report related to survey findings or follow-up activity.

Appealing Not Accredited or Preliminarily Nonaccredited Decisions

The hospital has 20 days from receipt of its *Official Accreditation Decision Report* to notify the Joint Commission, in writing, of its intent to appeal a decision to deny accreditation. A hospital that has received written notice from the Joint Commission of being preliminarily denied accreditation or provisional accreditation has 20 days to make a written request for a hearing.

Award Display and Use

The Joint Commission provides each accredited hospital with a certificate of accreditation. There is no charge for the initial certificate. Additional certificates may be purchased. Such requests should be sent to the Certificate Coordinator, Division of Accreditation Operations at the Joint Commission.

The certificate and all copies remain the Joint Commission's property. They must be returned if
- the hospital is issued a new certificate reflecting a name change; or
- the hospital's accreditation status is changed, withdrawn, or denied, for any reason.

A hospital accredited by the Joint Commission must be accurate in describing to the public the nature and meaning of its accreditation and its award.* On request, the Joint Commission's Department of Communications will supply a hospital receiving accreditation with appropriate guidelines for characterizing the accreditation award. Guidelines also cover accreditation with commendation awards.

Table 2. Types of Joint Commission Accreditation Decisions

The Joint Commission has seven accreditation decision categories. Each decision and the conditions that lead to it are described below.

Accreditation Decision Category	Conditions That Lead to this Type of Decision
Accreditation with Commendation	The highest accreditation decision that is awarded when a hospital has demonstrated exemplary performance in complying with Joint Commission standards. An organization is eligible for accreditation with commendation (1) if the summary grid score for all applicable programs is 90 or higher; (2) if no type I recommendations have been assigned; and (3) if all applicable programs of the organization that are eligible for survey have been surveyed and each applicable program meets criteria 1 and 2 stated above.
Accreditation without Type I Recommendations	An accreditation decision that results when a hospital has demonstrated acceptable compliance with Joint Commission standards in all performance areas.
Accreditation with Type I Recommendations	An accreditation decision that results when a hospital receives at least one recommendation addressing insufficient or unsatisfactory standards compliance in a specific performance area or a "Special Type I Recommendation" (for example, a special type I recommendation assigned when a requirement in the "Accreditation Participation Requirements" chapter is not met). Resolution of type I recommendations must be achieved within stipulated time frames (through a focused survey or a written progress report submitted by the hospital) to maintain accreditation.

continued on next page

Table 2. Types of Joint Commission Accreditation Decisions (continued)

Provisional Accreditation An accreditation decision that results when a hospital has demonstrated satisfactory compliance with the selected standards applied during the hospital's initial survey under the Early Survey Policy—Option 1. The second survey, or full survey, is conducted approximately six months later to allow the hospital sufficient time to demonstrate a track record of performance and results in the hospital's receiving one of the other official accreditation decisions.

Conditional Accreditation An accreditation decision that results when a hospital is not in substantial compliance with Joint Commission standards but is believed to be capable of achieving acceptable standards compliance within a stipulated time period. Findings of correction, which serve as the basis for further consideration of awarding full accreditation, must be demonstrated through a short-term follow-up survey.

Preliminary Nonaccreditation An accreditation decision that is assigned to a hospital when it is found to be in significant noncompliance with Joint Commission standards or when its accreditation is preliminarily withdrawn by the Joint Commission for other reasons (for example, falsification of documents) **prior** to the determination of the final decision (for example, Not Accredited). Preliminary nonaccreditation is an appealable accreditation decision.

continued on next page

Table 2. Types of Joint Commission Accreditation Decisions (continued)	
Not Accredited	An accreditation decision that results when a hospital is denied accreditation because of significant noncompliance with Joint Commission standards, when its accreditation is withdrawn by the Joint Commission for other reasons, or when the hospital voluntarily withdraws from the accreditation process. Not Accredited is an appealable accreditation decision.

A hospital may not engage in any false or misleading advertising of the accreditation award. Any such advertising may be grounds to deny accreditation. For example, a hospital may not represent its accreditation as being awarded by any of the Joint Commission's corporate members. These include the American College of Physicians, the American College of Surgeons, the American Dental Association, the American Hospital Association, and the American Medical Association. The Joint Commission has permission to reprint the seals of its corporate members on the certificates of accreditation. However, these seals must not be reproduced or displayed separately from the certificate.

Any organization that materially misleads the public about any matter relating to its accreditation must undertake corrective advertising of a degree acceptable to the Joint Commission in the same medium in which the misrepresentation occurred. If an organization fails to undertake the required corrective advertising following the communication of false or misleading advertising about its accreditation status, the organization may be subject to loss of accreditation.

The Joint Commission's logo is a registered trademark. An accredited hospital may use the logo if it follows these guidelines:
- The logo must remain in the same proportional relationship as provided and should not be displayed any larger than a hospital's own logo.
- The logo's format cannot be changed, the name may not be separated from the symbol, and they must be printed in the same color.
- Graphic devices such as seals, other words, or slogans cannot be added to the logo except for the words "Accredited by."

These guidelines apply for logo use on all print materials and promotional items, such as coffee mugs, T-shirts, and note pads. Contact the Department of Communications at the Joint Commission at 630/792-5631 for questions about using the Joint Commission logo.

---

* See Requirement 10 on page 46 in the Accreditation Participation Requirements chapter.

Before the Next Survey

This section provides information relevant to hospitals between Joint Commission surveys. Material includes the duration of an accreditation award; the process for continuing accreditation; how to notify the Joint Commission in the event of organizational changes including mergers, consolidations, and acquisitions; and unscheduled and unannounced surveys.

Duration of Accreditation Award

An accreditation award is valid for three years, unless revoked for cause or as otherwise outlined in this chapter. Accreditation is effective on the first day after the Joint Commission completes the hospital's survey. Hospitals may request a full accreditation survey more frequently than once every three years. The Joint Commission will, at its discretion and in accordance with its mission, determine whether to honor the request. Such requests should be sent to the hospital's accreditation service specialist.

Resolving Type I Recommendations. The Joint Commission requires a hospital receiving a type I recommendation to achieve substantial or significant compliance with the relevant standard(s) within a specific time frame. Failure to do so can result in a conditional accreditation or not accredited decision.

The Joint Commission monitors a hospital accredited with type I recommendations for their successful resolution. Monitoring and the time frame for demonstrating improvements depend on the nature of the type I recommendations. The potential impact on patient care is of particular concern. For many type I recommendations, the Joint Commission requires a hospital to submit a written progress report. Other type I recommendations require an on-site survey known as a focused survey. The number of surveyors and the length of the focused survey may depend on the number and nature of the type I recommendations.

During a focused survey, surveyors may need to address standards other than those cited with a type I recommendation(s) to fully address compliance with the cited standards. Also, hospitals are responsible for meeting the requirements of the most current standards—that is, the standards in effect at the time of the focused survey, which may be different from the standards that were in effect at the time the type I recommendation(s) was assigned.

Continuous Compliance. The Joint Commission expects an accredited hospital to be in continuous compliance with all applicable standards. It may ask a hospital to supply, in writing, information about standards compliance. Or it may survey a hospital at any time, with or without notice. The Joint Commission may perform such surveys in response to complaints, media coverage, or other information-raising questions about standards compliance or the adequacy of patient health and safety protections (see "Unscheduled and Unannounced Surveys" on page 40). The Joint Commission might also conduct a survey if a hospital fails to respond to a request for more information.

A hospital's failure to permit a survey can be viewed by the Joint Commission as grounds to deny accreditation or as withdrawal by the hospital from the accreditation process.*

Continuing Accreditation

The Joint Commission does not automatically renew a hospital's accreditation. A hospital seeking to continue its accreditation must apply for accreditation, undergo a full accreditation survey, and be found in compliance with the standards.

Accreditation Renewal Process. The Joint Commission sends a hospital an Application for Survey before the hospital's triennial accreditation due date. The hospital is responsible for completing and returning the Application for Survey to the Joint Commission.

---

* See Requirement 3 on page 42 in the Accreditation Participation Requirements chapter.

The Joint Commission schedules a survey to determine a hospital's eligibility to renew its accreditation award. This triennial survey occurs close to the end of the three-year accreditation cycle. Generally, the Joint Commission conducts a triennial survey in the time period between 45 days before the hospital's three-year survey due date and 45 days after the due date. The Joint Commission notifies the hospital of the survey date at least four weeks before the survey.

Accreditation Status During Triennial Survey. A hospital's previous accreditation status remains in effect until a decision is made either to accredit or to preliminarily nonaccredit the hospital.

Notification of Changes Made Between Surveys

Accreditation is neither automatically transferred nor continued if significant changes occur within the hospital. Such changes may necessitate an extension of accreditation survey of the hospital if the hospital has

- instituted a new service or program for which the Joint Commission has standards;
- changed ownership and there are a significant number of changes in the management and clinical staff or operating policies and procedures;
- offered at least 25% of its services at a new location or in a significantly altered physical plant;
- expanded its capacity to provide services by 25% or more as measured by beds, patient visits, pieces of equipment, or other relevant measures;
- provided a more intensive level of service (for example, from outpatient alcohol and drug use to residential alcohol and drug use); or
- merged with, consolidated with, or acquired an unaccredited site, service, or program for which there are applicable Joint Commission standards.

An extension of accreditation survey may also occur when

- the Joint Commission grants a hospital's request to continue its current accreditation beyond the conclusion of the three-year cycle;* or
- a hospital has merged, consolidated, or acquired an accredited hospital whose accreditation expiration date is within three months of the merger, consolidation, or acquisition, while its own accreditation expiration date is at least nine months away.

When any of these changes occur, the hospital must notify the Joint Commission in writing not more than 30 days after such change is made. When a hospital offers at least 25% of its services at a new location or in a significantly altered physical plant, the hospital must also fill out and submit to the Joint Commission Part 2: Basic Building Information of the Statement of Conditions™. Failure to provide timely notification to the Joint Commission of these changes may result in the loss of accreditation.

An extension of accreditation survey is conducted at an accredited hospital or at a site that is owned and operated by or that is publicly represented as being part of an accredited hospital if the accredited hospital's current accreditation is not due to expire for at least nine months and when at least one of the conditions above is met. The results of an extension of accreditation survey may affect the hospital's accreditation status.

Mergers, Consolidations, and Acquisitions. In the case of a merger, consolidation, or acquisition, the Joint Commission may decide that the hospital responsible for services must be resurveyed or initially surveyed. Barring exceptional circumstances, the Joint Commission continues the accreditation of the hospital undergoing the kind of changes described above until it determines whether an extension of accreditation survey is necessary.

---

* Such requests are granted only for unusual and compelling reasons.

Annual Update Process

All accredited health care organizations will be contacted by the Joint Commission on or around their triennial due date. Organizations will be contacted and asked to verify or correct key demographics maintained about their organization, including the selection of a performance measurement system and indicators as part of the ORYX Initiative. Once this demographic information is updated and verified, a certification form detailing the update will be sent to the health care organization. The organization will then be asked to verify and certify the information is correct and return it to the Joint Commission.

Unscheduled and Unannounced Surveys

The Joint Commission may perform either an unscheduled or unannounced survey when it becomes aware of potentially serious patient care or safety issues in an accredited hospital.* Either type of survey can take place at any point in a hospital's three-year accreditation cycle. The Joint Commission usually provides the hospital with 24 to 48 hours advance notice of an unscheduled survey.

No advance notice is provided for unannounced surveys. Reasons for unannounced surveys include occurrence of any event or series of events in an accredited organization that creates significant
- concern that there may be a continuing threat to the safety or care of patients;
- concern that there may be continuing serious and/or multiple significant standards compliance deficiency(ies); or
- suspicion that the organization is not or has not been in compliance with the Joint Commission's falsification policy.

Such a survey can either include all the hospital's services or only those areas where a serious concern may exist.

Results of any unannounced or unscheduled surveys may generate appropriate follow-up activities and can affect a hospital's current accreditation status. The Joint Commission may deny accreditation or conclude that the hospital has withdrawn from the accreditation process if the hospital does not let the Joint Commission conduct unscheduled or unannounced surveys.

Random Unannounced Surveys. The Joint Commission also conducts midcycle, unannounced surveys on a 5% random sample of accredited hospitals. The survey is generally conducted 18 months following the accreditation date (that is, the date after the last day of the survey) plus or minus 30 days. A hospital will receive a 24- to 48-hour notice of the random, unannounced survey. One surveyor conducts each such survey for one day.

The surveyor primarily assesses the five performance areas identified by the Joint Commission as the most troublesome in the previous year's aggregate survey data for the program to be surveyed and any additional performance areas as specified by the Accreditation Committee. These performance areas may change annually based on the previous year's data. Contact hospital accreditation services for a current list of performance areas.

In an effort to reduce duplication among surveying entities, those hospitals that have received an 18-month HCFA validation survey will be exempted from receiving a random unannounced survey for the current cycle.

---

* See Requirement 3 on page 42 in the Accreditation Participation Requirements chapter.

Accreditation Participation Requirements

This chapter includes specific requirements for participation in the accreditation process and for maintenance of an accreditation award. The requirements in this chapter differ from survey eligibility criteria in that the accreditation process may be initiated even when all accreditation participation requirements have not yet been met. Requirements 1 through 3 and Requirements 7 through 10 are existing accreditation policies within the Accreditation Cycle chapter (see pages 7 through 40) and are currently effective for accreditation purposes. Therefore, organizations must be in current compliance with each of these requirements. Each requirement is cross-referenced to the applicable section of the Accreditation Cycle chapter. By contrast, Requirements 4, 5, and 6 are new and will be implemented incrementally over the next few years. Requirements 4 and 5 became effective for accreditation purposes on January 1, 1998; Requirement 6 becomes effective on January 1, 1999.

For a hospital seeking accreditation for the first time, compliance with the accreditation participation requirements is assessed during the initial survey. For the accredited hospital, compliance with these requirements is assessed throughout the accreditation cycle through on-site surveys, written progress reports, periodic updates of hospital-specific data and information, and ad hoc communications. Starting January 1, 1998, when a hospital does not fully comply with an accreditation participation requirement, the hospital will usually be assigned a special type I recommendation. However, refusal to permit performance of an unscheduled or unannounced survey (Requirement 3) or falsification of information (Requirement 9), will immediately lead to preliminary nonaccreditation. Special type I recommendations can impact the accreditation decision, overall performance score, and follow-up requirements, as determined by established accreditation decision rules. Failure to resolve a special type I recommendation can ultimately lead to loss of accreditation.

Note: *Hospitals that have an average daily census (ADC) of less than 10 and an ambulatory population of less than 150 are not subject to Requirements 4, 5, and 6 until further notice. In addition, a field readiness study is being conducted by the Joint Commission for psychiatric hospitals. Therefore, performance measurement requirements for freestanding psychiatric hospitals are deferred for one year.*

Application for Survey

Requirement 1 The hospital provides the Joint Commission with all official records and reports of public or publicly recognized licensing (for example, a state license), examining, reviewing, or planning bodies.*

Requirement 2 The hospital immediately reports any changes in the information provided in the Application for Survey.†

A hospital that experiences a significant change in ownership or control, location, capacity, or the categories of services offered must notify the Joint Commission in writing not more than 30 days after such changes. The Joint Commission may decide that the hospital must be resurveyed when a significant merger or consolidation has taken place. The Joint Commission continues the hospital's accreditation until it determines whether a resurvey is necessary. Failure to provide timely notification to the Joint Commission of ownership, merger or consolidation, and service changes may result in interruption or loss of accreditation. When requested, the hospital is required to provide the Joint Commission with all official records and reports of public or publicly recognized licensing, examining, reviewing, or planning bodies.

Compliance with Requirement 1   ❏ Yes
                                    ❏ No

Compliance with Requirement 2   ❏ Yes
                                    ❏ No

Acceptance of Survey

Requirement 3 A hospital permits the performance of an unscheduled or unannounced survey‡ at the discretion of the Joint Commission.

The Joint Commission may perform either an unscheduled or unannounced survey when it becomes aware of potentially serious patient care or safety issues in a hospital. Either type of survey can take place at any point in a hospital's three-year accreditation cycle. An unscheduled or unannounced survey can either include all of the hospital's services or address only those areas where a serious concern may exist. In addition, the Joint Commission conducts unannounced surveys on a random sample of accredited hospitals at the approximate midpoint of their three-year accreditation cycles. A hospital's failure to permit an unscheduled or unannounced survey is grounds for withdrawal of accreditation.

Compliance with Requirement 3   ❏ Yes
                                    ❏ No

---

* See also page 23 in the Accreditation Cycle chapter.

† See also page 25 in the Accreditation Cycle chapter.

‡ See also page 40 in the Accreditation Cycle chapter. An explanation of the difference between an unscheduled and unannounced survey can be found on these pages. In addition, see the last paragraph of "Continuous Compliance" on page 38.

Accreditation Participation Requirements

Performance Measurement

Requirement 4 The hospital participates in a listed performance measurement system that has been found to be acceptable for use in the accreditation process.

Each hospital must select at least one performance measurement system that is listed by the Joint Commission as acceptable for use in the accreditation process. Each accredited hospital must notify the Joint Commission of its initial selection(s) prior to March 2, 1998. A hospital applying for initial survey must notify the Joint Commission of its selection(s) no later than the time of survey. Each hospital must notify the Joint Commission of any changes in its relationship with the selected performance measurement system(s) or the selection of a new or additional performance measurement system used to meet performance measurement reporting requirements.

Compliance with Requirement 4   ❏ Yes
               ❏ No

Requirement 5 The hospital selects and uses indicators from at least one listed performance measurement system.

The hospital identifies clinical indicators that meet Joint Commission requirements for the number of indicators and percentage of patient population covered. The number of indicators and percentage of patient population monitored will increase over time. The hospital submits data for its indicators to the performance measurement system(s) at least quarterly, and such submissions identify monthly data points. Each accredited hospital must notify the Joint Commission of its initial indicator selections prior to January 1, 1998. A hospital applying for initial survey must notify the Joint Commission of its indicator selection(s) at the time of survey. Each hospital must also notify the Joint Commission of any subsequent additions or changes to its indicator selections. An individual indicator must be used for at least four consecutive quarters. For purposes of reporting to the Joint Commission, a hospital will be expected to

- continue to use an indicator if the indicator data suggest an unstable pattern of performance or otherwise identify an opportunity for improvement; or
- change to a new indicator if the indicator data reflect continuing stable and satisfactory performance.

Note: Between the years 1997 and 2000, the minimum number of required measures and percentage of patient population monitored by the selected measures will increase according to the following schedule:

Year	Minimum Number of Clinical Measures	Minimum Percentage of Patient Population Monitored
1997	2	20%
1998	4	25%
1999	6	30%
2000	8	35%

Hospitals that have an ADC of less than 10 but more than 150 ambulatory visits per month may select ambulatory care measures in lieu of the required in-patient measures.

Compliance with Requirement 5   ❏ Yes
               ❏ No

Requirement 6 The hospital ensures that aggregate data for the selected indicators are submitted to the Joint Commission at least quarterly.

Hospital-specific aggregate data, which include monthly data points, must be submitted quarterly to the Joint Commission for use in the accreditation process. Findings based on the Joint Commission's analysis of the data may lead to subsequent intracycle monitoring activities. The quarterly data submissions must begin no later than the first quarter of 1999. The Joint Commission will define the type and format of performance measurement data to be submitted in a fashion consistent with nationally-recognized standards.

The submission of hospital-specific data will be performed by the performance measurement system(s) and will include comparative data for other hospitals that have selected these same performance measures.

Note: *Hospitals that have an ADC of 30 or fewer may report to their measurement systems quarterly (rather than monthly) indicator data points. Incremental measurement requirements over time for very small hospitals will be abated to the extent necessary to maintain statistically valid data point determinations on a quarterly basis.*

Compliance with Requirement 6

❑ Yes
❑ Data have not been submitted for one of four consecutive quarters
❑ Data have not been submitted for more than one of four consecutive quarters

Public Information Interviews

Requirement 7 The hospital provides notice of an upcoming full accreditation survey and of the opportunity for a public information interview.*

A hospital must provide an opportunity for the public to participate in a public information interview during a full survey. The public includes

- patients and their families;
- patient advocates;
- members of the community for whom services are provided; and
- hospital personnel.

To comply with the 30-day policy for notifying the public about the upcoming survey, the hospital is responsible for making the public information interview process widely known and effective as a source of compliance information in the accreditation process. The Joint Commission requires a hospital scheduled for a full survey to post announcements of the survey date and of the opportunity for a public information interview. To maximize participation, postings must be made throughout the hospital in the form provided by the Joint Commission. Hospitals should post notices in public eating areas, on bulletin boards near major entrances, and in treatment or residential areas. In addition, if all staff members are not likely to see such postings, the hospital must provide each staff member with a written announcement of the survey.

The hospital must also provide potential public information interview participants with sufficient advance notice. The Joint Commission requires hospitals to post public notices at least 30 days before the scheduled survey date. Notices must remain posted until the survey is completed.

The hospital should also promptly initiate community advertisement or other communications as soon as it receives notice of the survey date. Appropriate steps to take in notifying the community of the opportunity for public information interviews include

---

* See also pages 20 through 23 in the Accreditation Cycle chapter.

Accreditation Participation Requirements

- informing organized patient advocacy groups that have substantively communicated with the hospital in the previous 12 months;
- reaching other members of the community, for example through a classified advertisement in a local newspaper or newsletter; and
- informing individuals who inquire about the survey of the survey date(s) and opportunity to participate.

Compliance with Requirement 7 ❏ Yes
❏ No

Requirement 8 The hospital notifies the Joint Commission of any requests for a public information interview.*

The hospital must promptly forward to the Joint Commission all written requests to participate in a public information interview. Hospitals receiving an oral request should instruct the individual(s) to make the request in writing and mail it to the Joint Commission. The hospital should provide the individual(s) needing assistance in doing this with the necessary support. The hospital is responsible for notifying the interviewee(s) of the exact date, time, and place of the public information interview.

Compliance with Requirement 8 ❏ Yes
❏ No

Misrepresentation of Information

Requirement 9 The hospital does not misrepresent information in the accreditation process.[†]
Information provided by the hospital and used by the Joint Commission for the accreditation process must be accurate and truthful. Such information may
- be provided orally;
- be obtained through direct observation by Joint Commission surveyors;
- be derived from documents supplied by the hospital to the Joint Commission; and
- involve data submitted electronically by the hospital to the Joint Commission.

The Joint Commission requires each hospital seeking accreditation to engage in the accreditation process in good faith. Any hospital that fails to participate in good faith by falsifying information presented in the accreditation process may have its accreditation denied or removed by the Joint Commission.

For the purpose of this requirement, falsification is defined as the fabrication, in whole or in part, of any information provided by an applicant or accredited hospital to the Joint Commission. This includes any redrafting, reformatting, or content deletion of documents. However, the hospital may submit additional material that summarizes or otherwise explains the original information submitted to the Joint Commission. These additional materials must be properly identified, dated, and accompanied by the original documents.

Compliance with Requirement 9 ❏ Yes
❏ No

---

* See also page 28 in the Accreditation Cycle chapter.

[†] See also pages 15, 16, and 20 in the Accreditation Cycle chapter.

Requirement 10 The hospital does not publicly misrepresent its accreditation status or the scope of facilities and services to which the accreditation applies.*

Hospitals accredited by the Joint Commission must be accurate when describing to the public the nature and meaning of their accreditation. On request, the Joint Commission's Department of Communications will provide accredited hospitals with appropriate guidelines for characterizing the accreditation award. These guidelines also cover accreditation with commendation awards. A hospital may not engage in any false or misleading advertising with respect to the accreditation award. Any such advertising may be grounds for denying or revoking accreditation.

Compliance with Requirement 10   ❏ Yes
                                      ❏ No

---

* See also pages 15, 16, and 20 in the Accreditation Cycle chapter.

Patient Rights and Organization Ethics

Overview

The **goal** of the patient rights and organization ethics function* is to help improve patient outcomes by respecting each patient's rights and conducting business relationships with patients and the public in an ethical manner.

Patients have a fundamental right to considerate care that safeguards their personal dignity and respects their cultural, psychosocial, and spiritual values. These values often influence patients' perception of care and illness. Understanding and respecting these values guide the provider in meeting the patients' care needs and preferences.

A hospital's behavior towards its patients and its business practices has a significant impact on the patient's experience of and response to care. Thus, access, treatment, respect, and conduct affect patient rights. The standards in this chapter address the following processes and activities:
- Promoting consideration of patient values and preferences, including the decision to discontinue treatment;
- Recognizing the hospital's responsibilities under law;
- Informing patients of their responsibilities in the care process; and
- Managing the hospital's relationships with patients and the public in an ethical manner.

---

* **function** A goal-directed, interrelated series of processes, such as continuum of care or management of information.

Standards

The following is a list of all standards for this function. If you have a questions about a term used here, please check the Glossary, pages 281 through 307. Terms that are critical to the understanding of the standard are defined in the footnotes of the next section of this chapter.

RI.1 The hospital addresses ethical issues in providing patient care.

RI.1.1 The patient's right to treatment or service is respected and supported.

RI.1.2 Patients are involved in all aspects of their care.

RI.1.2.1 Informed consent is obtained.

RI.1.2.1.1 All patients asked to participate in a research project are given a description of the expected benefits.

RI.1.2.1.2 All patients asked to participate in a research project are given a description of the potential discomforts and risks.

RI.1.2.1.3 All patients asked to participate in a research project are given a description of alternative services that might also prove advantageous to them.

RI.1.2.1.4 All patients asked to participate in a research project are given a full explanation of the procedures to be followed, especially those that are experimental in nature.

RI.1.2.1.5 All patients asked to participate in a research project are told that they may refuse to participate, and that their refusal will not compromise their access to services.

RI.1.2.2 The family participates in care decisions.

RI.1.2.3 Patients are involved in resolving dilemmas about care decisions.

RI.1.2.4 The hospital addresses advance directives.

RI.1.2.5 The hospital addresses withholding resuscitative services.

RI.1.2.6 The hospital addresses forgoing or withdrawing life-sustaining treatment.

RI.1.2.7 The hospital addresses care at the end of life.

RI.1.3 The hospital demonstrates respect for the following patient needs:

RI.1.3.1 *confidentiality;*

RI.1.3.2 privacy;

Patient Rights and Organization Ethics

RI.1.3.3 security;

RI.1.3.4 resolution of complaints;

RI.1.3.5 pastoral care and other spiritual services;

RI.1.3.6 communication.

RI.1.3.6.1 When the hospital restricts a patient's visitors, mail, telephone calls, or other forms of communication, the restrictions are evaluated for their therapeutic effectiveness.

RI.1.3.6.1.1 Any restrictions on communication are fully explained to the patient and family, and are determined with their participation.

RI.1.4 Each patient receives a written statement of his or her rights.

RI.1.5 The hospital supports the patient's right to access protective services.

RI.2 The hospital implements policies and procedures, developed with the medical staffs' participation, for the procuring and donation of organs and other tissues.

RI.3 The hospital protects patients and respects their rights during research, investigation, and clinical trials involving human subjects.

RI.3.1 All consent forms address the information specified in RI.1.2.1.1 through RI.1.2.1.5; indicate the name of the person who provided the information and the date the form was signed; and address the participant's right to privacy, confidentiality, and safety.

RI.4 The hospital operates according to a code of ethical behavior.

RI.4.1 The code addresses marketing, admission, transfer and discharge, and billing practices.

RI.4.2 The code addresses the relationship of the hospital and its staff members to other health care providers, educational institutions, and payers.

RI.4.3 In hospitals with longer lengths of stay, the code addresses a patient's rights to perform or refuse to perform tasks in or for the hospital.

RI.4.4 The hospital's code of ethical business and professional behavior protects the integrity of clinical decision making, regardless of how the hospital compensates or shares financial risk with its leaders, managers, clinical staff, and licensed independent practitioners.

Standards and Intent Statements for Patient Rights

Standard

RI.1 The hospital addresses ethical issues in providing patient care.

Intent of RI.1

A mere listing of patient rights cannot guarantee that those rights are respected. Rather, a hospital demonstrates its support of patient rights through the processes by which staff members interact with and care for patients. These day-to-day interactions reflect a fundamental concern with and respect for patients' rights. All staff members are aware of the ethical issues surrounding patient care, the hospital's policies governing these issues, and the structures available to support ethical decision making.

The hospital establishes and maintains structures to support patient rights, and does so in a collaborative manner that involves the hospital's leaders and others. The structures are based on policies, procedures, and their philosophical basis, which makes up the framework that addresses both *patient care* and *organizational* ethical issues, including the following:
a. The patient's right to reasonable access to care;
b. The patient's right to care that is considerate and respectful of his or her personal values and beliefs;
c. The patient's right to be informed about and participate in decisions regarding his or her care;
d. The patient's right to participate in ethical questions that arise in the course of his or her care, including issues of conflict resolution, withholding resuscitative services, forgoing or withdrawal of life-sustaining treatment, and participation in investigational studies or clinical trials;
e. The patient's right to security and personal privacy and confidentiality of information;
f. The issue of designating a decision maker in case the patient is incapable of understanding a proposed treatment or procedure or is unable to communicate his or her wishes regarding care;
g. The hospital's method of informing the patient of these issues identified in this intent;
h. The hospital's method of educating staff about patient rights and their role in supporting those rights; and
i. The patient's right to access protective services.*

Standard

RI.1.1 The patient's right to treatment or service is respected and supported.

Intent of RI.1.1

A hospital provides care in response to a patient's request and need, so long as that care is within the hospital's capacity, its stated mission and philosophy, and relevant laws and regulations. When a hospital cannot provide the care a patient requests, staff fully inform the patient of his or her needs and the alternatives for care. If it is necessary and medically advisable, the hospital transfers the patient to another organization. The transfer has to be acceptable to the receiving organization.

---

* Protective services determine the need for protective intervention, correct hazardous living conditions or situations in which vulnerable adults are unable to care for themselves, and investigate evidence of neglect, abuse, or exploitation. Such services for children help families recognize the cause of any problems and strengthen parental ability to provide acceptable care. Protective services can include guardianship and advocacy services, conservatorship, state survey and certification agency, state licensure office, the state ombudsman program, the protection and advocacy network, and the Medicaid fraud control unit.

Patient Rights and Organization Ethics

Standard

RI.1.2 Patients are involved in all aspects of their care.

Intent of RI.1.2

Hospitals promote patient and family involvement in all aspects of their care through implementation of policies and procedures that are compatible with the hospital's mission and resources, have diverse input, and guarantee communication across the organization. Patients are involved in at least the following aspects of their care:
- Giving informed consent;
- Making care decisions;
- Resolving dilemmas about care decisions;
- Formulating advance directives;
- Withholding resuscitative services;
- Forgoing or withdrawing life-sustaining treatment; and
- Care at the end of life.

To this end, structures are developed, approved, and maintained through collaboration among the hospital's leaders and others.

Patients' psychosocial, spiritual, and cultural values affect how they respond to their care. The hospital allows patients and their families to express their spiritual beliefs and cultural practices, as long as these do not harm others or interfere with treatment.

Standard

RI.1.2.1 Informed consent is obtained.

Intent of RI.1.2.1

Staff members clearly explain any proposed treatments or procedures to the patient and, when appropriate, the family. The explanation includes
- potential benefits and drawbacks;
- potential problems related to recuperation;
- the likelihood of success;
- the possible results of nontreatment; and
- any significant alternatives.

Staff members also inform the patient of
- the name of the physician or other practitioner who has primary responsibility for the patient's care;
- the identity and professional status of individuals responsible for authorizing and performing procedures or treatments;
- any professional relationship to another health care provider or institution that might suggest a conflict of interest;
- their relationship to educational institutions involved in the patient's care;
- any business relationships between individuals treating the patient, or between the organization and any other health care, service, or educational institutions involved in the patient's care.

Standards

RI.1.2.1.1 All patients asked to participate in a research project are given a description of the expected benefits.

RI.1.2.1.2 All patients asked to participate in a research project are given a description of the potential discomforts and risks.

RI.1.2.1.3 All patients asked to participate in a research project are given a description of alternative services that might also prove advantageous to them.

RI.1.2.1.4 All patients asked to participate in a research project are given a full explanation of the procedures to be followed, especially those that are experimental in nature.

RI.1.2.1.5 All patients asked to participate in a research project are told that they may refuse to participate, and that their refusal will not compromise their access to services.

Intent of RI.1.2.1.1 Through RI.1.2.1.5
When patients are asked to participate in an investigational study or clinical trial, they need information upon which to base their decision. The hospital protects patients and respects their rights during research, investigation, and clinical trials involving human subjects by
- giving them information to make a fully informed decision;
- describing expected benefits;
- describing potential discomforts and risks;
- describing alternatives that might also help them;
- explaining procedures to be followed;
- explaining that they may refuse to participate, and that their refusal will not compromise their access to the hospital's services.

The hospital has policies and procedures for providing patients with this information.

Standard
RI.1.2.2 The family participates in care decisions.

Intent of RI.1.2.2
Care sometimes requires that people other than (or in addition to) the patient be involved in decisions about the patient's care. This is especially true when the patient does not have the mental or physical capacity to make care decisions, or when the patient is a child. When the patient cannot make decisions regarding his or her care, a surrogate decision maker* is identified. In the case of an unemancipated minor, the family or guardian is legally responsible for approving the care prescribed. The patient has the right to exclude any or all family members from participating in his or her care decisions.

Standard
RI.1.2.3 Patients are involved in resolving dilemmas about care decisions.

Intent of RI.1.2.3
Making decisions about care sometimes presents questions, conflicts, or other dilemmas for the hospital and the patient, family, or other decision makers. These dilemmas may arise around issues of

---

* **surrogate decision maker** Someone appointed to act on behalf of another. Surrogates make decisions only when an individual is without capacity or has given permission to involve others.

admission, treatment, or discharge. They can be especially difficult to resolve when the issues involve, for example, withholding resuscitative services or forgoing or withdrawing life-sustaining treatment. The hospital has a way of resolving such dilemmas and identifies those who need to be involved in the resolution.

Standard

RI.1.2.4 The hospital addresses advance directives.*

Intent of RI.1.2.4

The hospital determines whether a patient has or wishes to make advance directives. The hospital also ensures that health care professionals and designated representatives honor the directives within the limits of the law and the organization's mission, philosophy, and capabilities. For example, if a patient elects to donate organs at the end of life, the organization must have a process to honor that directive (see also IM.3.2.1). In the absence of the actual advance directive, the substance of the directive is documented in the patient's medical record. The lack of advance directives does not hamper access to care. The hospital, however, provides assistance to patients who do not have an advance directive but wish to formulate one.

Standards

RI.1.2.5 The hospital addresses withholding resuscitative services.

RI.1.2.6 The hospital addresses forgoing or withdrawing life-sustaining treatment.

Intent of RI.1.2.5 and RI.1.2.6

Decisions about withholding resuscitative services or forgoing or withdrawing life-sustaining treatment are among the most difficult choices facing patients, families, health care professionals, and hospitals. No single process can anticipate all of the situations in which such decisions must be made. All the more reason why it is important for the hospital to develop collaboratively a framework for making these difficult decisions.

The framework

- helps the hospital identify its position on initiating resuscitative services and using and removing life-sustaining treatment;
- ensures that the hospital conforms to the legal requirements of its jurisdiction;
- addresses situations in which these decisions are modified during the course of care;
- offers guidance to health professionals on the ethical and legal issues involved in these decisions and decreases their uncertainty about the practices permitted by the hospital.

The decision-making process is applied consistently, and the lines of accountability are clear. To ensure this, it is vital that a guiding process be formally adopted by the hospital's medical staff and approved by the governing body.

---

* **advance directive** A document or documentation allowing a person to give directions about future medical care or to designate another person(s) to make medical decisions if the individual loses decision-making capacity. Advance directives may include living wills, durable powers of attorney, do-not-resusitate (DNRs) orders, right to die, or similar documents expressing the individual's preferences as specified in the Patient Self-Determination Act.

Standard

RI.1.2.7 The hospital addresses care at the end of life.

Intent of RI.1.2.7
Dying patients have unique needs for respectful, responsive care. All hospital staff are sensitized to the needs of patients at the end of life. Concern for the patient's comfort and dignity should guide all aspects of care during the final stages of life.

The hospital's framework for addressing issues related to care at the end of life provide for
- providing appropriate treatment for any primary and secondary symptoms, according to the wishes of the patient or the surrogate decision maker;
- managing pain aggressively and effectively;
- sensitively addressing issues such as autopsy and organ donation;
- respecting the patient's values, religion, and philosophy;
- involving the patient and, where appropriate, the family in every aspect of care; and
- responding to the psychological, social, emotional, spiritual, and cultural concerns of the patient and the family.

Effective pain management is appropriate for all patients, not just for dying patients.

Standards

RI.1.3 *The hospital demonstrates respect for the following patient needs:*

RI.1.3.1 *confidentiality;*

RI.1.3.2 *privacy;*

RI.1.3.3 *security;*

RI.1.3.4 *resolution of complaints;*

RI.1.3.5 *pastoral care and other spiritual services;*

RI.1.3.6 *communication.*

RI.1.3.6.1 When the hospital restricts a patient's visitors, mail, telephone calls, or other forms of communication, the restrictions are evaluated for their therapeutic effectiveness.

RI.1.3.6.1.1 Any restrictions on communication are fully explained to the patient and family, and are determined with their participation.

Intent of RI.1.3 Through RI.1.3.6.1.1
Communication and information are important areas of rights and respect for patients. The hospital has a way of providing for
- effective communication* for each patient served, including the hearing and speech impaired;
- the patient's right to privacy and security;

---

* **effective communication** Any form of communication (for example, writing or speech) that leads to demonstrable understanding.

Patient Rights and Organization Ethics

- the patient's right to confidentiality of information; and
- the patient's right to voice complaints about his or her care, and to have those complaints reviewed and, when possible, resolved.

Generally, patients have the right to expect unrestricted access to communication. Sometimes, however, it may be necessary to restrict visitors, mail, telephone calls, or other forms of communication as a component of a patient's care (for example, to prevent injury or deterioration in the patient, damage to the environment, or infringement on the rights of others). The patient is included in any such decision.

Communication restrictions are explained in a language the patient understands. For an unemancipated minor or patient under guardianship, applicable law determines who is legally entrusted to act in the patient's best interest. Clinical justification of such restrictions is documented in the medical record.

For many patients, pastoral care and other spiritual services are an integral part of health care and daily life. The hospital is able to provide for pastoral care and other spiritual services for patients who request them.

Standard
RI.1.4 Each patient receives a written statement of his or her rights.

Intent of RI.1.4
Admission to the hospital can be a frightening and confusing experience for patients, making it difficult for them to understand and exercise their rights. A written copy of the hospital's statement of patients' rights is given to patients when they are admitted and is available to them throughout their stay. This statement is appropriate to the patient's age, understanding, and language.

The hospital may also post a copy of its patients' rights document in public areas accessible to patients and their visitors. When written communication is not effective (for example, the patient cannot read or the patient's language is rare in the patient population served), the patient is informed again of his or her rights after admission, in a manner that he or she can understand.

Standard
RI.1.5 The hospital supports the patient's right to access protective services.

Intent of RI.1.5
When the hospital serves a patient population that often needs protective services (that is, guardianship and advocacy services, conservatorship, and child or adult protective services), it has ways of helping patients' families and the courts determine a patient's need for special services, such as guardianship. An independent assessment ensures that the patient's best interests are of primary concern. When the services are especially pertinent to the population served by the hospital, the patient is given, in writing

- a list of names, addresses, and telephone numbers of pertinent state client advocacy groups such as the state survey and certification agency, the state licensure office, the state ombudsman program, the protection and advocacy network, and the Medicaid fraud control unit; and
- information regarding the patient's right to file a complaint with the state survey and certification agency if he or she has a concern about patient abuse, neglect, or about misappropriation of a patient's property in the facility.

The hospital has policies and procedures that address all the issues described above.

Standard

RI.2 The hospital implements policies* and procedures, developed with the medical staffs' participation, for the procuring and donation of organs and other tissues.

Intent of RI.2

Any hospital procuring human organs has an affiliation agreement with the appropriate organ procurement organization (OPO) and follows its rules and regulations. For nonfederal hospitals, this organization is the Organ Procurement and Transplantation Network (OPTN) established under section 372 of the Public Health Service Act. For Department of Defense hospitals, Veterans Affairs medical centers, and other federally administered health care facilities, the appropriate organizations are designated by the respective agency.

In addition, the hospital has an agreement with at least one tissue bank and at least one eye bank to cooperate in the retrieval, processing, preservation, storage, and distribution of tissues and eyes. This agreement is to assure that all usable tissues and eyes are obtained from potential donors, as long as it does not interfere with organ procurement.

Policies and procedures are written and implemented for organ and tissue procurement and donation include the following:

- The OPO with which the hospital is affiliated is identified;
- The hospital has procedures for notifying the OPO in a timely manner of individuals who have died, or whose death is imminent, in the hospital (that is, when an organ—specifically a heart, kidney, liver, lung, or pancreas—or other tissue potentially becomes available). In Department of Defense hospitals, Veterans Affairs medical centers, and other federally administered health care agencies, notification is carried out according to procedures approved by the respective agency;
- The OPO determines medical suitability for organ donation and, in the absence of alternative arrangements by the hospital, for tissue and eye donation;
- The hospital has procedures, developed in collaboration with the designated OPO, for notifying the family of each potential donor of the option to donate—or decline to donate—organs, tissues, or eyes. This notification is made by an organ procurement representative or the hospital's designated requestor;†
- Written documentation by the hospital's designated requestor shows that the patient or family accepts or declines the opportunity for the patient to become an organ or tissue donor;
- The hospital's staff exercises discretion and sensitivity to the circumstances, beliefs, and desires of the families of potential donors;
- The hospital maintains records of potential donors whose names have been sent to the OPO, as well as to tissue and eye banks;
- The hospital works cooperatively with the OPO, tissue, and eye banks in reviewing death records to improve identification of potential donors. In addition, the hospital works with these groups to maintain potential donors while the necessary testing and placement of potential donated organs, tissues, and eyes take place; and
- The hospital works cooperatively with the OPO, tissue, and eye banks in educating staff on donation issues.

---

* Effective January 1, 1999.

† A designated requestor is an individual who has completed a course offered or approved by the OPO, designed in conjunction with the tissue and eye bank community, that provides training in the methodology for approaching potential donor families and requesting organ and tissue donation.

Patient Rights and Organization Ethics

For Hospitals Performing Transplant Services
Hospitals transplanting human organs must be a member of the OPTN established under section 372 of the Public Health Service Act and abide by its rules. If requested, all organ-transplant-related data are provided to the OPTN, the Scientific Registry, or the hospital's designated OPO.

Standards

RI.3 The hospital protects patients and respects their rights during research, investigation, and clinical trials involving human subjects.

RI.3.1 *All consent forms address the information specified in RI.1.2.1.1 through RI.1.2.1.5; indicate the name of the person who provided the information and the date the form was signed; and address the participant's right to privacy, confidentiality, and safety.*

Intent of RI.3 and RI.3.1
A hospital that conducts research, investigations, or clinical trials involving human subjects knows that its first responsibility is to the health and well-being of the individual patient. To protect and respect patients' rights, the hospital always
- reviews all research protocols in relation to the hospital's mission statement, values, and other guidelines;
- weighs the relative risks and benefits to the subjects;
- obtains the subject's consent.

Because the patient's decision to participate in clinical trials or research needs to be based on his or her competency and sound information, the following items are documented in the patient's record:
- The name of the person who provided the information and
- The date the form was signed.

When research procedures are complete, the principal investigator does everything possible to eliminate any confusion, misinformation, stress, physical discomfort, or other harmful consequences the participant may have experienced as a result of the procedures.

Standards and Intent Statements for Organization Ethics

Standards

RI.4 The hospital operates according to a code of ethical behavior.*

RI.4.1 The code addresses marketing, admission, transfer and discharge, and billing practices.

RI.4.2 The code addresses the relationship of the hospital and its staff members to other health care providers, educational institutions, and payers.

---

* The hospital may have one code of ethical behavior or multiple codes addressing the issues identified in RI.4.1 through RI.4.2.

Intent of RI.4 Through RI.4.2

A hospital has an ethical responsibility to the patients and community it serves. Guiding documents, such as the hospital's mission statement and strategic plan, provide a consistent, ethical framework for its patient care and business practices.

But a framework alone is not sufficient. To support ethical operations and fair treatment of patients, a hospital has and operates according to a code of ethical behavior. The code addresses ethical practices regarding
- marketing;
- admission;
- transfer;
- discharge; and
- billing, and resolution of conflicts associated with patient billing.

The code ensures that the hospital conducts its business and patient care practices in an honest, decent, and proper manner.

Standard

RI.4.3 In hospitals with longer lengths of stay, the code addresses a patient's rights to perform or refuse to perform tasks in or for the hospital.

Intent of RI.4.3

Patients are encouraged to take responsibility for their own living quarters. In addition, patients may be offered the opportunity to perform work for the organization (for example, patient work therapy programs in grounds keeping or the library) that does not endanger the patient, other patients, or staff. If the hospital asks longer-stay patients to perform such tasks (work), the patient has the right to refuse. If the patient agrees to perform tasks for the organization
- the work is appropriate to the patient's needs and therapeutic goals;
- the organization documents the patient's desire for work in the plan of care;
- the plan specifies the nature of the services performed and whether the services are nonpaid or paid;
- compensation for paid services is determined based on the work performed, whether the work would be otherwise done by a paid employee, and the applicable wage and hourly standards in the community for the work; and
- the patient agrees to the work arrangement described in the plan of care.

The intent of this standard does not extend to the patient's care of his or her body, maintenance of his or her room or space, or the patient's preparation of his or her own meals.

Standard

RI.4.4 The hospital's code of ethical business and professional behavior protects the integrity of clinical decision making, regardless of how the hospital compensates or shares financial risk with its leaders, managers, clinical staff, and licensed independent practitioners.

Patient Rights and Organization Ethics

Intent of RI.4.4

To avoid compromising the quality of care, clinical decisions (including tests, treatments, and other interventions) are based on identified patient health care needs. The hospital's code of ethical business and professional behavior specifies that the hospital implements policies and procedures that address the relationship between the use of services and financial incentives. Policies and procedures addressing and information on this issue are available on request to all patients, clinical staff, licensed independent practitioners, and hospital personnel.

Assessment of Patients

Overview

The **goal** of the patient assessment function* is to determine what kind of care is required to meet a patient's initial needs as well as his or her needs as they change in response to care.

To provide patients with the right care at the time it is needed, qualified individuals in a hospital assess† each patient's care needs throughout the patient's contact with the hospital. The standards in this chapter address the following processes and activities:

- Collecting data.‡
  The hospital collects data about each patient's physical and psychosocial status and health history.
- Analyzing data.
  The hospital analyzes data to produce information§ about each patient's care needs, and to identify any additional information required.
- Making care decisions.
  The hospital bases care decisions on information developed about each patient's needs.

Hospitals meet the goal of this function by performing these processes and activities well.

---

* **function** A goal-directed, interrelated series of processes, such as continuum of care or management of information.

† **assess** To transform data into information by analyzing it.

‡ **data** Uninterpreted material, facts, or clinical observations.

§ **information** Interpreted set(s) of data that can assist in decision making.

Standards

The following is a list of all standards for this function. If you have a questions about a term used here, please check the Glossary, pages 281 through 307. Terms that are critical to the understanding of the standard are defined in the footnotes of the next section of this chapter.

PE.1 Each patient's physical, psychological, and social status are assessed.

PE.1.1 The scope and intensity of any further assessment are based on the patient's diagnosis, the care setting, the patient's desire for care, and the patient's response to any previous care.

PE.1.2 Nutritional status is assessed when warranted by the patient's needs or condition.

PE.1.3 Functional status is assessed when warranted by the patient's needs or condition.

PE.1.3.1 All patients referred for rehabilitation services receive a functional assessment.

PE.1.4 Diagnostic testing necessary for determining the patient's health care needs is performed.

PE.1.4.1 When a test report requires clinical interpretation, any relevant clinical information is provided with the request.

PE.1.5 The need for a discharge planning assessment is determined.

PE.1.6 Each admitted patient's initial assessment is conducted within a time frame specified by hospital policy.

PE.1.6.1 The patient's history and physical examination, nursing assessment, and other screening assessments are completed within 24 hours of admission as an inpatient.

PE.1.6.1.1 If a history and a physical examination have been performed within 30 days before admission, a durable, legible copy of this report may be used in the patient's medical record, provided any changes that may have occurred are recorded in the medical record at the time of admission.

PE.1.7 Before surgery, the patient's physical examination and medical history, any indicated diagnostic tests, and a preoperative diagnosis are completed and recorded in the patient's medical record.

PE.1.7.1 Any patient for whom anesthesia is contemplated receives a preanesthesia assessment.

PE.1.7.2 Before anesthesia, the patient is determined to be an appropriate candidate for the planned anesthesia.

PE.1.7.3 The patient is reevaluated immediately before anesthesia induction.

Assessment of Patients

PE.1.7.4 The patient's postoperative status is assessed on admission to and discharge from the postanesthesia recovery area.

PE.1.8 Possible victims of abuse are identified using criteria developed by the hospital.

PE.1.9 Pathology and clinical laboratory services and consultation are readily available to meet patients' needs.

PE.1.9.1 The hospital provides for prompt performance of adequate examinations in anatomic pathology, hematology, chemistry, microbiology, clinical microscopy, parasitology, immunohematology, serology, virology, and nuclear medicine related to pathology and clinical laboratory services.

PE.1.9.2 While the patient is under the hospital's care, all laboratory testing is done in the hospital's laboratories or approved reference laboratories.

PE.1.9.2.1 When organized central pathology and clinical laboratory services are not offered, the hospital identifies acceptable reference or contract laboratory services.

PE.1.9.2.2 Reference and contract laboratory services meet applicable federal standards for clinical laboratories.

Testing methods classified as waived testing under federal law and regulation must be in compliance with PE.1.10 through PE.1.14.2.

PE.1.10 The hospital defines the extent to which the test results are used in an individual's care (definitive or used only as a screen).

PE.1.11 The hospital identifies the staff members responsible for performing and supervising waived testing.

PE.1.12 Those performing tests have adequate, specific training and orientation to perform the tests, and demonstrate satisfactory levels of competence.

PE.1.13 Policies and procedures governing specific testing-related processes are current and readily available.

PE.1.14 Quality control checks, as defined by the hospital, are conducted on each procedure.

PE.1.14.1 At a minimum, manufacturers' instructions are followed.

PE.1.14.2 Appropriate quality control and test records are maintained.

PE.2 Each patient is reassessed at points designated in hospital policy.

PE.2.1 Reassessment occurs at regular intervals in the course of care.

PE.2.2 Reassessment determines a patient's response to care.

PE.2.3 Significant change in a patient's condition results in reassessment.

PE.2.4 Significant change in a patient's diagnosis results in reassessment.

PE.3 Staff members integrate the information from various assessments of the patient to identify and assign priorities to his or her care needs.

PE.3.1 Staff members base care decisions on the identified patient needs and care priorities.

PE.4 The hospital has defined patient assessment activities in writing.

PE.4.1 The hospital defines the scope of assessment performed by each discipline.

PE.4.2 A licensed independent practitioner with appropriate clinical privileges determines the scope of assessment and care for patients in need of emergency care.

PE.4.3 A registered nurse assesses the patient's need for nursing care in all settings where nursing care is provided.

PE.5 The assessment process for an infant, child, or adolescent patient is individualized.

PE.6 The special needs of patients who are receiving treatment for emotional or behavioral disorders are addressed by the assessment process.

PE.7 The special needs of patients who are receiving treatment for alcoholism or other drug dependencies are addressed by the assessment process.

PE.8 Patients who are possible victims of alleged or suspected abuse or neglect have special needs relative to the assessment process.

Assessment of Patients

Standards and Intent Statements for Initial Assessment

Standards

PE.1 Each patient's physical, psychological, and social status are assessed.

PE.1.1 The scope and intensity of any further assessment are based on the patient's diagnosis, the care setting, the patient's desire for care, and the patient's response to any previous care.

Intent of PE.1 and PE.1.1

When a patient enters a hospital service, staff members first need to find out the reason why the patient was admitted. The specific information the hospital requires at this stage, and the procedures for getting it, depend on the patient's needs and on the setting in which care is being provided. Hospital policy defines how this process works.

The initial assessment takes into account the patient's immediate and emerging needs, and considers those needs broadly—that is, not only physiological status but psychological and social concerns too. This initial assessment helps staff determine what care the patient needs as well as any further assessments. A patient's cultural and family* contexts and individual background are important factors in his or her response to illness and treatment; families can be of considerable help in these areas of assessment.

The information gathered at the first patient contact may indicate that the patient needs a broader or more detailed assessment. Precisely what further assessment is needed will depend, at least in part, on
- the patient's diagnosis;
- the care he or she is seeking;
- the care setting;
- the patient's response to any previous care; and
- his or her consent to treatment.

The hospital has a policy that addresses these issues and defines what areas to include in reassessments.

For dying patients, an assessment is made of the social, spiritual, and cultural variables that influence the perceptions and expressions of grief by the individual, family members, or significant other(s).

Standards

PE.1.2 Nutritional status is assessed when warranted by the patient's needs or condition.

PE.1.3 Functional status is assessed when warranted by the patient's needs or condition.

PE.1.3.1 All patients referred for rehabilitation services receive a functional assessment.

Intent of PE.1.2 Through PE.1.3.1

In its initial patient assessment, the hospital identifies patients at risk for nutritional problems, according to criteria developed by dietitians and other qualified professionals. The hospital refers such patients to a dietitian for further assessment.

---

* **family** The person(s) who plays a significant role in the individual's life. This may include a person(s) not legally related to the individual. This person(s) is often referred to as a surrogate decision maker if authorized to make care decisions for an individual should the individual lose decision-making capacity.

During the initial assessment, the hospital also identifies patients who require a functional assessment using criteria developed by rehabilitation specialists and other qualified professionals. This functional assessment, in turn, identifies any patients who will need rehabilitation services. Any patients who are currently receiving rehabilitation services at the hospital have had a functional assessment.

Some patients coming into the hospital setting may need special nutritional care and some patients may need rehabilitation services or other services addressing their ability to function. These patients will require specialized assessments. Therefore, it is important for the hospital to identify patients with special needs.

Standards

PE.1.4 Diagnostic testing* necessary for determining the patient's health care needs is performed.

PE.1.4.1 When a test report requires clinical interpretation, any relevant clinical information is provided with the request.

Intent of PE.1.4 and PE.1.4.1

Diagnostic testing is integral to the physical, psychological, and social assessment of the patient. Diagnostic testing covers operative and other procedures,[†] including laboratory, radiologic, electrodiagnostic, and other functional tests and imaging technologies. To appropriately care for patients, the results of these tests are used to determine the patient's health care or treatment needs. The hospital's clinical staff determines which of these tests, if any, will be performed when the patient enters the setting or service.

To be interpreted appropriately, some tests require additional clinical data or background information. A clinician who requests such a test provides, in writing, any information needed to perform and interpret the test properly.

Standard

PE.1.5 The need for a discharge planning assessment is determined.

Intent of PE.1.5

Continuity of care requires thoughtful preparation. When indicated, hospital staff identify when planning for a patient's post-hospital care and other needs is to be conducted. The hospital has a way of identifying those patients for whom discharge planning is critical.

Standards

PE.1.6 Each admitted patient's initial assessment is conducted within a time frame specified by hospital policy.

---

* **diagnostic testing** Laboratory and other invasive, diagnostic, and imaging procedures.

[†] **operative and other procedures** Includes operative, other invasive, and noninvasive procedures, such as radiotherapy, hyperbaric, CAT scan, and MRI, that place the patient at risk. The focus is on procedures and is not meant to include medications that place the patient at risk.

Assessment of Patients

PE.1.6.1 The patient's history and physical examination, nursing assessment, and other screening assessments are completed within 24 hours of admission as an inpatient.

PE.1.6.1.1 If a history and a physical examination have been performed within 30 days before admission, a durable, legible copy of this report may be used in the patient's medical record, provided any changes that may have occurred are recorded in the medical record at the time of admission.

Intent of PE.1.6 Through PE.1.6.1.1

The initial assessment of a patient is completed within a reasonable time frame, as defined by the hospital. Precisely what the time frame is will depend on a variety of factors, including the types of patients treated by the hospital, the complexity and duration of their care, and the dynamics of conditions surrounding their care. With that in mind, a hospital may establish different time frames for the initial assessment in different areas or services.

However, some elements of the assessment must be completed—by all hospitals and for all patients—within 24 hours of admission, even on weekends and holidays. These elements are
- medical history and physical examination;
- nursing care assessment; and
- other screening assessments, as needed.

Some of these elements may have been completed ahead of time, though no more than 30 days before the patient was admitted or readmitted, and only by the appropriate, qualified professionals. Specifically,
- a medical history and physical examination by a physician or oral and maxillofacial surgeon who is a member of the medical staff and
- a nursing care assessment completed by a qualified registered nurse.

Reports from these assessments may be used in place of new assessments, provided
- durable, legible copies (or originals) of the report are in the patient's record and
- any significant changes in the patient's condition since the report are recorded at the time of admission.

Standards

PE.1.7 Before surgery, the patient's physical examination and medical history, any indicated diagnostic tests, and a preoperative diagnosis are completed and recorded in the patient's medical record.

PE.1.7.1 Any patient for whom anesthesia* is contemplated receives a preanesthesia assessment.

PE.1.7.2 Before anesthesia, the patient is determined to be an appropriate candidate for the planned anesthesia.

PE.1.7.3 The patient is reevaluated immediately before anesthesia induction.

PE.1.7.4 The patient's postoperative status is assessed on admission to and discharge from the postanesthesia recovery area.

---

* See the "Care of Patients" chapter of this book for the scope of anesthesia to which these standards apply.

Intent of PE.1.7 Through PE.1.7.4

When a patient undergoes surgery or other procedure, hospital staff members evaluate the patient's status continuously before, during, and after the procedure. In an emergency, when there is no time to record the complete history and physical examination, a note on the preoperative diagnosis is recorded before surgery.

A preanesthesia assessment is an essential element of continuing evaluation for patients who will undergo anesthesia. Data collected during the assessment process provide information that clinicians need to determine risks and choose the most appropriate form of anesthesia, administer it safely, and interpret findings while monitoring the patient. A licensed independent practitioner with appropriate clinical privileges concurs with or makes this determination based on the preanesthesia assessment.

Note: *A licensed independent practitioner with appropriate clinical privileges concurs with the planned choice of anesthesia—general, regional, or sedation (with or without analgesia). The licensed independent practitioner (for example, a surgeon, obstetrician, or dentist) need not have privileges to actually administer the planned anesthesia.*

Standard

PE.1.8 Possible victims of abuse are identified using criteria developed by the hospital.

Intent of PE.1.8

Victims of abuse or neglect may come to a hospital through a variety of channels. The patient may be unable or reluctant to speak of the abuse, and it may not be obvious to the casual observer. Nevertheless, hospital staff members need to know if a patient has been abused, as well as the extent and circumstances of the abuse, to give the patient appropriate care.

The hospital has objective criteria for identifying and assessing possible victims of abuse and neglect, and they are used throughout the organization. Staff are to be trained in the use of these criteria.*

The criteria focus on observable evidence and not on allegation alone. They address at least the following situations:
a. Physical assault;
b. Rape or other sexual molestation;
c. Domestic abuse; and
d. Abuse or neglect of elders and children.

When used appropriately by qualified staff members, the criteria prevent any action or question that could create false memories of abuse in the individual being assessed.

Staff members are able to make appropriate referrals for victims of abuse and neglect. To help them do so, the hospital maintains a list of private and public community agencies that provide help for abuse victims.

In addition, the assessment of victims of alleged or suspected abuse or neglect is conducted consistent with standard PE.6 in this chapter.

---

* Consistent with standard HR.3 of this book.

Assessment of Patients

Standards and Intent Statements for Pathology and Clinical Laboratory Services—Waived Testing

Changes in federal regulations (CLIA '88) are incorporated into the standards published in the current edition of the *Comprehensive Accreditation Manual for Pathology and Clinical Laboratory Services* (*CAMPCLS*). If the hospital performs only limited laboratory testing (waived testing) or refers all testing to other organizations, then the standards in this section will apply. Hospitals that perform moderate- or high-complexity testing are surveyed under the *CAMPCLS*.

The following standards address the requirements that must be carried out when a hospital performs waived testing procedures. Waived tests are those that

- meet the Clinical Laboratory Improvement Amendments of 1988 (CLIA '88) requirements to be classified as waived tests;
- are cleared by the Food and Drug Administration (FDA) for home use;
- use methodologies that are so simple and accurate as to render the likelihood of erroneous results negligible; or
- pose no risk of harm to the patient if the test is performed incorrectly.

Standards

PE.1.9 Pathology and clinical laboratory services and consultation are readily available to meet patients' needs.

PE.1.9.1 The hospital provides for prompt performance of adequate examinations in anatomic pathology, hematology, chemistry, microbiology, clinical microscopy, parasitology, immunohematology, serology, virology, and nuclear medicine related to pathology and clinical laboratory services.

Intent of PE.1.9 and PE.1.9.1

The hospital has a system for providing laboratory services required by its patient population, services, and licensed independent practitioners. Laboratory services, including those required for emergencies, may be provided within the hospital, by agreement with another organization, or both. Laboratory results are provided on a timely basis to diagnose and treat individuals. This is particularly important for individuals with a critical health status.

Standards

PE.1.9.2 While the patient is under the hospital's care, all laboratory testing is done in the hospital's laboratories or approved reference laboratories.

PE.1.9.2.1 When organized central pathology and clinical laboratory services are not offered, the hospital identifies acceptable reference or contract laboratory services.

PE.1.9.2.2 Reference and contract laboratory services meet applicable federal standards for clinical laboratories.

Intent of PE.1.9.2 Through PE.1.9.2.2
Both in-house and reference labs provide the quality and accuracy necessary to support clinical and medical decisions. A hospital's services include those provided by a central laboratory and any ancillary, near-patient-testing, and point-of-care laboratories.

When reference or contract laboratories are used,
- they are selected based on evaluation of their past and current performance, acceptability as a source, and compliance with federal standards;
- the director(s) recommends reference laboratory services to the medical staff for acceptance; and
- a written agreement defines the responsibilities of the hospital and the laboratory when services are provided entirely by contract, and contracted services fulfill the hospital's needs.

Waived Testing
Testing methods classified as waived testing under federal law and regulation must be in compliance with PE.1.10 through PE.1.14.2.

Standard
PE.1.10 The hospital defines the extent to which the test results are used in an individual's care (definitive or used only as a screen).

Intent of PE.1.10
The hospital defines whether the results of waived testing will be considered definitive for purposes of care and diagnosis, or regarded as a screening tool, in which case they may be followed by confirmation testing. The hospital assesses all waived testing it performs, and specifies how each test will be used in diagnosis, care, and screening.

Standard
PE.1.11 The hospital identifies the staff members responsible for performing and supervising waived testing.

Intent of PE.1.11
The hospital identifies which staff members perform testing and which direct or supervise testing. These individuals may be employees of the hospital, contracted personnel, or employees of a contracted service.

Standard
PE.1.12 Those performing tests have adequate, specific training and orientation to perform the tests, and demonstrate satisfactory levels of competence.

Intent of PE.1.12
For waived tests to be performed properly, the individuals performing them must be qualified to do so. The hospital therefore ensures that those performing waived tests meet the following criteria:
a. They have had specific training in the tests. Such training may be acquired through hospital or other training programs, such as those provided by other health care organizations or by manufacturers.
b. They have had orientation that is specific to the hospital's needs.

c. They have shown current competence.

Skills are assessed at defined intervals, determined by the director or supervisor, based on the frequency that staff members perform tests and their technical backgrounds. The hospital emphasizes skills testing for individuals who perform testing infrequently.

Hospitals also consider the complexity of the test methodology and the consequences of an inaccurate result. Methods used to assess current skills can include
- performing a test on an unknown specimen;
- periodic observation of routine work by the supervisor or a delegate; and
- monitoring each user's quality control performance.

Standard

PE.1.13 Policies and procedures governing specific testing-related processes are current and readily available.

Intent of PE.1.13

Written policies and procedures address the following items (a through f):
a. Specimen collection;
b. Specimen preservation;
c. Instrument calibration;
d. Quality control and remedial action;
e. Equipment performance evaluation; and
f. Performing tests.

Policies and procedures are tailored to the hospital, but may refer to manufacturers' manuals. Policies and procedures are readily available at all times to staff members who perform tests.

Standards

PE.1.14 Quality control checks, as defined by the hospital, are conducted on each procedure.

PE.1.14.1 At a minimum, manufacturers' instructions are followed.

Intent of PE.1.14 and PE.1.14.1

The hospital's quality control plan includes a quality control program for testing. The plan specifies how procedures will be controlled for quality, establishes timetables, and explains the rationale for choice of procedures and timetables. The rationale is based on
- how the test is used;
- reagent stability;
- manufacturers' recommendations;
- the hospital's experience with the test; and
- currently accepted guidelines.

Quality control requirements for glucose meter testing include two levels of control for each instrument on each day of patient testing.

Standard

PE.1.14.2 Appropriate quality control and test records are maintained.

Intent of PE.1.14.2

Quality control test results are documented and test results may be located in the clinical record. Quality control records, instrument problems, and individual results are correlated. A log or other record is maintained to determine annual volume if required by other reporting agencies.

Standards and Intent Statements for Reassessment

Standards

PE.2 Each patient is reassessed at points designated in hospital policy.

PE.2.1 Reassessment occurs at regular intervals in the course of care.

PE.2.2 Reassessment determines a patient's response to care.

PE.2.3 Significant change in a patient's condition results in reassessment.

PE.2.4 Significant change in a patient's diagnosis results in reassessment.

Intent of PE.2 Through PE.2.4

Patient reassessment is key to understanding if care decisions are appropriate and effective. Patients are reassessed throughout the care process and at follow-up appointments. Hospital policy designates reassessment purposes and key reassessment points, including any specific time intervals.

Standards and Intent Statements for Care Decisions

Standards

PE.3 Staff members integrate the information from various assessments of the patient to identify and assign priorities to his or her care needs.

PE.3.1 Staff members base care decisions on the identified patient needs and care priorities.

Intent of PE.3 and PE.3.1

A patient may undergo many kinds of assessments from his or her physician and from several other disciplines. As a result, there may be a variety of data, analyses, and other information in the patient's record.

A patient benefits most when staff members work collaboratively to integrate this information into a comprehensive picture of his or her condition. From this collaboration, the patient's needs and their order of importance are identified, and appropriate care decisions are made.

Standards and Intent Statements for Structures Supporting the Assessment of Patients

Standards

PE.4 The hospital has defined patient assessment activities in writing.

PE.4.1 The hospital defines the scope of assessment performed by each discipline.

Intent of PE.4 and PE.4.1
To consistently assess patient needs, the hospital defines, in writing, the scope of assessments to be performed by each clinical discipline. Assessments are performed by each discipline within its scope of practice, state licensure laws, applicable regulations, or certification. The hospital defines assessment activities in policies and procedures, protocols, or other such documented guidelines, taking into account the different settings in which care or treatment is provided. Assessment policies and procedures define
- the data gathered to assess patient needs;
- the scope of assessment by each discipline;
- the processes used to analyze these data to determine the approach to meet patient care needs; and
- the framework for decision making based on the analysis of the information.

Standard

PE.4.2 A licensed independent practitioner with appropriate clinical privileges determines the scope of assessment and care for patients in need of emergency care.

Intent of PE.4.2
Patients coming into a hospital's emergency service area often need immediate care. A qualified, licensed independent practitioner is available, and is responsible for determining, as quickly as possible, what assessments the patient requires to care for his or her needs.

Standard

PE.4.3 A registered nurse assesses the patient's need for nursing care in all settings where nursing care is provided.

Intent of PE.4.3
The judgment and skill of a registered nurse are required to determine and set priorities on a patient's nursing care needs. Hospital policy therefore ensures that a registered nurse carries out these activities during a patient's initial assessment. The registered nurse may be assisted in any aspect of this process by other qualified nursing staff members—such as licensed practical nurses, licensed vocational nurses, mental health technicians, or nursing assistants—so long as their activities comply with applicable laws and regulations and with hospital policies and procedures.

1999 Hospital Accreditation Standards

Standards and Intent Statements for Additional Requirements for Specific Patient Populations

These standards address the assessment of patients who have special needs due to their age, disability, or condition. The assessment and reassessment of patients with special needs due to age, disability, or condition focus on data and information specific to the characteristics of each patient population or special situation.

Standard

PE.5 The assessment process for an infant, child, or adolescent patient is individualized.

Intent of PE.5

The assessment process for an infant, child, or adolescent is individualized to the patient's needs. The following are assessed and documented as appropriate to the patient's age and needs:
- Emotional, cognitive, communication, educational, social, and daily activity needs;
- The patient's developmental age, length or height, head circumference, and weight;
- The effect of the family or guardian on the patient's condition and the effect of the patient's condition on the family or guardian;
- The patient's immunization status; and
- The family's or guardian's expectations for and involvement in the patient's assessment, initial treatment, and continuing care.

Verification of immunization status may be obtained from a third party, such as the family physician, or school records. Documentation includes written evidence of immunization history or reliable oral verification that is subsequently documented by hospital staff.

Standard

PE.6 The special needs of patients who are receiving treatment for emotional or behavioral disorders are addressed by the assessment process.

Intent of PE.6

The content of the assessment and reassessment of patients receiving treatment for mental and behavioral disorders includes at least the following elements:
- A history of mental, emotional, behavioral, and substance use problems, their co-occurrence, and treatment;
- Current mental, emotional, and behavioral functioning, including a mental status examination;
- Maladaptive or problem behaviors; and
- A psychosocial assessment.

As appropriate to the patient's age and specific clinical needs, the psychosocial assessment includes information about the patient's
- environment and home;
- leisure and recreation;
- religion;
- childhood history;
- military service history;

Assessment of Patients

- financial status;
- the social, peer-group, and environmental setting from which the individual comes;
- sexual history, including abuse (either as the abuser or the abused);
- physical abuse (either as the abuser or the abused);
- the individual's family circumstances, including the constellation of the family group;
- the current living situation; and
- social, ethnic, cultural, emotional, and health factors.

Those responsible for the patient's care determine the need for family members to participate in the individual's care. When appropriate, the following additional assessments are conducted:

- Vocational or educational assessment and
- Legal assessment.

The community resources currently used by the individual (especially for patients with severe and persistent mental illness) are identified.

In addition, when indicated by the patient's age and specific clinical needs, the following are performed:

- A psychiatric evaluation;
- Psychological assessments, including intellectual, projective, neuropsychological, and personality testing; and
- Other functional evaluations of communication, self-care, and visual-motor functioning.

Standard

PE.7 The special needs of patients who are receiving treatment for alcoholism or other drug dependencies are addressed by the assessment process.

Intent of PE.7

Patients being treated for alcohol and other drug dependencies have specific needs that are consistently addressed in their assessment and reassessment, regardless of the setting or service in which the assessments take place. These areas include

- the patient's history of alcohol, nicotine, and other drug use, including age of onset, duration, intensity, patterns of use (for example, loss of control over amounts or frequencies of consumption, inability to consistently abstain from use, relapse), and consequences of use;
- the types of previous treatment and responses to that treatment;
- a history of mental, emotional, and behavioral problems; their co-occurrence with substance use problems; and their treatment;
- a history of biomedical complications associated with alcohol, nicotine, or other drug use, and the patient's level of awareness of the relationships between these behavioral conditions and the patient's pattern of substance use; and
- a psychosocial assessment.

As appropriate to the patient's age and specific clinical needs, the psychosocial assessment includes information about the patient's

- treatment acceptance or motivation for change;
- recovery environment features that serve as resources or obstacles to recovery, including the use of alcohol and other drugs by family members;
- the patient's religion and spiritual orientation;
- any history of physical or sexual abuse, as either the abuser or the abused; and
- the patient's sexual history and orientation;

- environment and home;
- leisure and recreation;
- childhood history;
- military service history;
- financial status;
- the social, peer-group, and environmental setting from which the patient comes;
- patient's family circumstances, including the constellation of the family group;
- the current living situation; and
- social, ethnic, cultural, emotional, and health factors.

Those responsible for the patient's care determine the need for family members to participate in the individual's care. When appropriate, the following additional assessments are conducted:
- Vocational or education assessment;
- Legal assessment; and
- Other functional evaluations of communication, self-care, and visual-motor functioning.

Hospital policy on patient assessment addresses these areas, and they are included in each patient's medical record.

Standard

PE.8 Patients who are possible victims of alleged or suspected abuse or neglect have special needs relative to the assessment process.

Intent of PE.8

As part of the initial screening and assessment process, information and evidentiary material(s) may be collected that could be used in future actions as part of the legal process. The hospital has specific and unique responsibilities for safeguarding such material(s).

Policies and procedures define the hospital's responsibility for collecting, retaining, and safeguarding information and evidentiary material(s). The following are documented in the patient's medical record:
- Consents from the patient, parent, or legal guardian, or compliance with other applicable law;
- Collecting and safeguarding evidentiary material released by the patient;
- Legally required notification and release of information to authorities; and
- Referrals made to private or public community agencies for victims of abuse.

Hospital policy defines these activities and specifies who is responsible for carrying them out.

Care of Patients

Overview

The **goal** of the care of patients function* is to provide individualized care in settings responsive to specific patient needs.

Patients deserve care that respects their choices, supports their participation in the care provided, and recognizes their right to experience achievement of their personal health goals. The goals of patient care are met when the following processes are performed well:
- Providing supportive care;
- Treating of a disease or condition;
- Rehabilitating physical or psychosocial impairment; and
- Promoting health.

The standards in this chapter address activities involved in these processes, including
- planning care;
- providing care;
- monitoring and determining the outcomes of care;
- modifying care; and
- coordinating follow-up.

These activities may be carried out by medical, nursing, pharmacy, dietetic, rehabilitation, and other types of providers. Each provider's role and responsibility are determined by their professional skills, competence, and credentials; the care or rehabilitation being provided; hospital policies; and relevant licensure, certification, regulation, privileges, scope of practice, or job description.

Note: *The first standard in this chapter outlines a process common to all patients receiving general care and addresses the core processes (that is, planning, providing, monitoring); thus, it applies to every hospital. Succeeding standards (Anesthesia Care through Rehabilitation Care and Services) address issues specific to certain types of care. Each standard or group of standards in these sections apply only when a hospital provides the type of care addressed by the standard(s).*

---

* **function** A goal-directed, interrelated series of processes, such as continuum of care or management of information.

Standards

The following is a list of all standards for this function. If you have a questions about a term used here, please check the Glossary, pages 281 through 307. Terms that are critical to the understanding of the standard are defined in the footnotes of the next section of this chapter.

TX.1 Care, treatment, and rehabilitation are planned to ensure that they are appropriate to the patient's needs and severity of disease, condition, impairment, or disability.

TX.1.1 Settings and services required to meet patient care goals are identified, planned, and provided if appropriate.

TX.1.1.1 When care is not planned to meet all identified needs, this is documented in the medical record.

TX.1.2 Care is planned and provided in an interdisciplinary, collaborative manner by qualified individuals.

TX.1.2.1 Patient care procedures (such as bathing) are performed in a manner that respects privacy.

TX.1.3 Patients' progress is periodically evaluated against care goals and the plan of care and when indicated, the plan or goals are revised.

TX.2 *A preanesthesia assessment is performed for each patient before anesthesia induction.*

TX.2.1 Each patient's anesthesia care is planned.

TX.2.2 Anesthesia options and risks are discussed with the patient and family prior to administration.

TX.2.3 Each patient's physiological status is monitored during anesthesia administration.

TX.2.4 *The patient's postprocedure status is assessed on admission to and before discharge from the postanesthesia recovery area.*

TX.2.4.1 Patients are discharged by a qualified licensed independent practitioner or according to criteria approved by the medical staff.

TX.3 *Medication use processes are organized and systematic throughout the hospital.*

TX.3.1 The organization identified an appropriate selection of medications available for prescribing or ordering.

TX.3.2 The organization addressed prescribing or ordering and procuring medications not available in the organization.

Care of Patients

TX.3.3 Policies and procedures support safe medication prescription or ordering.

TX.3.4 Preparing and dispensing medication(s) adhere to law, regulation, licensure, and professional standards of practice.

TX.3.5 Preparation and dispensing of medication(s) is appropriately controlled.

TX.3.5.1 A patient medication dose system is implemented.

TX.3.5.2 Pharmacists review all prescriptions or orders.

TX.3.5.3 When preparing and dispensing a medication(s) for a patient, important patient medication information is considered.

TX.3.5.4 Pharmacy services are available when the pharmacy department is closed or not available.

TX.3.5.5 Emergency medications are consistently available, controlled, and secure in the pharmacy and patient care areas.

TX.3.5.6 A medication recall system provides for retrieval and safe disposition of discontinued and recalled medications.

TX.3.6 Prescriptions or orders are verified and patients are identified before medication is administered.

TX.3.7 The organization has alternative medication administration systems.

TX.3.8 Investigational medications are safely controlled, administered, and destroyed.

TX.3.9 Medication effects on patients are continually monitored.

TX.4 Each patient's nutrition care is planned.

TX.4.1 An interdisciplinary nutrition therapy plan is developed and periodically updated for patients at nutritional risk.

TX.4.1.1 When appropriate to the patient groups served by a unit, meals and snacks support program goals.

TX.4.2 Authorized individuals prescribe or order food and nutrition products in a timely manner.

TX.4.3 Responsibilities are assigned for all activities involved in safe and accurate provision of food and nutrition products.

TX.4.4 Food and nutrition products are distributed and administered in a safe, accurate, timely, and acceptable manner.

1999 Hospital Accreditation Standards

TX.4.5 Each patient's response to nutrition care is monitored.

TX.4.6 The nutrition care service meets patients' needs for special diets and accommodates altered diet schedules.

TX.4.7 Nutrition care practices are standardized throughout the organization.

TX.5 The medical staff defines the scope of assessment for operative and other procedures.

TX.5.1 *Determining the appropriateness of a procedure for each patient is based, in part, on a review of*

TX.5.1.1 the patient's history;

TX.5.1.2 the patient's physical status;

TX.5.1.3 diagnostic data;

TX.5.1.4 the risks and benefits of procedures; and

TX.5.1.5 the need to administer blood or blood components.

TX.5.2 *Before obtaining informed consent, the risks, benefits, and potential complications associated with procedures are discussed with the patient and family.*

TX.5.2.1 Alternative options are considered.

TX.5.2.2 Discussions with the patient and family about the need for, risk of, and alternatives to blood transfusion when blood or blood components may be needed are considered.

TX.5.3 Plans of care are developed and documented in the patient's medical record before the operative or other procedure is performed.

TX.5.4 The patient is monitored during the postprocedure period.

TX.6 *Qualified professionals provide rehabilitation services, consistent with professional licensure laws, regulation, registration, and certification.*

TX.6.1 A rehabilitation plan, developed by qualified professionals and based on assessment of patient needs, guides provision of rehabilitation services.

TX.6.2 Qualified professionals implement the rehabilitation plan with the patient, and his or her family, social network, or support system.

TX.6.3 Rehabilitation restores, improves, or maintains the patient's optimal level of functioning, self-care, self-responsibility, independence, and quality of life.

Care of Patients

TX.6.4 The patient's readiness to end rehabilitation services is determined based on written discharge criteria.

TX.7 The hospital ensures that special procedures are safely and appropriately used.

TX.7.1 Restraint or seclusion use within the organization is limited to those situations with adequate, appropriate clinical justification.

TX.7.1.1 *Organization leaders support limited, justified use of restraint or seclusion through appropriate:*

TX.7.1.1.1 *Plans, policies, and priorities;*

TX.7.1.1.2 *Human resource planning;*

TX.7.1.1.3 *Staff orientation and education creating a culture emphasizing prevention and appropriate use and encouraging alternatives;*

TX.7.1.1.4 *Patient and, when appropriate, family education;*

TX.7.1.1.5 *Assessment processes that identify and, when appropriate, prevent potential behavioral risk factors;*

TX.7.1.1.6 *Design and delivery of patient care; and*

TX.7.1.1.7 The development and promotion of preventive strategies and use of safe and effective alternatives.

TX.7.1.2 Performance-improvement processes identify opportunities, when appropriate, to reduce restraint or seclusion use.

TX.7.1.3 When restraint or seclusion is used, organization policy and procedures guide appropriate and safe use.

TX.7.1.3.1 *Individual orders for restraint or seclusion are consistent with organization policy.*

TX.7.1.3.1.1 *Patient rights, dignity, and well-being are protected during restraint or seclusion use.*

TX.7.1.3.1.2 Restraint or seclusion use is based on the assessed needs of the patient.

TX.7.1.3.1.3 The least-restrictive safe and effective restraint or seclusion method is employed.

TX.7.1.3.1.4 *Restraint or seclusion is used correctly by competent, trained staff.*

TX.7.1.3.1.5 Patients in restraint or seclusion are monitored and reassessed appropriately.

TX.7.1.3.1.6 Patient needs are met during restraint or seclusion use.

TX.7.1.3.1.7 Restraint or seclusion use is ordered by a licensed independent practitioner.

TX.7.1.3.1.8 Orders for restraint or seclusion use define specific time limits.

TX.7.1.3.2 Documentation in medical records reflects organization policy.

TX.7.2 Electroconvulsive and other forms of convulsive therapy are used with adequate justification, documentation, and regard for patient safety.

TX.7.3 Psychosurgery or other surgical treatments for emotional, mental, or behavioral disorders are performed with adequate justification, documentation, and regard for patient safety.

TX.7.4 Use of behavior-management procedures conforms to the patient's treatment plan and hospital policy.

TX.7.4.1 Qualified staff review, evaluate, and approve all behavior-management procedures.

TX.7.5 The organization's leaders determine the organization's approach to the use of restraint in the care of nonpsychiatric patients, which limits its use to those situations where there is appropriate clinical justification.

TX.7.5.1 Performance-improvement processes seek to identify opportunities to reduce the risks associated with restraint use through the introduction of preventive strategies, innovative alternatives, and process improvements.

TX.7.5.2 Organization policy(ies) and procedure(s) guide appropriate and safe use of restraint.

TX.7.5.3 *Any use of restraint (to which these standards apply) is initiated pursuant to either an individual order (standard TX.7.5.3.1) or an approved protocol (standard TX.7.5.3.2).*

TX.7.5.3.1 Individual orders for initiation and renewal of restraint are consistent with organization policy(ies) and procedure(s), and are consistent with the patient's needs and clinical condition.

TX.7.5.3.2 Protocols for restraint use contain criteria to ensure only clinically justified use.

TX.7.5.4 Patients in restraint are monitored.

TX.7.5.5 Each episode of restraint use is documented in the patient's medical record, consistent with organization policy(ies) and procedure(s).

Care of Patients

Standards and Intent Statements for Planning and Providing Care

Certain activities are fundamental to providing patient care. These activities encompass planning and providing care, monitoring its results, modifying or completing care, and coordinating follow-up. Care planning is based on an assessment of the patient* who participates in care.† Staff members provide care according to their scope of practice, standards of practice, and hospital policies. Some care may be carried out by the patient, family,‡ or other caregivers following education. Monitoring and determining the outcomes of care involve assessing, or reassessing, the patient's progress throughout treatment, and reassessing to determine care outcomes. Any modifications, including a decision to terminate care, are based on a reassessment and patient need. Coordinating follow-up care§ helps ensure that the patient's care needs are met or referred.

Standard

TX.1 Care, treatment, and rehabilitation are planned to ensure that they are appropriate to the patient's needs and severity of disease, condition, impairment, or disability.

Intent of TX.1

Care is planned to respond to each patient's unique needs (including age-specific needs), expectations, and characteristics with effective, efficient, and individualized care. An essential element in the planning process is assessment of the severity of the patient's disease, condition, impairment, or disability.

Patients' care, treatment, and rehabilitation goals are identified as much as goals are at the heart of the care planning process. Written policies and procedures define when a program of regular dental care is required to meet oral health goals, based on length of stay.

Standard

TX.1.1 Settings and services required to meet patient care goals are identified, planned, and provided if appropriate.

Intent of TX.1.1

Acting on care goals requires deliberate planning. For most patients, meeting the goals requires a variety of services that often can be delivered in multiple settings. For each patient, the most appropriate setting(s) is selected and provided. Care begins when settings and services are identified and planned.

---

* See the "Assessment of Patients" chapter in this book.

† See the "Patient Rights and Organization Ethics" chapter in this book.

‡ **family** The person(s) who plays a significant role in the individual's life. This may include a person(s) not legally related to the individual. This person(s) is often referred to as a surrogate decision maker if authorized to make care decisions for an individual should the individual lose decision-making capacity.

§ See the "Continuum of Care" chapter in this book.

Standard

TX.1.1.1 When care is not planned to meet all identified needs, this is documented in the medical record.

Intent of TX.1.1.1

Because a patient's condition may be multidimensional and complex, multiple needs may be identified through assessment and reassessment. Qualified members of the patient's treatment team identify treatment priorities that will be addressed in the active plan of care, and may decide that other less urgent needs will not be included. Decisions not to address certain needs are justified in patient records.

Standard

TX.1.2 Care is planned and provided in an interdisciplinary, collaborative manner by qualified individuals.*

Intent of TX.1.2

A collaborative, interdisciplinary approach helps coordinate care and planning to meet patient care goals and achieve optimal outcomes. The mix of disciplines involved and the intensity of the collaboration will vary as appropriate to each patient. Collaborative care planning includes the family, as appropriate.[†]

Standard

TX.1.2.1 Patient care procedures (such as bathing) are performed in a manner that respects privacy.

Intent of TX.1.2.1

Patients who cannot care for themselves have the right to be cleaned and bathed in private. Incontinent patients are cleaned or bathed promptly after voiding or soiling with special consideration for their privacy.

Standard

TX.1.3 Patients' progress is periodically evaluated against care goals and the plan of care and when indicated, the plan or goals are revised.

Intent of TX.1.3

The frequency of evaluation is appropriate to the services provided and patients' needs.

---

* **qualified individual** An individual or staff member who is qualified to participate in one or all of the mechanisms outlined in Joint Commission standards by virtue of the following: education, training, experience, competence, registration or certification; or applicable licensure, law, or regulation.

[†] See RI.1.2.2 in the "Patient Rights and Organization Ethics" chapter of this book that addresses the family's involvement in the care of patients function.

Care of Patients

Standards and Intent Statements for Anesthesia Care

The standards for anesthesia care apply when patients, in any setting, receive, for any purpose, by any route,
1. general, spinal, or other major regional anesthesia or
2. sedation (with or without analgesia) which, in the manner used, may be reasonably expected to result in the loss of protective reflexes* as defined below.

Because sedation is a continuum, it is not always possible to predict how an individual patient receiving sedation will respond. Therefore, each organization develops specific, appropriate protocols for the care of patients receiving sedation that carries the risk of loss of protective reflexes. These protocols are consistent with professional standards and address at least the following:
- Sufficient qualified personnel present to perform the procedure and to monitor the patient (see TX.2 through TX.2.2, LD.2.7 and LD.2.9, and HR.1 and HR.2);
- Appropriate equipment for care and resuscitation (see LD.1.3.2 and EC.2.1.3);
- Appropriate monitoring of vital signs—heart and respiratory rates and oxygenation using pulse oximetry equipment (see TX.1 , TX.2 through TX.2.2, TX.3 through TX.3.9, and TX.5 through TX.5.4);
- Documentation of care (see IM.7.3 through IM.7.4); and
- Monitoring of outcomes (see the "Leadership" chapter and PI.3.1 through PI.3.1.3).

Standard

TX.2 *A preanesthesia assessment is performed for each patient before anesthesia induction.*

Intent of TX.2

Hospitals providing obstetric or emergency operative services can provide anesthesia services within approximately 30 minutes after anesthesia is deemed necessary.

Preanesthesia assessment considers data from other assessments and collects information needed to
- select and plan anesthesia care;
- safely administer anesthesia; and
- interpret findings of patient monitoring.

Standard

TX.2.1 Each patient's anesthesia care is planned.

Intent of TX.2.1

Because anesthesia carries a high level of risk, its administration is carefully planned. An anesthesia plan is developed to meet patient needs identified through preanesthesia assessment. Patients' anesthesia care needs are communicated among care providers.

Hospitals providing obstetric or emergency operative services can provide anesthesia services within approximately 30 minutes after anesthesia is deemed necessary.

---

* **loss of protective reflexes** An inability to handle secretions without aspiration or to maintain a patent airway independently.
  Note: *Indicators that the patient has retained protective reflexes include the patient's ability to respond appropriately to verbal commands and to respond purposefully to physical stimulation. There are special situations in which use of local anesthesia in the upper respiratory tract (with or without sedation or analgesia) may necessitate additional protective measures such as oropharyngeal protective screens, or other precautions as dictated by the nature of the procedure.*

Standard

TX.2.2 Anesthesia options and risks are discussed with the patient and family prior to administration.

Intent of TX.2.2

Patients' comfort with the anesthesia process depends on their understanding of anesthesia options and risks. Education is part of the full explanation of anesthesia options and risks. Only when patients have a complete understanding of anesthesia options and risks can they reach a level of comfort that enables them to provide informed consent.

Standard

TX.2.3 Each patient's physiological status is monitored during anesthesia administration.

Intent of TX.2.3

Physiological monitoring is often the only reliable source of assessment information for patients who have lost consciousness or protective reflexes. The patient's physiological status is measured and assessed throughout anesthesia to ensure appropriate physiological support. Monitoring methods depend on the patient's preprocedure status, anesthesia choice, and the complexity of the procedure.

Standards

TX.2.4 *The patient's postprocedure status is assessed on admission to and before discharge from the postanesthesia recovery area.*

TX.2.4.1 Patients are discharged by a qualified licensed independent practitioner or according to criteria approved by the medical staff.

Intent of TX.2.4 and TX.2.4.1

During postanesthesia recovery, patients move through levels of care to discharge as their status permits. Ongoing, systematic collection and analysis of patient status information is used to manage this process.

Organizations often quantify and standardize criteria for discharge from the postanesthesia recovery area. To ensure successful outcomes, compliance with discharge criteria is documented in the patient's medical record.

Standards and Intent Statements for Medication Use

Medications* are frequently potent agents for treating illness and often for moderating symptoms. While medications are often essential to patient care, their use and handling entail risks which must be managed. The following standards identify risk points and offer a system for managing them.

---

* **medication** Any substance, other than food or devices, that may be used on or administered to persons as an aid in the diagnosis, treatment, or prevention of disease or other abnormal condition.

Evaluation of patients' past and current drug treatments is conducted when pharmacological agents are indicated. Treatment efficacy, impact on current functioning, and side effects are reviewed, including evaluations from the patient, family, or caregivers.

Medication use is coordinated with psychosocial interventions, when appropriate, to alleviate side effects of dosage levels and responses that inhibit patient participation in psychosocial programming.

These standards address medication
- selection, procurement, and storage;
- prescribing or ordering;*
- preparation and dispensing;
- administration; and
- monitoring effects on the patient.

Standards

TX.3 *Medication use processes are organized and systematic throughout the hospital.*

TX.3.1 The organization identified an appropriate selection of medications available for prescribing or ordering.

TX.3.2 The organization addressed prescribing or ordering and procuring medications not available in the organization.

Intent of TX.3 Through TX.3.2

A list of medications that are always available within the organization is maintained. Medication selection is a collaborative process that considers patient need and safety as well as economics. Suggested criteria for selection include the following:
- Need, given the diseases and conditions treated;
- Effectiveness, in terms of
  - efficacy,
  - toxicity,
  - pharmacokinetic properties,
  - bioequivalence, if applicable,
  - pharmaceutical equivalence, if applicable,†
  - therapeutic equivalence; if applicable,‡
- Risks of
  - known incidence of adverse drug reactions;
  - potential for error in prescribing or ordering, preparation, dispensing, and administration; and
- Acquisition costs and cost impact.

---

* **prescribing or ordering** Directing the selection, preparation, or administration of medication(s).

† **pharmaceutical equivalence** The degree to which two formulations of the same medication are identical in strength, concentration, and dosage form.

‡ **therapeutic equivalence** The degree to which two formulations of different active ingredients are judged by the clinical staff to have acceptably similar therapeutic effects.

Standard

TX.3.3 Policies and procedures support safe medication prescription or ordering.

Intent of TX.3.3

Procedures supporting safe medication prescription or ordering address
- distribution and administration of controlled medications, including adequate documentation and record keeping required by law;
- proper storage, distribution, and control of investigational medications and those in clinical trial;
- situations in which all or some of a patient's medication orders must be permanently or temporarily canceled, and mechanisms for reinstating them;
- "as needed" (PRN) prescriptions or orders and times of dose administration;
- control of sample drugs;
- distribution of medications to patients at discharge;
- procurement, storage, control, and distribution of prepackaged medications obtained from outside sources;
- procurement, storage, control, distribution, and administration of radioactive medications;
- procurement, storage, control, distribution, administration, and monitoring of all
  - ❑ blood derivatives* and
  - ❑ radiographic contrast media.

Standard

TX.3.4 Preparing and dispensing medication(s) adhere to law, regulation, licensure, and professional standards of practice.

Intent of TX.3.4

The organization adheres to law, professional licensure, and practice standards governing the safe operation of pharmacy services.

Standards

TX.3.5 Preparation and dispensing of medication(s) is appropriately controlled.

TX.3.5.1 A patient medication dose system is implemented.

TX.3.5.2 Pharmacists review all prescriptions or orders.

Intent of TX.3.5 Through TX.3.5.2

Procedures are used to control all medications prepared by the pharmacy department or obtained elsewhere by the patient.† To ensure safe and accurate dispensing of medications
- pharmacists review each prescription or order for medication and contact the prescriber or orderer when questions arise (except when a licensed independent practitioner with appropriate clinical privileges controls prescription or ordering, preparation, and administration, as in

---

* **blood derivative** A pooled blood product, such as albumin, gamma globulin, or Rh immune globulin, whose use is considered significantly lower in risk than that of blood or blood components.

† See TX.3.5.4 regarding provision of medications when the pharmacy department is closed.

Care of Patients

endoscopy or cardiac catheterization laboratories, surgery, or during cardiorespiratory arrest, and for some emergency orders when time does not permit);
- all medications dispensed to inpatients or outpatients are appropriately and safely labeled using a standardized method; and
- medications are dispensed in the most ready-to-administer form possible to minimize opportunities for error.

Standard
TX.3.5.3 When preparing and dispensing a medication(s) for a patient, important patient medication information is considered.

Intent of TX.3.5.3
The pharmacist and appropriate staff receive important information about each patient's medication regimen to
- facilitate continuity of care;
- create an accurate medication history;
- supplement monitoring of medication adverse events;* and
- help provide safe administration of medications.

Standard
TX.3.5.4 Pharmacy services are available when the pharmacy department is closed or not available.

Intent of TX.3.5.4
To deliver consistent quality during all hours of service, the organization has a means of providing pharmacy services when the on-site pharmacy is closed or not available.

Standard
TX.3.5.5 Emergency medications are consistently available, controlled, and secure in the pharmacy and patient care areas.

Intent of TX.3.5.5
The intent of this standard is self-evident.

Standard
TX.3.5.6 A medication recall system provides for retrieval and safe disposition of discontinued and recalled medications.

Intent of TX.3.5.6
The intent of this standard is self-evident.

---
* See the "Improving Organization Performance" chapter.

Standard

TX.3.6 Prescriptions or orders are verified and patients are identified before medication is administered.

Intent of TX.3.6
The intent of this standard is self-evident.

Standard
TX.3.7 The organization has alternative medication administration systems.

Intent of TX.3.7
The hospital safely manages medications brought in by patients. The hospital supports the patient's safe self-administration of any such medications.

Standard
TX.3.8 Investigational medications are safely controlled, administered, and destroyed.

Intent of TX.3.8
The organization ensures that investigational or clinical medication studies are safely conducted. Those medications not administered during the study are safely destroyed.

Standard
TX.3.9 Medication effects on patients are continually monitored.

Intent of TX.3.9
Medication monitoring is a collaborative process. Input from the patient and various disciplines is used to evaluate, maintain, and improve the patient's medication regimen. Monitoring medication effects on patients is a collaborative process. Assessment of the medication's effect on the patient includes the patient's own perceptions and information from the patient's medical record and medication profile.

Standards and Intent Statements for Nutrition Care

These standards focus on provision of appropriate nutrition care,* including food and nutrition therapy, in a timely, effective, and efficient manner using all appropriate resources.

Like all patient care, nutrition care is an interdisciplinary process. Nutrition care is integrated with other aspects of patient care and involves the physician, registered dietitian, nurse, pharmacist, and other appropriate disciplines.

---

* **nutrition care** Interventions and counseling to promote appropriate nutrition intake, based on nutrition assessment and information about food, other sources of nutrients, and meal preparation consistent with the individual's cultural background and socioeconomic status. Nutrition therapy, a component of medical treatment, includes enteral and parenteral nutrition.

Care of Patients

Nutrition care consists of the following processes:
- Screening, assessing, and reassessing nutrition needs;*
- Developing the plan for nutrition therapy;
- Prescribing or ordering food and other nutrients;
- Preparing and distributing or administering food and other nutrients; and
- Monitoring patient response to nutrition care.

Nutrition screening[†] is conducted to determine the patient's need for a comprehensive nutrition assessment.[‡] Approved policies define the content of nutrition screening and may establish specific parameters for evaluating the patient's nutrition status, such as patient weight compared to height.

When indicated by results of the nutrition screen, a nutrition assessment[§] is completed and updated at specified intervals. This edition of the *HAS* does not require a written prescription or order for nutrition assessment.

Standard

TX.4 Each patient's nutrition care is planned.

Intent of TX.4

Based on the results of the nutrition screen and, when appropriate, nutrition assessment and reassessment, the nutrition therapy plan is implemented for all patients determined to be at nutritional risk. Patients at nutritional risk include
- patients with actual or potential malnutrition;
- patients on altered diets or diet schedules;
- patients with inadequate nutrition;
- lactating and pregnant women; and
- geriatric surgical patients.

Organization criteria guide development of the nutrition therapy plan. A nutrition therapy plan is not ordinarily developed for patients receiving only a regular diet by mouth.

All patients, regardless of their nutritional status or need, receive a prescription or order for food or other nutrients.** The food or other nutrients ordered can range from nothing by mouth (NPO orders), to regular diets, to parenteral or enteral tube nutrition.

Standard

TX.4.1 An interdisciplinary nutrition therapy plan is developed and periodically updated for patients at nutritional risk.

---

* See also PE.1.2 in the "Assessment of Patients" chapter in this book.

[†] **nutrition screening** The process of using characteristics known to be associated with nutrition problems in order to determine if patients are malnourished or at high nutrition risk for malnourishment.

[‡] See the "Assessment of Patients" chapter in this book for a description of the nutrition screening process.

[§] **nutrition assessment** A comprehensive process for defining an individual's nutrition status using medical, nutrition, and medication intake histories, physical examination, anthromorphic measurements, and laboratory data.

** **nutrients** Protein, carbohydrates, lipids, vitamins, electrolytes, minerals, and water.

Intent of TX.4.1
A more intensive plan for nutrition therapy may be indicated for patients at high nutritional risk. The plan identifies measurable goals and actions to achieve them. The patient's physician, the registered dietitian, nursing, and pharmaceutical services staff participate in developing the plan, and their roles in implementation are clearly defined.

Standard
TX.4.1.1 When appropriate to the patient groups served by a unit, meals and snacks support program goals.

Intent of TX.4.1.1
Depending on the types or ages of patients served, some units may provide snacks or meals for special occasions or recreational activities. For example, on a child or adolescent service, the child learns to select appropriate snacks according to a plan for nutrition care. When appropriate, facilities that permit patient involvement are available for preparing and serving meals and snacks. Staff members assist patients when necessary and ensure that each patient receives an adequate amount and variety of food.

Standard
TX.4.2 Authorized individuals prescribe or order food and nutrition products in a timely manner.

Intent of TX.4.2
Food and nutrition products are administered only when prescribed or ordered by medical staff, authorized house staff, or other individuals with appropriate clinical privileges. Consistent with medical staff rules and regulations, verbal prescriptions or orders for food and nutrition products are accepted by designated personnel. Verbal prescriptions and orders are authenticated by the initiator within a defined time frame. All prescription orders are documented in the patient's medical record before any food or other nutrient is administered to the patient. A prescription or order for food or other nutrient is accepted by designated personnel. Such orders are documented in the patient's medical record before any food or other nutrient is administered to the patient.

Standard
TX.4.3 Responsibilities are assigned for all activities involved in safe and accurate provision of food and nutrition products.

Intent of TX.4.3
Staff responsibilities for preparation, storage, distribution, and administration of food and nutrition products are clearly defined to ensure safety and accuracy.

Standard
TX.4.4 Food and nutrition products are distributed and administered in a safe, accurate, timely, and acceptable manner.

Care of Patients

Intent of TX.4.4
Food is distributed in a timely manner to preserve nutrient value and serving temperature and provide nutrition that is appetizing and palatable. Food and nutrition products are distributed and administered to the patients for whom they were prescribed or ordered.

Standard
TX.4.5 Each patient's response to nutrition care is monitored.

Intent of TX.4.5
Ongoing patient monitoring is essential to effective, appropriate, and continuous nutrition care. Nutrition care monitoring is a collaborative process that may involve
- a formal nutrition care team;
- representatives from multiple disciplines conducting patient care rounds;
- communication among the various disciplines; or
- integration of nutrition care with the patient care team.

Standard
TX.4.6 The nutrition care service meets patients' needs for special diets and accommodates altered diet schedules.

Intent of TX.4.6
Food and nutrition services include processes for
- meeting special diet or diet schedule needs;
- providing food or nutrition products at times other than the regular delivery schedule;
- accommodating personal dietary requests; and
- storing, handling, and controlling food or nutrition products obtained from outside sources.

Standard
TX.4.7 Nutrition care practices are standardized throughout the organization.

Intent of TX.4.7
The medical staff, the nutrition care service or department, and other disciplines (for example, nursing) collaborate in developing and maintaining standardized approaches to nutrition care. Approaches are communicated and used throughout the organization.

Standards and Intent Statements for Operative and Other Procedures

The standards in this section apply whenever an operative or other procedure may result in a significant (as defined by the hospital) physiological effect, whether or not anesthesia is administered. They focus on operative and other procedures for

- diagnosis;
- cure;
- reduction or prevention of impairment or disability;
- restoration or improvement of function; and
- relief of symptoms.

These standards relate to the processes of
- selecting appropriate procedures;
- preparing patients for procedures;
- performing procedures and patient monitoring; and
- providing postprocedure care.

Standards

TX.5 The medical staff defines the scope of assessment for operative and other procedures.

TX.5.1 *Determining the appropriateness of a procedure for each patient is based, in part, on a review of*

TX.5.1.1 the patient's history;

TX.5.1.2 the patient's physical status;

TX.5.1.3 diagnostic data;

TX.5.1.4 the risks and benefits of procedures; and

TX.5.1.5 the need to administer blood or blood components.

Intent of TX.5 Through TX.5.1.5

Patients undergoing operative and other invasive procedures are assessed according to medical staff guidelines. Assessment provides information necessary to
- select the appropriate procedure and the optimal time;
- perform procedures safely; and
- interpret findings of patient monitoring.

Standards

TX.5.2 Before obtaining informed consent, the risks, benefits, and potential complications associated with procedures are discussed with the patient and family.

TX.5.2.1 Alternative options are considered.

TX.5.2.2 Discussions with the patient and family about the need for, risk of, and alternatives to blood transfusion when blood or blood components may be needed are considered.

Care of Patients

Intent of TX.5.2 Through TX.5.2.2
Patients receive adequate information to participate in care decisions and provide informed consent. If the patient's condition does not allow for such interaction, appropriate documentation is provided in the medical record.

Standard
TX.5.3 Plans of care are developed and documented in the patient's medical record before the operative or other procedure is performed.

Intent of TX.5.3
Adequate preoperative assessment and planning helps meet patients' needs with an appropriate level of safe and effective care. To ensure optimal patient care and safety, the following are developed or performed before the procedure is performed:
a. A nursing plan of care;
b. A plan for the operative or other procedure;
c. A postprocedure plan of care;
d. Assessment of the need for additional diagnostic data;
e. Initial assessment of patient acuity to determine the appropriate level of postprocedure care; and
f. Initial assessment of the patient's physical, mental, and neurological status and needs.

Plans of care are developed and documented in the patient's medical record before the operative or other procedure is performed. During the procedure, the patient's physiological status is monitored at a level consistent with the procedure's potential effect and a registered nurse supervises perioperative nursing care.

Standard
TX.5.4 The patient is monitored during the postprocedure period.

Intent of TX.5.4
The patient is monitored continuously during the postprocedure period. The following items are monitored:
a. Physiological and mental status;
b. Status of or findings related to pathological conditions, such as drainage from incisions;
c. Intravenous fluids and drugs administered, including blood and blood components;
d. Impairments and functional status; and
e. Unusual events or postoperative complications and their management.

Results of monitoring trigger key decisions, such as transfer to an alternative level of care due to a precipitous drop in vital signs, or discharge.

Standards and Intent Statements for Rehabilitation Care and Services

Rehabilitation is designed to achieve an optimal level of functioning, self-care, self-responsibility, independence, and quality of life. Achieving the patient's optimal level of function means restoring, improving, or maintaining the patient's assessed level of functioning. Rehabilitation services aim to minimize symptoms, exacerbation of chronic illnesses, impairments, and disabilities.

Qualified professionals provide rehabilitation services consistent with professional standards of practice. All interventions encourage the patient to make choices, to sustain a sense of achievement about treatment progress, and if necessary, to modify participation in the rehabilitation process.

Assessment* identifies the patient's physical, cognitive, behavioral, communicative, emotional, and social status and identifies facilitating factors that may influence attainment of rehabilitation goals. Problems may include
- substance use disorders;
- emotional, behavioral, and mental disorders;
- cognitive disorders;
- communicative disorders;
- developmental disabilities;
- vision and hearing impairments and disabilities; and
- physical impairments and disabilities.

Assessment also helps identify services and accommodations helpful to increasing the patient's readiness for rehabilitation.

The rehabilitation plan identifies goals and services and interventions to meet them. Rehabilitation provides patients with skills and supports to function in an environment with as much independence and choice and as little supervision and restrictiveness as possible. Decisions are based on regular reassessment and reliable measures of patient needs, strengths, symptoms, behavioral patterns, and goal achievement. The patient and clinician agree on care choices.

Rehabilitation provides access to community resources and services that promote continued goal achievement and independence after rehabilitation concludes.

Note: *These standards do not apply to psychiatric and addiction programs that do not have a rehabilitation mission (for example, psychiatric programs with an average length of stay less than thirty [30] days).*

Standard

TX.6 *Qualified professionals provide rehabilitation services, consistent with professional licensure laws, regulation, registration, and certification.*

Intent of TX.6
Rehabilitation services are provided by competent professionals who are qualified by education, professional licensure, regulation, registration, certification, training, and experience.

---

* Described in the "Assessment of Patients" chapter of this book.

Standard

TX.6.1 A rehabilitation plan, developed by qualified professionals and based on assessment of patient needs, guides provision of rehabilitation services.

Intent of TX.6.1

Based on assessment of the patient's physical, cognitive, emotional, and social status, a written treatment plan is developed that identifies the patient's rehabilitation needs. The rehabilitation plan incorporates, at least
a. the patient's personal goals for rehabilitation;
b. rehabilitation goals and objectives related to activities of daily living, learning, and working;
c. measures and time frames for achievement of rehabilitation goals and objectives; and
d. factors that may influence use of services or goal achievement.

The rehabilitation plan is designed to provide the skills, support, education, practice, experience, and treatment necessary to help the patient reach reasonable personal rehabilitation goals. The plan describes
- long-term rehabilitation goals and short-term skill development objectives, in functional terms and developed in collaboration with the patient and family;
- strategies and time frames for achieving rehabilitation goals;
- who will help the patient and monitor progress;
- measures of
  - rehabilitation goal attainment,
  - successful role performance,
  - changes in the patient's level of functioning,
  - efficiency of resource supports;
- barriers other than the patient's primary problem;
- criteria for transition to more independent, less restrictive environments and successful adaptation in natural community settings; and
- patient skill and support requirements for living, learning, and working with optimal independence and choice.

Rehabilitation services are provided to meet patients' needs according to the plan.

Standard

TX.6.2 Qualified professionals implement the rehabilitation plan with the patient, and his or her family, social network, or support system.

Intent of TX.6.2

Qualified professionals develop and implement the rehabilitation plan and involve patients, families, and their social support systems. Patients are encouraged to make choices about their participation in rehabilitation and develop a sense of achievement in progress. Patients and members of their support systems participate in implementing the rehabilitation plan, including
a. identifying interventions to reach reasonable goals;
b. coordinating and collaborating on rehabilitation interventions;
c. documenting the patient's treatment choices, response to interventions, progress toward goals and objectives, and changes in the patient's condition; and
d. advocating to enhance patients' social support systems, facilitate environmental modifications, and create new support systems.

Patients and family receive information about potential benefits and risks of rehabilitation services in order to make informed decisions. Their expectations are considered and documented in the rehabilitation plan.

The plan identifies activities, services, and interventions the patient will use to reach rehabilitation goals. An interdisciplinary team implements and coordinates planned treatment and services. The service provider advocates for patient needs and improvements in the system.

Standard

TX.6.3 Rehabilitation restores, improves, or maintains the patient's optimal level of functioning, self-care, self-responsibility, independence, and quality of life.

Intent of TX.6.3

Consistent with treatment plan goals, rehabilitation services help patients meet skill and support requirements for living, learning, and work activities. Patients learn to apply skills gained in rehabilitation to their housing, vocational, educational, recreational, and social environments.

Standard

TX.6.4 The patient's readiness to end rehabilitation services is determined based on written discharge criteria.

Intent of TX.6.4

Discharge planning is initiated early in treatment based on continuing assessments and stated expectations for achieving treatment goals and objectives. Criteria for discharge or termination of services may vary based on age, disability, treatment setting, and the organization's bylaws, rules and regulations, and written plan for professional services.

Standards and Intent Statements for Special Procedures

These standards address interventions that call for special sensitivity to patient rights and risk management, such as aversive therapies, electroconvulsive therapy, and restraint and seclusion. Clinicians take special precautions to ensure these interventions are warranted and do not endanger patients.

Standard

TX.7 The hospital ensures that special procedures are safely and appropriately used.

Intent of TX.7

Policies and procedures for the use of special interventions are developed through an interdisciplinary process and approved by medical staff and administration. Staff roles and responsibilities in the use of special procedures are identified for all appropriate disciplines. Requirements for documenting the justification and use of these procedures are defined.

Care of Patients

Standards for the Use of Restraint and Seclusion for Behavioral Health Patients*†

Introduction to the Restraint and Seclusion Standards TX.7.1 through TX.7.1.3.2 for Psychiatric Hospitals, Patients in Psychiatric Units in Acute Care Organizations, and Patients Receiving Behavioral Health Services in Designated Beds in Acute Care Hospitals

See also "Introduction to the Restraint Standards in Acute Medical and Surgical (Nonpsychiatric) Care" on page 107.

Creating a physical, social, and cultural environment limiting restraint and seclusion use to clinically appropriate and adequately justified situations or that actually reduces their use through preventive or alternative strategies helps organization staff focus on the patient's well-being. The leaders' role is to help create such an environment. This requires planning and, frequently, new or reallocated resources, thoughtful education, and performance improvement. The result is an organization approach to restraint and seclusion that protects the patient's health and safety and preserves his or her dignity, rights, and well-being.

Restraint or seclusion may be used in response to emergent, dangerous behavior; addictive disorders; as an adjunct to planned care; as a component of an approved protocol; or, in some cases, as part of standard practice. Because restraint or seclusion may be necessary for certain patients, health care organizations and providers need to be aware of the associated risks of both use and nonuse. They also need to be able to use restraint or seclusion when essential to protect patients from harming themselves, other patients, or staff.

In its broadest context, *restraint* is any method of physically restricting a person's freedom of movement, physical activity, or normal access to his or her body. In the context of these standards, restraint is considered involuntary use as either part of an approved protocol, or as indicated by individual orders. *Seclusion* refers to the involuntary confinement of a person alone in a room where the person is physically prevented from leaving.

Restraint and seclusion have the potential to produce serious consequences, such as physical and psychological harm, loss of dignity, violation of an individual's rights, and even death. Because of the associated risks and consequences of use, organizations are increasingly exploring ways to decrease restraint and seclusion use through effective preventive strategies or the use of alternatives. For some organizations, a restraint- and seclusion-free environment is appropriate to their patient populations and clinical services and is achievable now or in the future. But, for many organizations, restraint or seclusion use may continue to be necessary in clinically justified situations and in the foreseeable future, given the organization's patient populations and clinical services, the current state of knowledge, and available effective alternatives.

These standards for restraint and seclusion address processes and activities that
- identify areas of organization leadership and action that will limit restraint and seclusion use to clinically justified situations and may, when appropriate, seek to reduce restraint use through performance improvement;
- guide an organization's efforts to prevent the need to restrain or seclude patients; and
- provide a patient-focused framework to guide any actual restraint or seclusion use through clinical protocols or individual orders.

Standard(s)
- TX.7.1.1 through TX.7.1.1.7 address limiting restraint and seclusion use;
- TX.7.1.2 addresses reducing restraint and seclusion use as part of performance improvement;
- TX.7.1.3 addresses the policies and procedures associated with restraint and seclusion use;

---

* Effective January 1, 1999.

† See also "Introduction to the Restraint Standards in Acute Medical and Surgical (Nonpsychiatric) Care" on page 107.

99

- TX.7.1.3.1 through TX.7.1.3.1.8 address restraint and seclusion use initiated through individual orders; and
- TX.7.1.3.2 addresses medical record documentation.

Many of these standards for restraint and seclusion parallel or duplicate existing standards found in other chapters of this book. Those standards are scored in those appropriate chapters. They appear here, however, to provide a complete perspective on all the requirements.

Applicability of These Restraint and Seclusion Standards

Standards TX.7.1 through TX.7.1.3.2 are applicable to any organization where restraint or seclusion use is initiated by individual orders for patients receiving behavioral health services in psychiatric hospitals or in psychiatric units or designated beds in acute care hospitals.

The standards do **not** apply to

- standard practices that include *temporary* immobilization or limitation of mobility related to medical, dental, diagnostic, or surgical procedures and the related post-procedure care processes (for example, surgical positioning, IV armboards, radiotherapy procedures, protection of surgical and treatment sites in pediatric patients);
- adaptive support in response to assessed patient need (for example, postural support, orthopedic appliances, tabletop chairs);
- therapeutic holding or comforting of children or to a time-out when the person to whom it is applied is physically prevented from leaving a room for 15 minutes or less and when its use is consistent with the behavior management standards; or
- forensic and correction restrictions used for security purposes. However, restraint or seclusion use related to the clinical care of an individual under forensic or correction restrictions is surveyed under these standards.

Standard

TX.7.1 Restraint or seclusion use within the organization is limited to those situations with adequate, appropriate clinical justification.

Intent of TX.7.1

Limiting the use of restraint or seclusion to clinically justified situations requires clear policies and procedures, well-trained staff, and the support of the organization's leaders and culture.

Clinical justification can be guided by clear criteria present in practice guidelines, practice parameters, pathways of care, or other standardized care processes from relevant professional organizations. When not available, the qualified staff of an organization establishes criteria or otherwise guides justification for the patient population served and clinical services provided by the organization.

Standards

TX.7.1.1 *Organization leaders support limited, justified use of restraint or seclusion through appropriate:*

TX.7.1.1.1 *Plans, policies, and priorities;*

TX.7.1.1.2 *Human resource planning;*

TX.7.1.1.3 Staff orientation and education creating a culture emphasizing prevention and appropriate use and encouraging alternatives;

TX.7.1.1.4 Patient and, when appropriate, family education;

TX.7.1.1.5 Assessment processes that identify and, when appropriate, prevent potential behavioral risk factors;

TX.7.1.1.6 Design and delivery of patient care; and

TX.7.1.1.7 The development and promotion of preventive strategies and use of safe and effective alternatives.

Intent of TX.7.1.1 Through TX.7.1.1.7
Limiting the use of restraint or seclusion to those situations with appropriate and adequate clinical justification requires
- effective leadership to shape the culture of the organization;
- supportive plans, policies, and priorities;
- an understanding of the human resource implications of limited use and choices related to reduced use;
- ongoing staff orientation and education;
- patient and, when appropriate, family education; and
- the integration of restraint and seclusion into the organization's performance-improvement activities.

In particular, attention is directed toward
- refining behavioral health*, diagnostic patient assessment processes to identify earlier the potential risk of dangerous patient behavior and the prevention, when appropriate, of those behaviors;
- reviewing and, when necessary, redesigning patient care processes associated with restraint and seclusion use; and
- identifying, developing, and promoting preventive strategies and the use of safe and effective alternatives.

Standard
TX.7.1.2 Performance-improvement processes identify opportunities, when appropriate, to reduce restraint or seclusion use.

Intent of TX.7.1.2
Restraint and seclusion are high risk and problem prone and thus are a logical component of an organization's performance-improvement program. The measurement and assessment process related to restraint and seclusion seeks to understand the root cause of their use and incorporates this understanding into the organization's plans and priorities to evaluate and, if appropriate, reduce their use. This understanding is advanced by the assessment of aggregate data on restraint and seclusion

---

* Behavioral health services is the contemporary term for a broad array of mental health, chemical dependency, and mental retardation/developmental disabilities services provided in settings such as acute, long term, and ambulatory care.

episodes from all units, for all shifts, and for all purposes for which restraint and seclusion are used. Particular attention is paid to instances of multiple episodes of use for individual patients and the frequency of restraint use by type(s) of staff.

Standard

TX.7.1.3 When restraint or seclusion is used, organization policy and procedures guide appropriate and safe use.

Intent of TX.7.1.3

Several essential elements govern how an organization uses restraint and seclusion in a way that is appropriate to the population and individuals served. These elements focus on the patient and are described in organization policy(ies) and procedure(s) and include appropriate details as to how the organization

- protects and preserves the patient's rights, dignity, and well-being during use;
- bases use on the patient's assessed needs;
- makes decisions about least-restrictive methods;
- assures safe application and removal by competent staff;
- monitors and reassesses the patient during use;
- meets patient needs during use;
- limits individual orders to licensed independent practitioners;
- time-limits orders; and
- documents in the medical record when restraint or seclusion is used, or individual orders written.

These essential elements assure that any use of restraint or seclusion protects and preserves the patient and his or her rights, dignity, and well-being. Appropriate staff approve policy(ies) and procedure(s) related to restraint and seclusion.

Standard

TX.7.1.3.1 *Individual orders for restraint or seclusion are consistent with organization policy.*

Intent of TX.7.1.3.1

Individual orders are the most common source for initiating restraint or seclusion, especially in behavioral health settings. Who is authorized to order restraint or seclusion, how orders are conveyed, the details provided in an order (for example, those related to time limits), and who is authorized to carry out the order are all essential aspects of processes to protect the individual patient, other patients, and staff.

Standard

TX.7.1.3.1.1 Patient rights, dignity, and well-being are protected during restraint or seclusion use.

Intent of TX.7.1.3.1.1

Each patient has a right to respectful care that maintains his or her dignity. Restraint and seclusion have the potential to significantly restrict these rights and can have serious adverse impact on the patient's well-being. Thus, each episode of use considers how the intervention will affect the patient including whether

- the application or initiation respects the patient as an individual;

Care of Patients

- the environment is safe and clean;
- the patient is able to continue his or her care and participate in care processes; and
- modesty, visibility to others, and comfortable body temperature are maintained.

Standard
TX.7.1.3.1.2 Restraint or seclusion use is based on the assessed needs of the patient.

Intent of TX.7.1.3.1.2
Single episodes of use or continued use of restraint or seclusion is based on patient needs as identified in the initial assessment process or by qualified staff in emergent situations that pose the risk of injury to self or others. Thus, there is clinical justification for each episode of use, including emergency use when a licensed independent practitioner is not available.

Use is not based solely on prior history of use or history of dangerous behavior. Rather, use is based on the patient's needs in the immediate care environment and the interaction of the patient and staff with other patients in that environment. The organization does not permit any other use, such as for punishment or staff convenience.

Use appropriate to the needs of patients is assured by
- the training and skill of those who decide to apply restraint or initiate seclusion for emergency reasons in the absence of a licensed independent practitioner;
- clinical oversight by a licensed independent practitioner;
- review and evaluation of multiple episodes of use or continuous use; and
- organization policy.

Standard
TX.7.1.3.1.3 The least-restrictive safe and effective restraint or seclusion method is employed.

Intent of TX.7.1.3.1.3
The choice of restraint or seclusion method is guided by policy. The choice of a safe, effective, and least-restrictive method is determined by the patient's assessed needs and the effective or ineffective methods previously used on the patient. In the absence of previous experience, policy describes whether and how least-restrictive methods are to be tried first. Once employed, monitoring and reassessment of the patient assures that less-restrictive methods are used when possible and their use is discontinued as soon as possible. Patient and staff safety are considered in making these decisions.

Standard
TX.7.1.3.1.4 *Restraint or seclusion is used correctly by competent, trained staff.*

Intent of TX.7.1.3.1.4
Competent staff is essential to the safe and effective use of restraint or seclusion and to the protection of patients during use. Appropriate use of restraint or seclusion is essential if the patient's rights are to be respected and harm to the patient avoided. The organization identifies, educates, and determines the competency of those staff members who apply or remove restraint or who initiate or terminate seclusion. Frequently repeated in-service education, including an understanding of manufacturer's instructions for use of restraint devices, helps assure safe use.

If possible, and as appropriate to the patient population and methods used, the insights of former patients who have experienced being placed in restraints are included to help staff better understand all aspects of their use.

Standard

TX.7.1.3.1.5 Patients in restraint or seclusion are monitored and reassessed appropriately.

Intent of TX.7.1.3.1.5

Patients can experience harm, unintentional limitation of their rights and dignity, deterioration in well-being, and feelings of isolation when restraint or seclusion methods are used. Monitoring is essential to prevent or reduce such occurrences. Patient reassessment during monitoring permits the reduction in or early termination of restraint or seclusion.

Organization policy defines the monitoring frequency as continuous or no less frequent than every 15 minutes and defines the nature and extent of appropriate monitoring by observation and direct, face-to-face interaction with the patient.

Reassessment associated with monitoring is used primarily to determine the patient's well-being. Reassessment associated with time-limited orders is used primarily to determine the continuing need for the restraint or seclusion.

Standard

TX.7.1.3.1.6 Patient needs are met during restraint or seclusion use.

Intent of TX.7.1.3.1.6

A patient's physical and emotional needs are considered while the patient is in restraint or seclusion. The basic rights of human dignity and respect are maintained and physical well-being is preserved through adequate exercise, nourishment, and personal care.

Standard

TX.7.1.3.1.7 Restraint or seclusion use is ordered by a licensed independent practitioner.*

Intent of TX.7.1.3.1.7

Licensed independent practitioners have the responsibility for overseeing how their patients' assessed needs are met. This requires knowledge about and involvement in any use of restraint and seclusion. Each licensed independent practitioner can best carry out his or her responsibility when he or she
- provides verbal or written orders for initial use or to reauthorize continuing emergency use;
- participates in daily reviews of restraint and seclusion use related to his or her patients; and
- participates in measuring and assessing use for all patients within the organization.

Organization policy identifies who (in accordance with state law) is authorized by the organization to give verbal or written orders for restraint or seclusion and who may receive, record, and initiate verbal orders. Organization policy also identifies the process for reviewing and reauthorizing emergency restraint or seclusion use.

---

* **licensed independent practitioner** Any individual permitted by law and by the organization to provide care and services without direction or supervision, within the scope of the individual's license and consistent with individually granted clinical privileges.

The organization may authorize an individual who is not a licensed independent practitioner to order emergency restraint or seclusion use in response to a patient who poses an immediate danger to himself or herself or to others. However, a licensed independent practitioner is called within one hour. Continued use depends on authorization by a licensed independent practitioner.

Standard
TX.7.1.3.1.8 Orders for restraint or seclusion use define specific time limits.

Intent of TX.7.1.3.1.8
Time-limited orders. Written orders for restraint or seclusion are limited to
- 4 hours for adults;
- 2 hours for children and adolescents ages 9 to 17; or
- 1 hour for patients under age 9.

Early release. Staff can use criteria to guide early restraint or seclusion termination. When restraint or seclusion is terminated early and the same behavior is still evident, the original order can be reapplied if alternatives remain ineffective.

Continuation of orders. After the original order expires, the patient receives a face-to-face reassessment by a licensed independent practitioner. The licensed independent practitioner writes a new order if restraint or seclusion is going to be continued. Organization policy and the original order may permit a licensed, qualified, and authorized individual (such as a registered nurse) to perform the reassessment and make a decision to continue the original order for an additional
- 4 hours for adults up to a maximum of 24 hours;
- 2 hours for children and adolescents ages 9 to 17 up to a maximum of 24 hours; or
- 1 hour for children under age 9 for periods up to a maximum of 24 hours.

Standard
TX.7.1.3.2 Documentation in medical records reflects organization policy.

Intent of TX.7.1.3.2
The use of restraint or seclusion is recorded in the patient's medical record. The purpose and focus of an entry(ies) is on the patient.

Each episode of use is recorded and includes
- clinical justification for use;
- orders for restraint or seclusion that meet the requirements described in organization policy; and
- measures taken to protect the rights, dignity, and well-being of the patient including monitoring, reassessment, and attention to patient needs.

Standard
TX.7.2 Electroconvulsive and other forms of convulsive therapy are used with adequate justification, documentation, and regard for patient safety.

Intent of TX.7.2
Written policies regulate the use of electroconvulsive and other forms of convulsive therapy. Whenever convulsive therapy is used, the procedure is adequately justified and documented in the patient's medical record.

Before initiating electroconvulsive therapy for a child or adolescent, two qualified, experienced child psychiatrists who are not directly involved in treating the patient
- examine the patient;
- consult with the psychiatrist responsible for the patient; and
- document their concurrence with the treatment in the patient's medical record.

Standard
TX.7.3 Psychosurgery or other surgical treatments for emotional, mental, or behavioral disorders are performed with adequate justification, documentation, and regard for patient safety.

Intent of TX.7.3
Written policies and procedures regulate the use of psychosurgery or other surgical treatments for mental, emotional, or behavioral disorder. Whenever these procedures are used, they are adequately justified and documented in the patient's medical record.

Standards
TX.7.4 Use of behavior-management procedures conforms to the patient's treatment plan and hospital policy.

TX.7.4.1 Qualified staff review, evaluate, and approve all behavior-management procedures.

Intent of TX.7.4 and TX.7.4.1
The hospital defines staff roles and responsibilities for all appropriate disciplines involved in using special procedures. When behavior-management procedures are used, they are included in the patient's plan of treatment. Policies describe
- under what conditions specific behavior management* procedures can be used and when they should not be used, and
- requirements for approval of behavior management procedures in a patient's plan of treatment.

The hospital uses educational and positive reinforcement techniques (for example, alternative adaptive behaviors) wherever possible. When more restrictive techniques are clinically necessary, the least restrictive alternative is used to avoid harm to the patient. Time-out and procedures using restraining devices or aversive techniques are used only consistent with the patient's plan of treatment, policies and procedures, and state and federal laws. The hospital protects the patient's nutritional status and physical safety (for example, from corporal punishment).

Other patients may assist in implementing a patient's behavior management program only if
- it is conducted as part of a structured treatment plan;
- it is conducted under the supervision of qualified staff;
- it is limited to empowering patients to provide positive reinforcement; and
- it does not become abusive.

---

* **behavior management** The use of basic learning techniques, such as biofeedback, reinforcement, or aversion therapy, to manage and improve an individual's behavior.

Introduction to the Restraint Standards in Acute Medical and Surgical (Nonpsychiatric) Care*

In its broadest context, *restraint* is any physical method of restricting a person's freedom of movement, physical activity, or normal access to his or her body. Restraint may be used in response to emergent, dangerous behavior; as an adjunct to planned care; as a component of an approved protocol; or, in some cases, as part of standard practice. Because restraint may be necessary for certain patients, health care organizations and providers need to be able to use restraint when essential to protect patients from harming themselves, other patients, or staff. They also need to be aware of the associated risks of both its use and nonuse.

Restraint has the potential to produce serious consequences, such as physical or psychological harm, loss of dignity, violation of an individual's rights, and even death. Because of the associated risks and consequences of use, organizations are increasingly exploring ways to decrease restraint use through effective preventive strategies or the use of alternatives. For some organizations, a restraint free environment is appropriate to their patient populations and clinical services and is achievable now or in the future. But for many organizations, restraint use may continue to be necessary in clinically justified situations and in the foreseeable future, given the organization's populations and clinical services, the current state of knowledge, and available effective alternatives.

A physical, social, and organizational environment that limits restraint use to clinically appropriate and adequately justified situations and that seeks to identify opportunities to reduce the risks associated with restraint use through the introduction of preventive strategies, innovative alternatives, and process improvements is an environment that helps organization staff focus on the patient's well-being. The leaders' role is to help create such an environment. This requires planning and, frequently, new or reallocated resources, thoughtful education, and performance improvement. The result is an organization approach to restraint that protects the patient's health and safety and preserves his or her dignity, rights, and well-being.

Applicability of these Restraint Standards in Acute Medical and Surgical (Nonpsychiatric) Care†

Standards TX.7.5 through TX.7.5.5 apply to the use of restraint in the care of medical and surgical patients, which includes patients receiving pediatric, obstetrical, or rehabilitation care. This includes patients of any age who are

- *hospitalized in an acute care hospital on other than a psychiatric unit in order to receive medical or surgical services,*
- *in the emergency department for the purpose of assessment, stabilization, or treatment, even if awaiting transfer to a psychiatric hospital or psychiatric unit,*
- *awaiting transfer from a nonpsychiatric unit to a psychiatric hospital or psychiatric unit after receiving medical or surgical care,*
- *in medical observation beds,*
- *receiving subacute services, unless, at the request of the hospital, such subacute services are surveyed under the Joint Commission protocol for subacute programs,*
- *undergoing same-day surgical or other ambulatory health care procedures, or*
- *undergoing rehabilitation as an outpatient or inpatient.*

The specific nature of the device used to restrain a patient does not in itself determine whether these standards are to be applied. Rather, it is the device's intended use (ie, physical restriction), its involuntary application, and/or the identified patient need that determines whether the device use triggers the application of these standards. Therefore, these standards do not apply to

---

* Effective January 1, 1999.

† Effective January 1, 1999.

- standard practices that include limitation of mobility or temporary immobilization related to medical, dental, diagnostic, or surgical procedures and the related post-procedure care processes (for example, surgical positioning, IV armboards, radiotherapy procedures, protection of surgical and treatment sites in pediatric patients);
- adaptive support in response to assessed patient need (for example, postural support, orthopedic appliances, tabletop chairs);
- helmets;
- therapeutic holding or comforting of children, or adolescents, or pediatric behavior management methods (to which the behavior management standards in this book apply—TX.7.4 and TX.7.4.1);
- restraint for patients hospitalized on psychiatric units or for psychiatric purposes (to which the restraint standards in this manual for psychiatric patients apply); or
- forensic and correction restrictions used for security purposes.

Organizational Oversight of Restraint Use

Standard

TX.7.5 The organization's leaders determine the organization's approach to the use of restraint in the care of nonpsychiatric patients, which limits its use to those situations where there is appropriate clinical justification.

Intent of TX.7.5

Limiting the use of restraint to clinically justified situations requires clear policies and procedures, well-trained staff, and the support of the organization's leaders.

Clinical justification can be guided by clear criteria present in practice guidelines, practice parameters, pathways of care, or other standardized care processes developed by relevant professional organizations. When not available, the qualified staff of an organization establishes criteria or otherwise guides justification for the patient population served and clinical services provided by the organization.

Limiting the use of restraint to those situations with appropriate clinical justification requires
- the organization's leaders to determine the organization's approach to the use of restraint in the care of nonpsychiatric patients;
- supportive plans, policies, and priorities;
- understanding of the staffing needs associated with alternatives to restraint;
- ongoing staff orientation and education; and
- patient and, when appropriate, family education.

In particular, attention is directed toward
- refining medical, dental, surgical, and diagnostic patient assessment processes to identify earlier the potential risk of dangerous patient behavior and the prevention, when appropriate, of those behaviors;
- reviewing and, when necessary, redesigning patient care processes associated with restraint use;
- developing policy(ies), procedure(s), and protocols for the proper use of restraints; and
- identifying, developing, and promoting preventive strategies and the use of safe and effective alternatives.

Standard

TX.7.5.1 Performance-improvement processes seek to identify opportunities to reduce the risks associated with restraint use through the introduction of preventive strategies, innovative alternatives, and process improvements.

Intent of TX.7.5.1
The measurement and assessment process related to restraint seeks to understand why it is used and incorporates this understanding into the organization's plans and priorities to evaluate and, if appropriate, reduce its use. This understanding can be advanced by an initial baseline assessment of aggregate data on restraint episodes, followed by targeted monitoring.

Standard
TX.7.5.2 Organization policy(ies) and procedure(s) guide appropriate and safe use of restraint.

Intent of TX.7.5.2
Several essential elements govern how an organization uses restraint in a way that is appropriate to the population and individuals served. These elements focus on the patient and are described in organization policy(ies) and procedure(s) and include appropriate details as to how the organization
Group A Elements
- protects the patient and preserves the patient's rights, dignity, and well-being during use;
- bases use on the patient's assessed needs;
- makes decisions about least-restrictive methods;
- assures safe application and removal by qualified staff;
- monitors and reassesses the patient during use, using qualified staff;
- meets patient needs during use;

Group B Elements
- addresses risk associated with vulnerable patient populations, such as emergency, pediatric, and cognitively or physically limited patients;
- makes efforts to discuss the issue of restraint, when practical, with the patient and family around the time of its use;
- when orders are needed, limits individual orders to licensed independent practitioners (see standards TX.7.5.3.1 and TX.7.5.3.2);
- requires renewal of orders in accordance with applicable state law; and
- documents restraint episodes in the medical record (see standard TX.7.5.5).

These essential elements assure that any use of restraint, whether initiated by an individual order or through the use of a protocol, protects the patient and preserves his or her rights, dignity, and well-being.

The organization policy(ies) and procedure(s) are developed by appropriate staff and approved by the medical staff, nursing leadership, and, when appropriate, others.

Restraint Use by Individual Order or Protocol
Standards
TX.7.5.3 *Any use of restraint (to which these standards apply) is initiated pursuant to either an individual order (standard TX.7.5.3.1) or an approved protocol (standard TX.7.5.3.2).*

TX.7.5.3.1 Individual orders for initiation and renewal of restraint are consistent with organization policy(ies) and procedure(s), and are consistent with the patient's needs and clinical condition.

Intent of TX.7.5.3 and TX.7.5.3.1
Restraint of an acute medical or surgical patient (to which these standards apply) is only used pursuant to either an individual order or an approved protocol.

Individual orders provide the framework for ensuring clinical justification of restraint use and for protecting the rights, dignity, and well-being of the patient.

Individual Orders for Restraint (except for restraint initiated under a protocol as described in standard TX.7.5.3.2);
- Restraint (to which these standards apply) is used upon the order of a licensed independent practitioner.
  - If a licensed independent practitioner is not available to issue such an order, restraint use is initiated by a registered nurse based on an appropriate assessment of the patient. In that case, a licensed independent practitioner is notified within 12 hours of the initiation of restraint and a verbal or written order is obtained from that practitioner and entered into the patient's medical record. If the initiation of restraint is based on a significant change in the patient's condition, the registered nurse immediately notifies a licensed independent practitioner. A written order, based on an examination of the patient by a licensed independent practitioner, is entered into the patient's medical record within 24 hours of the initiation of restraint.
- Continued use of restraint beyond the first 24 hours is authorized by a licensed independent practitioner renewing the original order or issuing a new order if restraint use continues to be clinically justified. Such renewal or new order is issued no less often than once each calendar day and is based upon an examination of the patient by the licensed independent practitioner.

Content of Individual Orders
- The individual order is consistent with organization policy(ies) and procedure(s).
- The individual order identifies any variation from organization policy(ies) and procedure(s) for monitoring of the patient and for release from restraint before the order expires.

Standard
TX.7.5.3.2 Protocols for restraint use contain criteria to ensure only clinically justified use.

Intent of TX.7.5.3.2
During the treatment of certain specific conditions (eg, post-traumatic brain injury) or the use of certain specific clinical procedures (eg, intubation) restraint may often be necessary in order to prevent significant harm to the patient. For specified conditions or procedures, protocols for the use of restraint may be established, based upon the frequent presentation in those conditions or procedures of behavior by patients that seriously endangers the patient or seriously compromises the effectiveness of the procedure. Such restraint protocols include guidelines for assessing the patient, criteria for applying restraint, criteria for monitoring the patient and reassessing the need for restraint, and criteria for terminating restraint. Authorized staff can initiate, maintain, and terminate restraint in accordance with these criteria, based on the individual patient's need and appropriate clinical justification, without obtaining an order from a licensed independent practitioner. The initiation of restraint in the absence of such a protocol requires the order of a licensed independent practitioner (see standard TX.7.5.3.1). The criteria for use of restraint that are incorporated into such a protocol reflect the organization policy(ies) and procedure(s) on the appropriate and safe use of restraint, and are approved by the medical staff, nursing leadership, and, when appropriate, others.

Care of Patients

Patient Monitoring

Standard

TX.7.5.4 Patients in restraint are monitored.

Intent of TX.7.5.4

Organization policy(ies) and procedure(s), applicable state law, protocols, individual orders, the setting (eg, emergency department, outpatient surgery, endoscopy suite), and individual patient needs are used to establish the frequency, nature, and extent of monitoring of a patient in restraints. At a minimum, a patient in restraints is monitored every two hours. Monitoring is accomplished by observation, interaction with the patient, or related direct examination of the patient by qualified staff. Monitoring determines
- the physical and emotional well-being of the patient;
- that the patient's rights, dignity, and safety are maintained;
- whether less restrictive methods are possible;
- changes in the patient's behavior or clinical condition needed to initiate the removal of restraints;
- whether the restraint has been appropriately applied, removed, or reapplied.

Note: *Documentation of monitoring is in accordance with organization policy(ies) and procedure(s) (see standard TX.7.5.5). Documentation is scored at standard TX.7.5.5.*

Documentation

Standard

TX.7.5.5 Each episode of restraint use is documented in the patient's medical record, consistent with organization policy(ies) and procedure(s).

Intent of TX.7.5.5

Organization policy(ies) and procedure(s) establish the frequency, format (if appropriate), and content of entries in the patient's record relative to each episode of restraint use. The purpose of the entry is to provide clinical justification for use and document clinical oversight. Such documentation includes relevant orders for use, results of patient monitoring, reassessment, and significant changes in the patient's condition. When restraint is used as part of a protocol, the patient's record contains the protocol or references the protocol.

Education

Overview

The **goal** of patient and family* education function† is to improve patient health outcomes by promoting healthy behavior and involving the patient in care and care decisions.

Education promotes healthy behaviors, supports recovery and a speedy return to function, and enables patients to be involved in decisions about their own care. The goals of patient and family education are met when a hospital performs the following processes well:
- Assessing organizationwide patient education programs and activities;
- Formulating patient education program goals;
- Allocating resources for patient education;
- Determining and prioritizing specific patient educational needs; and
- Providing education to meet identified patient needs.

The standards in this chapter address activities involved in these processes, including
- promoting interactive communication between patients and providers;
- improving patients' understanding of their health status, options for treatment, and the anticipated risks and benefits of treatment;
- encouraging patient participation in decision making about care;
- increasing the likelihood that patients will follow their therapeutic plans of care;
- maximizing patient self-care skills;
- increasing the patient's ability to cope with his or her health status;
- enhancing patient participation in continuing care;
- promoting healthy life-styles; and
- informing patients about their financial responsibilities for treatment when known.

Psychosocial, spiritual, and cultural values also affect patients' responses to care and their willingness to participate actively in care and education.‡ Recognizing the impact these values have, a hospital supports its patients' involvement in their care and the educational process. The hospital makes sure its education process supports ongoing interaction between patients and staff.

Note: *While the standards in this chapter recommend a systematic approach to education, they do not require any specific structure, such as an education department, a patient education committee, or the employment of an educator. More important is a philosophy that views the educational function as an interactive one in which both parties are learners. These standards help the hospital focus on how education is consistent with the patient's plan of care, level of care, the educational setting, and continuity of care.*

---

* **family** The person(s) who plays a significant role in the individual's life. This may include a person(s) not legally related to the individual. This person(s) is often referred to as a surrogate decision maker if authorized to make care decisions for an individual should the individual lose decision-making capacity.

† **function** A goal-directed, interrelated series of processes, such as continuum of care or management of information.

‡ This aspect of patient education relates to standard RI.1.2 in the "Patient Rights and Organization Ethics" chapter of this book.

Standards

The following is a list of all standards for this function. If you have a questions about a term used here, please check the Glossary, pages 281 through 307. Terms that are critical to the understanding of the standard are defined in the footnotes of the next section of this chapter.

PF.1 The patient's learning needs, abilities, preferences, and readiness to learn are assessed.

PF.1.1 The assessment considers cultural and religious practices, emotional barriers, desire and motivation to learn, physical and cognitive limitations, language barriers, and the financial implications of care choices.

PF.1.2 When called for by the age of the patient and the length of stay, the hospital assesses and provides for patients' academic education needs.

PF.1.3 Patients are educated about the safe and effective use of medication, according to law and their needs.

PF.1.4 Patients are educated about the safe and effective use of medical equipment.

PF.1.5 Patients are educated about potential drug-food interactions, and provided counseling on nutrition and modified diets.

PF.1.6 Patients are educated about rehabilitation techniques to help them adapt or function more independently in their environment.

PF.1.7 Patients are informed about access to additional resources in the community.

PF.1.8 Patients are informed about when and how to obtain any further treatment the patient may need.

PF.1.9 The hospital makes clear to patients and families what their responsibilities are regarding the patient's ongoing health care needs, and gives them the knowledge and skills they need to carry out their responsibilities.

PF.1.10 With due regard for privacy, the hospital teaches and helps patients maintain good standards for personal hygiene and grooming, including bathing, brushing teeth, caring for hair and nails, and using the toilet.

PF.2 Patient education is interactive.

PF.3 When the hospital gives discharge instructions to the patient or family, it also provides these instructions to the organization or individual responsible for the patient's continuing care.

PF.4 The hospital plans, supports, and coordinates activities and resources for patient and family education.

Education

PF.4.1 The hospital identifies and provides the educational resources required to achieve its educational objectives.

PF.4.2 The patient and family educational process is collaborative and interdisciplinary, as appropriate to the plan of care.

Standards and Intent Statements for Patient and Family Education and Responsibilities

Standards

PF.1 The patient's learning needs, abilities, preferences, and readiness to learn are assessed.

PF.1.1 The assessment considers cultural and religious practices, emotional barriers, desire and motivation to learn, physical and cognitive limitations, language barriers, and the financial implications of care choices.

PF.1.2 When called for by the age of the patient and the length of stay, the hospital assesses and provides for patients' academic education needs.

PF.1.3 Patients are educated about the safe and effective use of medication, according to law and their needs.

PF.1.4 Patients are educated about the safe and effective use of medical equipment.

PF.1.5 Patients are educated about potential drug-food interactions, and provided counseling on nutrition and modified diets.

PF.1.6 Patients are educated about rehabilitation techniques to help them adapt or function more independently in their environment.

PF.1.7 Patients are informed about access to additional resources in the community.

PF.1.8 Patients are informed about when and how to obtain any further treatment the patient may need.

Intent of PF.1 Through PF.1.8

Hospitals offer education to patients and families to give them the specific knowledge and skills they need to meet the patient's ongoing health care needs. Clearly, such instruction needs to be presented in ways that are understandable to those receiving them.

Openness and flexibility are important elements in patient education, and can make a critical difference in whether the patient follows instructions. In assessing a patient's needs, abilities, and readiness for education, staff members take into account such variables as

- the patient's and family's beliefs and values;
- their literacy, educational level, and language;
- emotional barriers and motivations;
- physical and cognitive limitations;
- the financial implications of care choices.

When school-age children or adolescent patients are hospitalized for long periods of time, state or local laws may specify the requirements for meeting the child's schooling needs. Although the hospital may not provide school teachers directly, it is responsible for providing access to schooling, according to state education law.

In addition, the hospital uses guidelines in educating patients on the following topics:
- Safe and effective use of medication;
- Safe and effective use of medical equipment;
- Diet and nutrition;
- Rehabilitation;
- Educational resources in the community; and
- Follow-up care.

The appropriate disciplines are involved in developing these guidelines.

Standard

PF.1.9 The hospital makes clear to patients and families what their responsibilities are regarding the patient's ongoing health care needs, and gives them the knowledge and skills they need to carry out their responsibilities.

Intent of PF.1.9

Hospitals are entitled to reasonable and responsible behavior on the part of patients and their families—always keeping in mind, of course, the nature of the illness and the constraints it imposes. To facilitate such behavior, hospital staff members clearly identify for patients and families what their responsibilities are, and educate them accordingly. Hospital policies and procedures make clear how and by whom this is done.

Patient responsibilities generally include at least the following:
- **Providing information.** The patients and family are responsible for providing, to the best of their knowledge, accurate and complete information about present complaints, past illnesses, hospitalizations, medications, and other matters relating to the patient's health. They are responsible for reporting unexpected changes in the patient's condition to the responsible practitioner.
- **Asking questions.** The patient and family are responsible for asking questions when they do not understand what they have been told about the patient's care or what they are expected to do.
- **Following with instructions.** The patient and family are responsible for following the treatment plan developed with the practitioner. They should express any concerns they have about their ability to follow the proposed course of treatment; the hospital, in turn, makes every effort to adapt the treatment plan to the patient's specific needs and limitations. Where such adaptations are not recommended, the patient and family should understand the consequences of failing to follow the recommended course of treatment, or of using other treatments.
- **Accepting the consequences of not following instructions.** If the patient or family refuses treatment or fails to follow the practitioner's instructions, they are responsible for the outcomes.
- **Following hospital rules and regulations.** The patient and family are responsible for following the hospital's rules and regulations concerning patient care and conduct.
- **Acting with consideration and respect.** Patients and families are expected to be considerate of other patients and hospital personnel by not making unnecessary noise, smoking, or causing distractions. Patients and families are responsible for respecting the property of other persons and that of the hospital.

Standard

PF.1.10 With due regard for privacy, the hospital teaches and helps patients maintain good standards for personal hygiene and grooming, including bathing, brushing teeth, caring for hair and nails, and using the toilet.

Intent of PF.1.10

Personal hygiene and grooming is maintained or even improved during a hospital stay. The patient has a primary responsibility for these activities; however, the hospital supports, encourages, and provides education when necessary to help the patient.

Standard

PF.2 Patient education is interactive.

Intent of PF.2

Interactive patient education is an integral part of patient care. An "interactive" education process is one in which hospital staff, while imparting information to patients and families, continuously elicits feedback to ensure that the information is understood, and that it is appropriate, useful, and usable in practical terms. There are several crucial steps in this process:

- Identifying the patient's learning needs. This depends on many factors, including not only the patient's medical diagnosis but also the anticipated length of stay, tasks the patient can or cannot accomplish, resources available to the patient in the community, and the patient's own preferences regarding education. It also depends on the ability of the patient and family to understand and implement the education provided.
- Setting priorities on individual learning needs. Staff should understand that not all patients need education concerning their plan of care, and that particular elements of education should be given when the patient is ready to receive them.
- Implementing the education plan, including feedback to make sure it is understood and effective.

Standard

PF.3 When the hospital gives discharge instructions to the patient or family, it also provides these instructions to the organization or individual responsible for the patient's continuing care.

Intent of PF.3

The purpose of discharge planning is to help develop a workable plan for care following the patient's release from the hospital. Education as well as continuity of care are integral to effective discharge planning. Education in preparation for the patient's discharge includes several elements:

- Helping the patient and family understand the patient's treatment and the need for continuing care;
- Teaching the patient and family what they need to know about care after discharge;
- Making life-style changes; and
- Managing continuing care, whether it is carried out at home (with or without home health care services) or at another facility.

Instructions for care after discharge are given not only to the patient and family, but to anyone responsible for the patients' health care needs so that ongoing education can be provided as necessary. For example, the hospital forwards a copy of the discharge summary and instructions to the patient's primary care provider.

Standard

PF.4 The hospital plans, supports, and coordinates activities and resources for patient and family education.

Education

Intent of PF.4

Within the context of its mission and scope of services, the hospital plans for and provides patient education. In this planning, the hospital considers two major factors:
- The types of patients who will need education, including their illnesses, ages, and sociocultural backgrounds, and the community resources that will be available to them to support life-style changes and
- The settings in which patients will be educated, including outpatient and inpatient settings.

While the primary goal of patient education is to promote and maintain patients' health, it may also contribute to other hospital activities and patient outcomes, such as risk management, obtaining informed consent, and patient satisfaction.

Planning can be an informal process; it does not require a written plan. However, a well-planned patient education strategy will encompass these steps:
- Establish an environment that encourages patients and families to ask questions, learn, and participate in decision making and care.
- Provide for the competency of staff members who provide patient and family education.
- Establish processes and procedures to identify and respond to individual learning needs, requests, abilities, and resources. (This includes the identification of community resources.)
- Help staff members think about and understand the environment in which the patient will apply the education they provide.
- Provide for appropriate, available, effective, and efficacious educational resources.
- Provide for the delivery of education in a continuous, safe, timely, efficient, caring, and respectful manner.
- Ensure that explanations and instructions are understandable to the patient and family, and that they take into consideration the patient and family's culture, religion, language, age, abilities, resources, and physical disabilities.
- Assess and improve educational systems and outcomes as part of the hospital's performance improvement process.

Standard

PF.4.1 The hospital identifies and provides the educational resources required to achieve its educational objectives.

Intent of PF.4.1

As part of its commitment to patient and family education, the hospital selects and makes available a variety of educational resources, based on the learning needs of its patient population. These resources may include
- direct teaching by appropriate members of the health care team;
- educational materials such as pamphlets and videotapes;
- materials and resources that accommodate persons with disabilities (for example, braille, audiotape, or large print for the sight impaired);
- community resources for education; and
- referrals to programs that can meet special needs.

Standard

PF.4.2 The patient and family educational process is collaborative and interdisciplinary, as appropriate to the plan of care.

Intent of PF.4.2

When health care professionals understand one another's contributions to patient education, they can collaborate more effectively. Collaboration, in turn, ensures that the information patients and families receive is comprehensive, consistent, and as effective as possible.

Collaboration is not always necessary or appropriate. Sometimes patient education is best provided by a single discipline—for example, the physician or the nurse—in the hospital or a private office. However, when patient education is *multidisciplinary*—involving, for example, the physician, nurse, and physical therapist—it should be *interdisciplinary,* that is, coordinated among the various disciplines involved.

Continuum of Care

Overview

The **goal** of the continuum of care function* is to define, shape, and sequence the following processes and activities to maximize coordination of care† within this continuum of care.

Over time, patients may receive a range of care in multiple settings from multiple providers. For this reason it is important for a hospital to view the patient care it provides as part of an integrated system of settings, services, health care practitioners, and care levels that make up a continuum of care.‡

Before Admission
- The hospital identifies and uses available information sources about the patient's needs.
- The hospital communicates with other care settings and organizations.

During Admission
- The hospital's services are consistent with its mission, population served, and settings.
- The hospital makes arrangements with other organizations and settings to facilitate the patient's admission.
- Patients are referred and transferred§ to meet their needs based on intensity, risk, and staffing level.
- Clinical consultants and contractual arrangements are used for referrals and transfers, when appropriate.

In the Hospital
- Services flow continuously from assessment through treatment and reassessment.
- The patient's care is coordinated among practitioners.

Before Discharge
- The patient's status and need for continuing care** are assessed.
- Education prepares the patient for discharge.

---

* **function** A goal-directed, interrelated series of processes, such as continuum of care or management of information.

† **coordination of care or services** The process of coordinating care or services provided by a healthcare organization, including referral to appropriate community resources and liaison with others (such as the individual's physician, other health care organizations, or community services involved in care or services) to meet the ongoing identified needs of individuals, to ensure implementation of the plan of care, and to avoid unnecessary duplication of services.

‡ **continuum of care** Matching an individual's ongoing needs with the appropriate level and type of medical, psychological, health, or social care or services within an organization or across multiple organizations.

§ **transfer (within an organization)** The formal shifting of responsibility for the care of an individual (1) from one patient care unit to another, (2) from one clinical service to another, (3) from the care of one licensed independent practitioner to another, or (4) from one organization to another.

** **continuing care** Care provided over an extended time, in various settings, spanning the illness-to-wellness continuum.

At Discharge

- The patient is directly referred to practitioners, settings, and organizations to meet his or her continuing needs.
- The use and value of continuing care to meet the patient's needs are reassessed.
- The hospital provides information or data to help others meet the patient's continuing care needs.

A hospital meets the goal of this function by performing these processes and activities well.

Note: *While the standards in this chapter address a systematic approach to continuum of care, they do not require a specific way of carrying out the function, such as a department, position, or service. Instead, the standards encourage the hospital to define its individual role in the continuum of health care services available to its patients in its geographic area.*

Continuum of Care

Standards

The following is a list of all standards for this function. If you have a questions about a term used here, please check the Glossary, pages 281 through 307. Terms that are critical to the understanding of the standard are defined in the footnotes of the next section of this chapter.

CC.1 Patients have access to the appropriate type of care.

CC.2 When the hospital accepts a patient for entry into a particular service or setting, its decision to do so is based on the outcomes of its assessment procedures.

CC.2.1 Criteria define the patient information necessary to determine the appropriate care setting or services.

CC.3 Patients and families receive information about proposed care during the entry process.

CC.4 The hospital ensures continuity over time among the phases of service to a patient.

CC.5 The hospital ensures coordination among the health professionals and services or settings involved in a patient's care.

CC.6 The hospital provides for referral, transfer, or discharge of the patient to another level of care, health professional, or setting, based on the patient's assessed needs and the hospital's capacity to provide the care.

CC.6.1 The discharge process provides for continuing care based upon the patient's assessed needs at the time of discharge.

CC.7 The hospital ensures that appropriate patient care and clinical information is exchanged when patients are admitted, referred, transferred, or discharged.

CC.8 An established procedure(s) is used to resolve denial-of-care conflicts over care, services, or payment.

Standards and Intent Statements for Continuum of Care

Standard
CC.1 Patients have access to the appropriate type of care.

Intent of CC.1
Individuals are screened at their first point of contact with the hospital. This may occur during emergency transport to the hospital, or when the patient comes in for urgent or elective care (either inpatient or ambulatory), or when the patient is referred or transferred to the hospital. The hospital can use various means to match individuals' identified needs with the organization, the available setting, and the services best able to meet the patients' needs. The hospital may use various mechanisms to facilitate and support this process, so long as it is carried out in a timely and appropriate manner.

The hospital's decision to provide a specific setting and service is based on its mission and capability to provide the requisite staffing, facilities, and services.

Standard
CC.2 When the hospital accepts a patient for entry into a particular service or setting, its decision to do so is based on the outcomes of its assessment* procedures.

Intent of CC.2
To facilitate appropriate, effective care, the entry process includes assessment of
- patients' needs;
- the proper care setting; and
- the hospital's ability to provide necessary services and settings.

Standard
CC.2.1 Criteria define the patient information necessary to determine the appropriate care setting or services.

Intent of CC.2.1
To ensure that patients are cared for in appropriate settings and services, criteria define
- the care provided;
- the specific needs that care meets;
- the patient information that determines eligibility for the setting; and
- acceptance of referrals.
    When care is provided in a short-stay unit, the hospital also determines
- the scope of services it can provide;
- the patient populations appropriate for admission, based on physiological parameters approved by professional staff; and
- the specific circumstances under which such patients will be admitted.

---

* **assessment** (1) For purposes of performance improvement, the systematic collection and review of patient-specific data. (2) For purposes of patient assessment, the process established by an organization for obtaining appropriate and necessary information about each individual seeking entry into a health care setting or service. The information is used to match an individual's need with the appropriate setting, care level, and intervention.

Standard

CC.3 Patients and families* receive information about proposed care during the entry process.

Intent of CC.3

During the entry process, patients and their families receive sufficient information to make a knowledgeable decision about seeking care. Information is also provided about the nature, goals, and availability of care. Costs of care are ascertained and discussed on entry.

Standards

CC.4 The hospital ensures continuity over time among the phases of service to a patient.

CC.5 The hospital ensures coordination among the health professionals and services or settings involved in a patient's care.

Intent of CC.4 and CC.5

Care is coordinated throughout
- entry;
- assessment;
- diagnosis;
- planning;
- treatment; and
- transfer or discharge.

Throughout all phases, patient needs are matched with appropriate resources within the continuum (for example, special care units, skilled nursing facility, or community services). Transitions between levels of care are smooth. Coordination of services may involve promoting communication to facilitate family support, social work, nursing care, consultation or referral, primary physician care, or other follow-up. Communication and transfer of information between and among the health care professionals is essential to a seamless process.

Standard

CC.6 The hospital provides for referral, transfer, or discharge of the patient to another level of care, health professional, or setting, based on the patient's assessed needs and the hospital's capacity to provide the care.

Intent of CC.6

Consultation, referral, and transfer procedures address
- how responsibility is shifted between providers and settings;
- reason(s) for transfer (for example, need for definitive care rather than emergent or urgent care);
- conditions under which transfer can occur (for example, acceptance by the receiving organization and patient stabilization);
- who has responsibility for the patient during transfer; and

---

* **family** The person(s) who plays a significant role in the individual's life. This may include a person(s) not legally related to the individual. This person(s) is often referred to as a surrogate decision maker if authorized to make care decisions for an individual should the individual lose decision-making capacity.

- mechanisms for internal and external referral, including formal affiliations and informal arrangements.

Standard

CC.6.1 The discharge process provides for continuing care based upon the patient's assessed needs at the time of discharge.

Intent of CC.6.1

Discharge planning focuses on meeting patients' health care needs after discharge. Discharge planning identifies patients' continuing physical, emotional, housekeeping, transportation, social, and other needs, and arranges for services to meet them.

Discharge services may include
- adult foster care;
- case management;
- home health services;
- hospice;
- long-term care facilities;
- ambulatory care;
- support groups;
- rehabilitation services; and
- community mental health.

Discharge planning involves the patient, the family, the practitioner primarily responsible for the patient, nursing and social work professionals, and other appropriate staff. Staff members help the patient and family adapt to the plan of care.

Standard

CC.7 The hospital ensures that appropriate patient care and clinical information is exchanged when patients are admitted, referred, transferred, or discharged.

Intent of CC.7

To ensure continuity of care among settings, organizations, and providers, appropriate patient information is communicated whenever patients are admitted, referred for consultation or treatment, transferred, or discharged. Consistent patient care information facilitates service coordination within and among organizations and within the community. Patient information shared with other providers consists of relevant information, including
- the reason for transfer, referral, or discharge;
- the patient's physical and psychosocial status;
- a summary of care provided and progress toward goals; and
- community resources or referrals provided to the patient.

Standard

CC.8 An established procedure(s) is used to resolve denial-of-care conflicts over care, services, or payment.

Intent of CC.8

Once a patient requests or presents for care, the hospital is professionally and ethically responsible for providing care that is within its capability, mission, and the applicable law and regulation. At times, indications for such care may be in conflict with the recommendations of an external entity doing utilization review (for example, peer review organizations, insurance companies, managed care reviewers). If such a conflict arises, treatment and discharge decisions must be made in response to the care required by the patient, regardless of the external agency's recommendation.

Improving Organization Performance

Overview

The **goal** of the improving organization performance function is to ensure that the organization designs processes well and systematically monitors, analyzes, and improves its performance to improve patient outcomes. Value in health care is the appropriate balance between good outcomes, excellent care and services, and costs. To add value to the care and services provided, organizations need to understand the relationship between perception of care, outcomes, and costs and how these three issues are affected by processes carried out by the organization. An organization's performance of important functions significantly affects the quality and value of its services.

The organization's approach to improving its performance includes the following essential processes:
- Designing processes,
- Monitoring performance through data collection,
- Analyzing current performance, and
- Improving and sustaining improved performance.

This approach is anchored in the real work of health care professionals and in the real improvements that can be achieved to benefit patients and others.

Because most organizations identify more improvement opportunities than they can act on, priorities have to be set. Criteria are helpful in setting priorities and can include
- the expected impact on performance;
- the selecting high-risk, high-volume, or problem-prone processes to monitor;
- the relationship of the potential improvement to the dimensions of performance and functions in this book; and
- the organization's resources.

All relevant disciplines participate in testing or implementing improvement strategies. After such implementation, the success of the new strategy is again measured.

Continuously monitoring, analyzing, and improving performance of clinical and other processes are the heart of this function and what the standards in this chapter address. Leaders* and staff carry out these activities. Examples of improvement efforts include designing a new service, flowcharting a clinical process, collecting data about performance measures or patient outcomes, comparing the organization's performance to that of other organizations, selecting areas for priority attention, and even experimenting with new ways of carrying out a function. Leadership also empowers and assigns an individual to lead the improvement by providing time and resources necessary to make the improvement throughout the organization.

---

* **leaders** The leaders described in the leadership function include at least the leaders of the governing body; the chief executive officer and other senior managers; department leaders; the elected and the appointed leaders of the medical staff and the clinical departments and other medical staff members in organizational administrative positions; and the nurse executive and other senior nursing leaders.

Dimensions of Performance

Performance is *what* is done and *how well* it is done to provide health care. The level of performance in health care is
- the degree to which *what* is done is *efficacious* and *appropriate* for the individual patient; and
- the degree to which it is *available* in a *timely* manner to patients who need it, *effective*, *continuous* with other care and care providers, *safe*, *efficient*, and *caring* and *respectful* of the patient.

Characteristics of *what* is done and *how well* it is done are called *dimensions of performance*:
- The degree to which an organization does the right things and does them well is influenced strongly by its design and operation of a number of important functions—many of which are described in this book.
- The effect of an organization's performance of these functions is reflected in patient outcomes and in the cost of its services.
- Patients and others judge the quality of the health care based on patient health outcomes (and sometimes on their perceptions of what was done and how it was done).
- Patients and others may also judge the value of the health care by comparing their judgments about quality with the cost of the health care.

The dimensions of performance are defined in Table 1 (below).

Table 1. Dimensions of Performance

I. Doing the Right Thing

The **efficacy** of the procedure or treatment in relation to the patient's condition
> The degree to which the patient's care and services have been shown to accomplish the desired or projected outcome(s)

The **appropriateness** of a specific test, procedure, or service to meet the patient's needs
> The degree to which the care and services provided are relevant to the patient's clinical needs, given the current state of knowledge

II. Doing the Right Thing Well

The **availability** of a needed test, procedure, treatment, or service to the patient who needs it
> The degree to which appropriate care and services are available to meet the patient's needs

The **timeliness** with which a needed test, procedure, treatment, or service is provided to the patient
> The degree to which the care and services are provided to the patient at the most beneficial or necessary time

The **effectiveness** with which tests, procedures, treatments, and services are provided
> The degree to which the care and services are provided in the correct manner, given the current state of knowledge, to achieve the desired or projected outcome for the patient

continued on next page

Table 1. Dimensions of Performance (continued)

The **continuity** of the services provided to the patient with respect to other services, practitioners, and providers and over time

> The degree to which the patient's care is coordinated among disciplines, among organizations, and over time

The **safety** of the patient and others to whom the services are provided

> The degree to which the risk of an intervention and risk in the care environment are reduced for the patient and others, including the health care provider

The **efficiency** with which care and services are provided

> The relationship between the outcomes (results of care) and the resources used to deliver patient care and services

The **respect and caring** with which care and services are provided

> The degree to which those providing care and services do so with sensitivity and respect for the patient's needs, expectations, and individual differences

> The degree to which the patient or a designee is involved in his or her own care and service decisions

Standards

The following is a list of all standards for this function. If you have a questions about a term used here, please check the Glossary, pages 281 through 307. Terms that are critical to the understanding of the standard are defined in the footnotes of the next section of this chapter.

PI.1 *The leaders establish a planned, systematic, organizationwide approach to process design and performance measurement, analysis, and improvement.*

PI.1.1 *The activities are planned in a collaborative and interdisciplinary manner.*

PI.2 New or modified processes are designed well.

PI.2.1 Performance expectations are established for new and modified processes.

PI.2.2 The performance of new and modified processes is measured.

PI.3 *Data are collected to monitor the stability of existing processes, identify opportunities for improvement, identify changes that will lead to improvement, and sustain improvement.*

PI.3.1 The organization collects data to monitor its performance.

PI.3.1.1 The organization collects data to monitor the performance of processes that involve risks or may result in sentinel events.

PI.3.1.2 The organization collects data to monitor performance of areas targeted for further study.

PI.3.1.3 The organization collects data to monitor improvements in performance.

PI.4 Data are systematically aggregated and analyzed on an ongoing basis.

PI.4.1 Appropriate statistical techniques are used to analyze and display data.

PI.4.2 The organization compares its performance over time and with other sources of information.

PI.4.3 Undesirable patterns or trends in performance and sentinel events are intensively analyzed.

PI.4.4 The organization identifies changes that will lead to improved performance and reduce the risk of sentinel events.

PI.5 Improved performance is achieved and sustained.

Standards and Intent Statements for Design

Leadership Role in Improving Organization Performance
If an organization is to initiate and maintain improvement, leadership and planning are essential. This is especially critical for uniting existing and new improvement activities into a systematic, organizationwide approach. These standards point to the importance of leadership's role in planning an approach to improvement. In conjunction with standards in the "Leadership" chapter, the leaders also ensure that necessary processes and structures are in place to carry out performance-improvement activities and that all services and disciplines collaborate to carry out that approach.

Standards

PI.1 *The leaders establish a planned, systematic, organizationwide approach to process design and performance measurement, analysis, and improvement.*

PI.1.1 *The activities are planned in a collaborative and interdisciplinary manner.*

Intent of PI.1 and PI.1.1
Performance-improvement activities are most effective when they are planned, systematic, and organizationwide and when all appropriate individuals and professions work collaboratively to plan and implement them. At times, performance-improvement efforts occur within specific departments, units, or disciplines. This happens when the organization is small in size or when the services of only one distinct discipline are provided. However, when the disciplines representing the scope of care and services across the organization are included in performance-improvement activities, complex problems and processes can be improved. The ongoing mutual support that develops among interdisciplinary groups provides the momentum necessary to complete long-term improvement projects. Collaboration on performance-improvement activities enables an organization to create a culture focused on performance improvement and to plan and provide systematic and organizationwide improvement.

Designing Processes and Performance Measures Into Processes
Organizations often establish new services, extend product lines, occupy a new facility, or design or redesign functions or systems. The following key questions can help the organization design more effective processes, functions, or services:
- Is the process, function, or service consistent with the organization's mission, vision, and other plans?
- What do the organization's staff, individuals served, and other customers expect from the process, function, or service, and how do they think it should work?
- What do scientific and professional experts and other reliable sources say about the design of the process, function, or service?
- Is new technology available that will affect the design of the process, function, or service, and how exactly will the new technology affect the design?
- What information is available about the performance of similar processes, functions, or services in other organizations, and how can the information benefit the design?

The answers to these questions assist the organization in developing a basic set of performance expectations that guide process design as well as measurement and assessment of the process, function, or service. These data, in turn, guide performance-improvement activities over time.

Standard

PI.2 New or modified processes are designed well.

Intent of PI.2

When processes, functions, or services are designed well, they draw on a variety of information sources. Good process design
a. is consistent with the organization's mission, vision, values, goals and objectives, and plans;
b. meets the needs of individuals served, staff, and others;
c. is clinically sound and current (for instance, use of practice guidelines, information from relevant literature, and clinical standards);
d. is consistent with sound business practices;
e. incorporates available information from other organizations about the occurrence of sentinel events* to reduce the risk of similar sentinel events; and
f. incorporates the results of performance-improvement activities.

The organization incorporates information related to these elements, when available and relevant, in the design or redesign of processes, functions, or services.

Standards

PI.2.1 Performance expectations are established for new and modified processes.

PI.2.2 The performance of new and modified processes is measured.

Intent of PI.2.1 and PI.2.2

Performance expectations† are identified during the design or redesign phase of a function, process, or service.

A performance measure‡ is used to determine whether the process, function, or service is actually performing according to the identified performance expectations and the way it was designed. Performance measures can be developed by the organization or be adopted or adapted from measure sets used in existing databases, which will enable data collection and comparison between or among locations or organizations.

The organization uses criteria to define its own performance measures or to select performance measures from an external system. The criteria help ensure that the data collected are appropriate for monitoring performance. The criteria include the following:
- The measure can identify the events it was intended to identify;
- The measure has a documented numerator and a denominator statement or description of the population to which the measure is applicable;
- The measure has defined data elements and allowable values;

---

* **sentinel event** An unexpected occurrence involving death or serious physical or psychological injury, or the risk thereof. Serious injury specifically includes loss of limb or function. The phrase "or risk thereof" includes any process variation for which a recurrence would carry a significant chance of a serious adverse outcome.

† **Performance expectations** are attributes or dimensions (such as timeliness, effectiveness, and efficiency) which describe expected performance of a function, process, or service. They define how something is expected to work.

‡ **Performance measure** (also referred to as a process or outcome measure) is a quantitative tool that provides an indication of an organization's performance in relation to a specified process or outcome.

- The measure can detect changes in performance over time;
- The measure allows for comparison over time within the organization or between the organization and other entities (this may require risk adjustment);
- The data intended for collection are available; and
- Results can be reported in a way that is useful to the organization and other interested stakeholders.

The performance measures are the benchmarks or statistical measures to be used for comparison.

Standards and Intent Statements for Data Collection

Monitoring Performance Through Data Collection

Monitoring performance through data collection is the foundation of all performance-improvement activities. Collecting data about current performance provides for such information and allows the organization to

- make informed judgments about the stability* of existing processes (for example, undesirable process variation);
- identify opportunities for incrementally improving processes;
- identify the need to redesign processes; and
- decide whether improvements or redesign of processes meet objectives.

Because most organizations have limited resources, they cannot collect data to monitor everything they want to monitor. Leaders must therefore decide which processes to monitor and which data to collect. Leaders determine the importance of the organization's processes in relation to its mission, available resources, and functions, as well as concerns of the individuals served, their families, staff, payers, and other customers.

Data collection focuses on

- processes, particularly those that are high-risk, high-volume, or problem prone;
- outcomes;
- targeted areas of study;
- comprehensive performance measures (indicators);
- other gauges of performance, such as
  - clients' and others' needs, expectations, and feedback,
  - results of ongoing infection control activities,
  - safety of the environment, and
  - quality control and risk-management findings; and
- the dimensions of performance (such as efficiency and timeliness) that are important to a process or an outcome.

The organization's leaders decide the scope and focus of performance monitoring and data collection activities. In determining the scope, the leaders identify and consider the important care and services and organization functions performed. The important functions common to all health care organizations are identified by the chapter titles in this book and represent logical starting points. The leaders determine the focus of data collection monitoring when they set priorities for monitoring. When setting priorities, they consider and are guided by various concerns, such as identified high-risk

---

* A stable process can have very large common-cause variation or can fail to produce the desired results. So it is possible to have a process that is stable, yet incapable of performing satisfactorily.

or problem-prone processes or results from regulatory or accreditation reports. An organizationwide approach to monitoring performance will, over time, include measures that relate to each of the important functions described in this book.

Once they determine the scope and focus of monitoring and data collection, the leaders decide
- how to organize those activities into a systematic approach;
- the frequency and intensity of data collection;
- the relevant dimensions of performance to be monitored; and
- the incorporation of data collection activities into daily work processes.

The standards in this chapter allow each organization to develop its own approach and are therefore equally applicable to approaches that organize monitoring and data collection around diagnosis-related groups (DRGs), CLIA requirements, medication review, clinical paths, product lines, or important functions. Finally, some processes are measured on a periodic, ongoing basis whereas other processes are measured more intensively.

Standard

PI.3 *Data are collected to monitor the stability of existing processes, identify opportunities for improvement, identify changes that will lead to improvement, and sustain improvement.*

Intent for PI.3

Collected data help the organization evaluate outcomes or determine the performance of a function or process. When data collection is systematic, it can be used to
- establish a performance baseline;
- describe process performance or stability;
- describe the dimensions of performance relevant to functions, processes, and outcomes;
- identify areas for more focused data collection; and
- sustain improvement.

The leaders use the judgments made about stability or performance to identify and prioritize issues for more focused data collection and analysis (see LD.1.4, LD.4.2, and LD.4.3 for the leaders using criteria to prioritize data collection for improvement).

Standard

PI.3.1 The organization collects data to monitor its performance.

Intent for PI.3.1

Performance monitoring and improvement are data driven. The stability of important processes can provide the organization with information about its performance. Every organization must choose which processes and outcomes (and thus which types of data) are important to monitor based on its mission and the scope of care and services it provides. The leaders prioritize data collection based on the organization's mission, care and services provided, and populations served (see LD.4.2 for priority setting). Data that the organization considers for collection to monitor performance include the following:
- Performance measures related to accreditation and other requirements;
- Risk management;
- Utilization management;
- Quality control;

- Staff opinions and needs;
- Behavior management* procedures, if used;
- Outcomes of processes or services;
- Autopsy results, when performed;
- Performance measures from acceptable databases;
- Customer demographics and diagnoses;
- Financial data;
- Infection control surveillance and reporting;
- Research data; and
- Performance data identified in various chapters of this book.

Organizations are required to collect data about the needs, expectations, and satisfaction of individuals and organizations served. Individuals served and their family members can provide information that will give an organization insight about process design and functioning. The organization asks them about
- their specific needs and expectations;
- their perceptions[†] of how well the organization meets these needs and expectations; and
- how the organization can improve.

The organization can use a number of ways to get input from these groups, including satisfaction surveys, regularly scheduled meetings held with these groups, and focus groups.

Standard

PI.3.1.1 The organization collects data to monitor the performance of processes that involve risks or may result in sentinel events.

Intent of PI.3.1.1

Organizations select processes that are known to be high-risk, high-volume, problem-prone areas related to the care and services provided. This information is correlated with the listing of frequently occurring sentinel events published by the Joint Commission, the organization's risk-management data, or information about problem-prone processes generated by field-specific or professional organizations.

Organizations select performance measures for processes that are known to jeopardize the safety of the individuals served or associated with sentinel events in similar health care organizations. At a minimum, the organization identifies performance measures related to the following processes, as appropriate to the care and services provided:
- Medication use;
- Operative and other procedures[‡] that place patients at risk:
- Use of blood and blood components;
- Restraint use;

---

* The use of basic learning techniques, such as biofeedback, reinforcement, or aversion therapy, to manage and improve an individual's behavior.

† To better measure the performance of organizations on how well they meet the needs, expectations and concerns of individuals, the Joint Commission is moving from the term *satisfaction* toward the more inclusive term *perception of care and service*. By using this term, the organization will be prompted to assess not only individuals' and/or families' satisfaction with care or treatment, but also whether their needs and expectations are met by the organization.

‡ Includes operative, other invasive, and noninvasive procedures, such as radiotherapy, hyperbaric treatment, CAT scan, and MRI, that place the patient at risk. In this context, the focus is on procedures and is not meant to include medications that place the patient at risk.

- Seclusion when it is part of the care or services provided; and
- Care or services provided to high-risk populations.

The detail and frequency of data collection have been determined and are appropriate for monitoring high-risk, problem-prone processes. Data are collected at the frequency and with the detail identified by the organization.

The performance measure data are used to evaluate outcomes or performance of problem-prone processes.

Standard

PI.3.1.2 The organization collects data to monitor performance of areas targeted for further study.

Intent of PI.3.1.2

A specific area for further study is identified by considering the information provided by the data about process stability, risks, and sentinel events, and priorities set by the leaders. Narrowing the focus of study allows the organization to better describe processes related to the area of study, allows data collection to occur as processes are carried out, and allows the organization to identify potential changes that can lead to more significant improvement. The area targeted for further study can be a specific population, a specific diagnosis, a specific service provided, or an organization management issue, and is time limited. Performance measures are chosen that address the topic area.

The detail and frequency of data collection are determined as appropriate for monitoring targeted areas of study. Data are collected at the frequency and with the detail identified by the organization. The data collected about the performance measures help focus change or improvement activities for that specific area of study.

Standard

PI.3.1.3 The organization collects data to monitor improvements in performance.

Intent of PI.3.1.3

When planning for improvement, the organization identifies those areas needing improvement and identifies the desired changes (see PI.4.4). Performance measures are then identified to determine whether the change results in an improvement and value is increased. Data on the performance measures are collected. The data are analyzed to determine the effectiveness of the change. Performance measures are used on a continuing basis to ensure continued improvement once the change is fully implemented. Data are collected for a period of time that allows the organization to ensure that sustained improvement continues.

If a process is redesigned as part of an improvement activity, then data are collected for the performance measures that were developed as part of the redesign activity.

The detail and frequency of data collection have been determined and are appropriate for monitoring improvements in performance. For example, data collection may be ongoing or time limited. Data are collected at the frequency and with the detail identified by the organization.

Standards and Intent Statements for Aggregation and Analysis

Aggregating and Analyzing Data to Support Performance Improvement

Aggregating and analyzing data means transforming data into information. The organization can use this information to draw conclusions about its performance of a process or the nature of the outcome. Data analysis can answer questions such as the following:
- What is our current level of performance?
- How stable are our current processes?
- Are there areas that could be improved?
- Was a strategy to stabilize or improve performance effective?
- Did we meet design specifications for processes?

The goal is to develop an analysis process that incorporates four basic comparisons: with self, with other comparable organizations, with standards, and with best practices. How often the organization aggregates and analyzes data depends on the process being measured and the organization's priorities. For example, an organization might analyze data about the medication reactions every month and data about staff education needs every six months.

Conclusions about current performance based on data analysis may indicate a need for targeted study or more intense analysis of processes or outcomes. Such conclusions are based on comparison with
- pre-established criteria;
- sentinel events;
- control limits;*
- review of all occurrences; or
- other interpretation methods.

Data analysis is interdisciplinary when appropriate for the process or outcome under review. When the analysis focuses on an individual's clinical performance, the organization takes appropriate action.

Standard

PI.4 Data are systematically aggregated and analyzed on an ongoing basis.

Intent of PI.4

The frequency with which data are aggregated has been determined and is appropriate to the activity or area being studied. Aggregation of data at points in time enables the organization to judge a particular process's stability or a particular outcome's predictability in relation to performance expectations. Aggregated data are analyzed to make judgments about
- whether design specifications for processes were met;
- the level of performance and stability of important existing processes;
- opportunities for improvement;
- actions to improve the performance of processes; and
- whether changes in processes resulted in improvement.

---

* **control limits** In statistics, an expected limit of common-cause variation, sometimes referred to as either an upper or lower limit. Variation beyond a control limit is evidence that special causes are affecting a process. Control limits are calculated from process data and are not to be confused with engineering specifications or tolerance limits. Control limits are typically plotted on a control chart.

Standard

PI.4.1 Appropriate statistical techniques are used to analyze and display data.

Intent of PI.4.1

Understanding statistical techniques is helpful both in assessing variation and in studying a process to determine where the improvement needs to occur. By understanding the type and cause of variation through the use of statistical tools and methods, the organization can focus its attention and resources on making improvement changes to the processes that will result in better outcomes. Some of the types of statistical tools that could be considered are
- run charts, which display summary and comparative data;
- control charts, which display variation and trends over time;
- histograms;
- Pareto charts;
- cause-and-effect or fishbone diagrams; and
- other statistical tools, as appropriate.

Standard

PI.4.2 The organization compares its performance over time and with other sources of information.

Intent of PI.4.2

Performance can be evaluated from three perspectives:
- Performance compared internally over time;
- Performance compared to performance of similar processes in other organizations; and
- Performance compared to external sources of information.

These comparisons are used to determine if there is excessive variability or unacceptable levels of performance of processes and outcomes.

External sources are as up-to-date as possible and include
- recent scientific, clinical, and management literature;
- well-formulated practice guidelines or parameters;
- performance measures;
- reference databases; and
- standards that are periodically reviewed and revised.

Reference databases are excellent sources of performance information. They permit comparison with like processes and outcomes in other organizations and may lead to identifying best practices. Organizations that collect long-term data about the individuals served use the data, as appropriate, to improve themselves.

Standard

PI.4.3 Undesirable patterns or trends in performance and sentinel events are intensively analyzed.

Intent of PI.4.3

When the organization detects or suspects significant undesirable performance or variation, it initiates intense analysis to determine where best to focus changes for improvement. The organization initiates intense analysis when the comparisons show that

- levels of performance, patterns, or trends vary significantly and undesirably from those expected;
- performance varies significantly and undesirably from that of other organizations;
- performance varies significantly and undesirably from recognized standards; or
- when a sentinel event has occurred.

When monitoring performance of specific clinical processes, certain events always elicit intense analysis. Based on the scope of care or services provided, intense analysis is performed for the following:
- Confirmed transfusion reactions;
- Significant adverse drug reactions; and
- Significant medication errors.*

Intense analysis should also occur for those topics chosen by the leaders as performance-improvement priorities or when undesirable variation occurs that changes the priorities. Intense analysis involves studying a process to learn in greater detail about how it is performed or how it operates.

A root cause analysis[†] is performed when a sentinel event occurs. An intense analysis is also performed for the following:
- Major discrepancies, or patterns of discrepancies, between preoperative and postoperative (including pathologic) diagnoses, including those identified during the pathologic review of specimens removed during surgical or invasive procedures; and
- Significant adverse events associated with anesthesia use.

Standard

PI.4.4 The organization identifies changes that will lead to improved performance and reduce the risk of sentinel events.

Intent of PI.4.4

The organization uses the information from the data analysis to identify changes that will improve performance or reduce the risk of sentinel events. Changes are identified based on the analysis of data from targeted study or from analysis of data from ongoing monitoring. A change is selected, and the organization plans to implement the change on a pilot test basis or across the organization. Performance measures are selected that help determine the effectiveness of the change and whether it resulted in an improvement (see PI.3.1.1, PI.3.1.2, and PI.3.1.3) once the change is implemented.

---

* **significant adverse drug reactions and significant medication errors** Unintended, undesirable, and unexpected effects of prescribed medications or medication errors that require discontinuing a medication or modifying the dose, require initial or prolonged hospitalization, result in disability, require treatment with a prescription medication, result in cognitive deterioration or impairment, are life threatening, result in death, or result in congenital anomalies.

[†] **root cause analysis** A process for identifying the basic or causal factor(s) that underlie variation in performance, including the occurrence or possible occurrence of a sentinel event.

Standards and Intent Statements for Performance Improvement

Performance Improvement

The purpose of the performance improvement function is to improve existing processes and outcomes and then sustain the improved performance. This can be accomplished by incrementally improving existing processes, redesigning an existing process, or designing an essentially new process (for example, re-engineering).

Leaders recognize and celebrate improvement successes. To sustain improvements, leaders support one-on-one discussions of successful changes among professionals and other staff. Change is managed and implemented incrementally.

Standard

PI.5 Improved performance is achieved and sustained.

Intent of PI.5

Once performance-improvement priorities are identified, the organization uses appropriate resources and involves those individuals, disciplines, and departments closest to the process, function, or service identified for improvement. Changes to improve performance are identified, planned, and tested. Effective changes are incorporated into standard operating procedure.

The organization sustains improvement through education of key staff about the redesigned process(es) or other changes being implemented. The input of key staff is obtained as they begin to carry out the process to identify additional opportunities for improvement. Performance measures are used (see PI.2.2, PI.3.1.2, and PI.3.1.3) to determine whether the improvement is being sustained. Data are collected as part of performance monitoring. Feedback is provided to staff and leaders on a regular basis.

The organization reduces the risk of sentinel events by using available information about sentinel events known to occur with significant frequency in health care organizations that provide similar care and services. This is done so that the organization can design or redesign care and services to prevent the event from occurring in its organization.

Leadership

Overview

The **goal** of the leadership function* is for the hospital's leaders† to use a framework to establish health care services that respond to community and patient needs.

Providing excellent patient care in a hospital requires effective leadership. The standards in this chapter provide the framework for planning, directing, coordinating, providing, and improving health care services.

Effective leadership depends on the performance of the following processes and their related activities:

- *Planning and designing services*
  Leadership provides a collaborative process to develop a mission that is reflected in long-range, strategic, and operational plans; service design; resource allocation; and organizational policies.
- *Directing services*
  Leadership provides organization, direction, and staffing for patient care and support services according to the scope of services offered.
- *Integrating and coordinating services*
  Leadership communicates objectives and coordinates efforts to integrate patient care and support services throughout the hospital.
- *Improving performance*
  Leadership establishes expectations, plans, and priorities, and manages the performance improvement process. It ensures implementation of processes to measure, assess, and improve the performance of the hospital's governance, management, clinical, and support processes.

The standards in this chapter address these processes and activities.

Leadership is what individuals provide collectively and individually to a hospital, and can be carried out by any number of individuals in the hospital. Building on the hospital's mission, effective leadership creates a clear vision for the future and defines the values that underlie the day-to-day activities carried out throughout the hospital. Effective leadership

- is inclusive, not exclusive;
- encourages staff participation in shaping the hospital's vision and values;
- develops leaders at every level who help to fulfill the hospital's mission, vision, and values;
- accurately assesses the needs of patients and other users of the hospital's services; and
- develops an organizational culture that focuses on continuously improving performance to meet these needs.

To realize the hospital's vision and values, leadership plays a role in teaching and coaching staff; thus, staff education is an essential leadership function.

Note: *These standards do not require or suggest any particular leadership style, structure, or method.*

---

* **function** A goal-directed, interrelated series of processes, such as continuum of care or management of information.

† **leaders** The leaders described in the leadership function include at least the leaders of the governing body; the chief executive officer and other senior managers; department leaders; the elected and the appointed leaders of the medical staff and the clinical departments and other medical staff members in organizational administrative positions; and the nurse executive and other senior nursing leaders.

1999 Hospital Accreditation Standards

Standards

The following is a list of all standards for this function. If you have a questions about a term used here, please check the Glossary, pages 281 through 307. Terms that are critical to the understanding of the standard are defined in the footnotes of the next section of this chapter.

LD.1 *The leaders provide for hospital planning.*

LD.1.1 Planning includes defining a mission, a vision, and values for the hospital and creating the strategic, operational, programmatic, and other plans and policies to achieve the mission and vision.

LD.1.1.1 Planning addresses at least those important patient care and hospitalwide functions identified by the chapter titles in this book.

LD.1.1.2 The leaders of hospitals that belong to a multihospital system participate in systemwide policy decisions affecting the hospital.

LD.1.1.3 The hospital plans for the appropriate care of patients under legal or correctional restrictions.

LD.1.2 The leaders communicate the hospital's mission, vision, and plans.

LD.1.3 The plan(s) includes patient care services based on identified patient needs and is consistent with the hospital's mission.

LD.1.3.1 The leaders, and, as appropriate, community leaders and the leaders of other organizations, collaborate to design services.

LD.1.3.2 The design of hospitalwide patient care services is appropriate to the scope and level of care required by the patients served.

LD.1.3.3 Services are designed to respond to patient and family needs and expectations.

LD.1.3.3.1 *The leaders are responsible for gathering, assessing, and acting on information regarding patient and family satisfaction with the services provided.*

LD.1.3.4 The hospital provides services in a timely manner to meet patients' needs.

LD.1.3.4.1 Patient care services are provided either directly or through referral, consultation, contractual arrangements, or other agreements.

LD.1.3.4.2 The medical staff approves sources of patient care provided outside the hospital.

LD.1.4 The planning process provides for setting performance-improvement priorities and identifies how the hospital adjusts priorities in response to unusual or urgent events.

Leadership

LD.1.5 The leaders develop an annual operating budget and long-term capital expenditure plan, including a strategy to monitor the plan's implementation.

LD.1.5.1 The governing body approves the annual operating budget and long-term capital expenditure plan.

LD.1.5.2 The budget review process considers the appropriateness of the hospital's plan for providing care to meet patient needs.

LD.1.5.3 An independent public accountant conducts an annual audit of the hospital's finances, unless otherwise provided by law.

LD.1.6 The leaders provide for the uniform performance of patient care processes.

LD.1.7 The scope of services provided by each department is defined in writing and is approved by the hospital's administration, medical staff, or both, as appropriate.

LD.1.7.1 Each department provides patient care according to its written goals and scope of services.

LD.1.8 The leaders and other relevant personnel collaborate in decision making.

LD.1.9 The leaders develop programs for recruitment, retention, development, and continuing education of all staff members.

LD.1.9.1 The leaders implement programs to promote staff members' job-related advancement and educational goals.

LD.2 Each hospital department has effective leadership.

LD.2.1 Directors integrate their department's services with the hospital's primary functions.

LD.2.2 Directors coordinate and integrate services within their department and with other departments.

LD.2.3 Directors develop and implement policies and procedures that guide and support the provision of services.

LD.2.4 Directors recommend a sufficient number of qualified and competent persons to provide care.

LD.2.5 Directors determine the qualifications and competence of department personnel who provide patient care services and who are not licensed independent practitioners.

LD.2.6 *Directors continuously assess and improve their department's performance.*

LD.2.7 Directors maintain appropriate quality control programs.

LD.2.8 Directors provide for orientation, in-service training, and continuing education of all persons in the department.

LD.2.9 Directors recommend space and other resources needed by the department.

LD.2.10 Directors participate in selecting outside sources for needed services.

LD.2.11 Departments that are not medical staff services that provide patient care are directed by one or more qualified professionals.

LD.2.11.1 Responsibility for administrative direction and clinical direction is defined in writing.

LD.2.11.2 A qualified professional with appropriate clinical training and experience is responsible for the clinical direction of patient care.

LD.2.11.3 When a department has more than one director, the responsibilities of each are clearly defined in writing.

LD.3 Patient care services are integrated throughout the hospital.

LD.3.1 The hospital's plan for the provision of patient care services describes the organization and functional relationships of departments.

LD.3.2 The leaders foster communication and coordination among individuals and departments.

LD.3.3 The leaders communicate with the leaders of health care delivery organizations corporately or functionally related to the hospital.

LD.3.4 All departments develop policies and procedures in collaboration with associated departments.

LD.4 The hospital's leaders set expectations, develop plans, and manage processes to measure, assess, and improve the quality of the hospital's governance, management, clinical, and support activities.

LD.4.1 The leaders understand the approaches to and methods of performance improvement.

LD.4.2 The leaders adopt an approach to performance improvement.

LD.4.3 Leaders ensure that important processes and activities are measured, assessed, and improved systematically throughout the hospital.

LD.4.3.1 All leaders participate in interdisciplinary, interdepartmental performance-improvement activities.

LD.4.3.2 Relevant information is forwarded to leaders and coordinators of hospitalwide performance-improvement activities.

LD.4.3.3 Responsibility for acting on recommendations generated through performance-improvement activities is assigned and defined in writing.

LD.4.3.4 Leaders ensure that the processes for identifying and managing sentinel events are defined and implemented.

LD.4.4 *The leaders allocate adequate resources for measuring, assessing, and improving the hospital's performance.*

LD.4.4.1 The leaders assign personnel needed to participate in performance-improvement activities.

LD.4.4.2 The leaders provide adequate time for personnel to participate in performance-improvement activities.

LD.4.4.3 The leaders provide information systems and data management processes for ongoing performance improvement.

LD.4.4.4 The leaders provide for staff training in the basic approaches to and methods of performance improvement.

LD.4.5 The leaders measure and assess the effectiveness of their contributions to improving performance.

Standards and Intent Statements for Planning

Standards

LD.1 *The leaders provide for hospital planning.*

LD.1.1 Planning includes defining a mission, a vision, and values for the hospital and creating the strategic, operational, programmatic, and other plans and policies to achieve the mission and vision.

LD.1.1.1 Planning addresses at least those important patient care and hospitalwide functions identified by the chapter titles in this book.

Intent of LD.1 Through LD.1.1.1

Effective leadership creates a framework for planning the hospital's health care services. The leaders develop and implement a planning process for defining timely and clear goals. The leaders direct activities to achieve the hospital's goals and ensure the allocation of sufficient human, space, equipment, and other resources.

An effective planning process first defines and communicates the hospital's mission and vision. In light of the mission, leaders assess patients' needs, plus those of other external and internal customers. To meet these needs, administrative and medical staff leaders collaborate on long-range, strategic, and operational plans; budgets; priorities for resource allocation; and policies. The planning process continually monitors activities to ensure consistency with the hospital's mission.

Planning and design of patient care and support services consider the arrangement and allocation of space to promote efficient and effective patient care. Accessibility issues are addressed. The leaders conduct planning and design activities in the manner that best meets the hospital's needs. The Joint Commission's standards for planning and design do not require a computer-assisted process.

The leaders create a written plan for providing interior and exterior space suitable to the clinical services offered and the ages and other characteristics of the patient population served. Planning also provides for the safe use, maintenance, accessibility, and supervision of grounds, equipment, and special activity areas.

The planning process addresses at least the important patient care and hospitalwide functions that are carried and identified by chapter titles in this book. (The term *important function* refers to a group of interdependent processes that affect patient health outcomes significantly.)

Standard

LD.1.1.2 The leaders of hospitals that belong to a multihospital system participate in systemwide policy decisions affecting the hospital.

Intent of LD.1.1.2

If the hospital belongs to a multihospital system, hospital leaders identify how they interact with corporate levels of the system (for example, with regional staff, the system's governing body, or corporate office staff) in making policy decisions that affect the hospital's patient care services.

Regardless of how the relationship between hospital and system leadership is defined, at least the following three patient care policy issues must be addressed:

- The scope and degree of the leaders' involvement, authority, and responsibility in corporate-level policy decisions;

Leadership

- The mechanism for introducing information from performance-improvement and other activities to improve patient care; and
- How conflicts are resolved between the hospital and the corporate body.

Standard

LD.1.1.3 The hospital plans for the appropriate care of patients under legal or correctional restrictions.

Intent of LD.1.1.3

The hospital plans for and addresses in writing those special issues that arise in caring for patients who are prisoners or wards of the legal system. The hospital orients and educates staff working with these patients consistent with standards HR.3 and HR.3.1 in "Management of Human Resources." Leaders develop mechanisms to coordinate administrative and clinical decisions on at least the following issues:

- Use of seclusion and restraint for nonclinical purposes;
- Imposition of disciplinary restrictions;
- Length of stay;
- Restriction of rights;
- Plan for discharge and continuing care.

Standard

LD.1.2 The leaders communicate the hospital's mission, vision, and plans.

Intent of LD.1.2

Once the hospital develops its mission, vision, and plans, the leaders clearly communicate them throughout the hospital. Effective communication guides staff members in their day-to-day activities. It also promotes innovation and motivates staff members to implement the hospital's strategic, operational, programmatic, and other plans. Communication effectiveness may be measured by the degree to which all individuals throughout the hospital understand the hospital's mission, vision, and plans.

Standard

LD.1.3 The plan(s) includes patient care services based on identified patient needs and is consistent with the hospital's mission.

Intent of LD.1.3

Patient care services, including education, are planned and designed to respond to the needs of the patient population. Patient needs are identified as part of the planning process. Hospitalwide plans describe the care and services to be provided. Care provided is consistent with the hospital's mission. As leaders set priorities during the planning process, human and material resources are considered for educational activities. The mission and resources (both human and material) also are considered before undertaking research activities.

Standard

LD.1.3.1 The leaders, and, as appropriate, community leaders and the leaders of other organizations, collaborate to design services.

Intent of LD.1.3.1
The leaders and staff who are most familiar with service(s) collaborate in service planning. Relevant community leaders and provider hospitals are involved in planning of services to respond to community needs.

Standard
LD.1.3.2 The design of hospitalwide patient care services is appropriate to the scope and level of care required by the patients served.

Intent of LD.1.3.2
The leaders plan the scope and level of care provided throughout the hospital to satisfy the patient population's particular level of health care needs and accepted standards of practice. A systematic process designs services to ensure that patients receive care that meets their projected identified level of needs.

Standards
LD.1.3.3 Services are designed to respond to patient and family needs and expectations.

LD.1.3.3.1 *The leaders are responsible for gathering, assessing, and acting on information regarding patient and family satisfaction with the services provided.*

Intent of LD.1.3.3 and LD.1.3.3.1
The hospital makes an ongoing effort to determine whether it is meeting its patient care mission, goals, and objectives. This effort includes regular assessment of patient and family expectations, and patient and family satisfaction with the care, including patient education, that is provided. The hospital draws on the information derived from these activities to improve its plans and performance.

Standards
LD.1.3.4 The hospital provides services in a timely manner to meet patients' needs.

LD.1.3.4.1 Patient care services are provided either directly or through referral, consultation, contractual arrangements, or other agreements.

LD.1.3.4.2 The medical staff approves sources of patient care provided outside the hospital.

Intent of LD.1.3.4 Through LD.1.3.4.2
A hospital demonstrates a commitment to its community by providing essential services in a timely manner. Through the planning process, leaders determine, first, what diagnostic, therapeutic, rehabilitative and other services are essential to the community; second, which of these services the hospital will provide directly and which through referral, consultation, contractual arrangements, or other agreements; and third, time frames for providing patient care.

Essential services include at least the following:
- Diagnostic radiology;
- Dietetic;
- Emergency;

- Nuclear medicine*;
- Nursing care;
- Pathology and clinical laboratory;
- Pharmaceutical;
- Physical rehabilitation†;
- Respiratory care‡; and
- Social work.

In addition, the hospital has at least one of the following acute care clinical services:
- Medicine;
- Obstetrics and gynecology§;
- Pediatrics;
- Surgery**;
- Child, adolescent, or adult psychiatry; and
- Substance use treatment.

The hospital's leaders are responsible for ensuring the availability of services to meet the needs of its patient population. Services may be provided directly or through referral, consultation, or contractual arrangement. Any outside source providing patient care services provides for the consistent performance of patient care processes according to the standards in this book. The hospital defines time frames within which select patient care services will be provided and communicates these time frames to the community and to outside providers of care. Thus, the hospital defines what constitutes timely care.

A written agreement defines the nature and scope of the care provided by an outside source(s). The medical staff requires outside sources to provide timely care that meets applicable standards in this book.

Standard

LD.1.4 The planning process provides for setting performance-improvement priorities and identifies how the hospital adjusts priorities in response to unusual or urgent events.

Intent of LD.1.4

The planning process provides the framework or criteria for establishing performance-improvement priorities. The planning process gives priority consideration to:
- Processes that affect a large percentage of patients;
- Processes that place patients at risk if not performed well, if performed when not indicated, or if not performed when indicated; and
- Processes that have been or are likely to be problem prone.

The hospital's priority setting is sensitive to emerging needs such as those identified through data collection and assessment, changing regulatory requirements, significant patient and staff needs, changes in the environment of care, or changes in the community.

---

* Not required for hospitals that provide only psychiatric and substance-use services.

† Not required for hospitals that provide only psychiatric and substance-use services.

‡ Not required for hospitals that provide only psychiatric and substance-use services.

§ When the hospital provides surgical or obstetric services, anesthesia services are also available.

** When the hospital provides surgical or obstetric services, anesthesia services are also available.

Standards

LD.1.5 The leaders develop an annual operating budget and long-term capital expenditure plan, including a strategy to monitor the plan's implementation.

LD.1.5.1 The governing body approves the annual operating budget and long-term capital expenditure plan.

LD.1.5.2 The budget review process considers the appropriateness of the hospital's plan for providing care to meet patient needs.

Intent of LD.1.5 Through LD.1.5.2

Fiscal pressures present a major challenge to hospitals and the health professionals who practice in them. Hospitals are complex organizations in which many disciplines bring unique expertise to patient care. Standards LD.1.5 through LD.1.5.2 help to ensure appropriate representation in budgetary and other decisions that affect the provision of care within various disciplines and departments.

It is essential that leaders and other representatives from disciplines and services whose ability to provide patient care are affected directly or indirectly by the following:
- Strategic plans;
- Revenue and capital, expense, and personnel budgets, and any other plans for allocation of fiscal or other resources;
- Operational plans;
- Policies that have a bearing on resource allocation and the provision of patient care.

Leaders accomplish this by participating in meetings, forums, or other activities to develop the items listed above.

The hospital's budget quantifies the hospital's goals and objectives. The hospital develops both an annual operating budget and a long-term capital expenditure plan that, at a minimum, meets applicable legal and regulatory requirements and includes a strategy to monitor implementation.

Department budgets are developed in collaboration with staff from the respective services involved and are consistent with the hospital's budget. Regardless of the process used or the persons who develop the budget, documentation shows that the following factors are considered in preparing department budgets:
- The assumptions on which the budget is built;
- Applicable data and information from
   - ongoing review of the system for determining patients' need for care,
   - ongoing review of hospital staffing plans,
   - performance-improvement activities, including risk management and utilization management,
   - other sources that address the adequacy of fiscal and other resource allocations for meeting patient needs;
- Any information from the hospital's strategic planning process that indicates a need to refine the fiscal resources allocated for providing patient care;
- The process used for measuring department performance relative to the approved budget, including the methods for measuring and acting on variances as defined by the hospital.

Standard

LD.1.5.3 An independent public accountant conducts an annual audit of the hospital's finances, unless otherwise provided by law.

Leadership

Intent of LD.1.5.3
The intent of this standard is self-evident.

Note: *For hospitals that are part of a multihosipital system, the intent of this standard can be met if (1) an annual audit of the hospital's finances is conducted by the corporate entity, and (2) an annual audit of the system's finances, including validation of a sample of the system's audits of its member hospitals, is conducted by an independent public accountant.*

Standard
LD.1.6 The leaders provide for the uniform performance of patient care processes.

Intent of LD.1.6
Patients with the same health problems and care needs have a right to receive the same quality of care throughout the hospital. The principle of "one level of quality of care" is reflected in the following:
- Access to and appropriateness of care and treatment does not depend on a patient's ability to pay or source of payment;
- Acuity of the patient's condition determines the resources allocated to meet the patient's needs;
- The level of care provided to patients who have been administered anesthesia in areas outside the operating room is comparable to that provided in the operating room;
- Patients with the same nursing care needs receive comparable levels of nursing care throughout the hospital.

Standard
LD.1.7 The scope of services provided by each department is defined in writing and is approved by the hospital's administration, medical staff, or both, as appropriate.

LD.1.7.1 Each department provides patient care according to its written goals and scope of services.

Intent of LD.1.7 and LD.1.7.1
Documents prepared by each department define its goals, as well as the scope of current and planned services. Departmental documents describe the kinds of care patients can expect to receive—that is, what the staff does to, for, or with patients and their significant others to provide care consistent with the hospital's and department's mission.

Departmental policies and procedures reflect the department's goals and scope of services, as well as the staff's knowledge and skill. At a minimum, policies and procedures describe how the department assesses and meets the care needs of patients and patient populations. It also addresses the care provided to patients and their families. The process for developing departmental policies and procedures considers at least the following elements:
a. Types and ages of patients served;
b. Methods used to assess and meet patients' care needs;
c. Scope and complexity of patients' care needs;
d. The appropriateness, clinical necessity, and timeliness of support services provided directly by the hospital or through referral contacts;
e. The availability of necessary staff;
f. The extent to which the level of care or service provided meets patients' needs;
g. Recognized standards or practice guidelines, when available.

The hospital's administration or medical staff, or both, as appropriate, approve departmental documents defining goals, scope of services, policies and procedures.

Standard

LD.1.8 The leaders and other relevant personnel collaborate in decision making.

Intent of LD.1.8

The hospital's leaders and directors of relevant departments collaborate in:
- Development of hospitalwide patient care programs, policies, and procedures that describe how patients' care needs are assessed and met;
- Development and implementation of the hospital's plan for providing patient care;
- Decision-making structures and processes;
- Implementation of an effective and continuous program to measure, assess, and improve performance.

Standards

LD.1.9 The leaders develop programs for recruitment, retention, development, and continuing education of all staff members.

LD.1.9.1 The leaders implement programs to promote staff members' job-related advancement and educational goals.

Intent of LD.1.9 and LD.1.9.1

A hospital's ability to care for patients is directly related to its ability to attract and retain qualified, competent staff. The hospital's leaders consider at least the following factors when developing programs that promote the recruitment, retention, development, and continuing education of staff members:
a. The hospital's mission;
b. The case mix of patients the hospital or department serves and the degree and complexity of care required by patients and their families;
c. The technology used in providing patient care;
d. The patient care expectations of the hospital and medical staff, patients and their families;
e. Staff learning needs, whether stated, inferred, or otherwise identified;
f. Recognizing the expertise and performance of staff members engaged in patient care; and
g. Staff-identified issues that influence the decision to continue employment with the hospital.

Because hospitals find that retention, rather than recruitment, activities provide the greatest long-term benefit, it is incumbent on leaders to promote staff educational and advancement goals that relate to the hospital's mission. At a minimum, leaders collaborate to develop and implement programs that enable and encourage staff to pursue job-related advancement and educational goals.

Leadership

Standards and Intent Statements for Directing Departments

Standard

LD.2 Each hospital department has effective leadership.

Intent of LD.2

Department-level leadership is as important as the hospital's senior leadership. Department leaders embrace common qualities of effective leadership shared by all hospital leaders. Specifically, department leaders help create an environment or culture that enables a hospital to fulfill its mission and meet or exceed its goals.

Department leaders clearly convey the hospital's mission to all staff. They support staff and encourage in them a sense of ownership of their work processes. They also hold staff accountable for their performance. Department leaders motivate staff to improve their performance continuously, thereby improving the hospital's performance.

Ultimately, department directors are responsible for the operation of their department, and for the measurement, assessment, and continuous improvement of the department's performance. The best evidence of effective leadership is a department that operates effectively and efficiently.

Patient care services are organized, directed, and staffed in keeping with the scope of services offered.

Standards

LD.2.1 Directors integrate their department's services with the hospital's primary functions.

LD.2.2 Directors coordinate and integrate services within their department and with other departments.

LD.2.3 Directors develop and implement policies and procedures that guide and support the provision of services.

LD.2.4 Directors recommend a sufficient number of qualified and competent persons to provide care.

LD.2.5 Directors determine the qualifications and competence of department personnel who provide patient care services and who are not licensed independent practitioners.*

LD.2.6 *Directors continuously assess and improve their department's performance.*

LD.2.7 Directors maintain appropriate quality control programs.

LD.2.8 Directors provide for orientation, in-service training, and continuing education of all persons in the department.

---

* **licensed independent practitioner** Any individual permitted by law and by the organization to provide care and services without direction or supervision, within the scope of the individual's license and consistent with individually granted clinical privileges.

LD.2.9 Directors recommend space and other resources needed by the department.

LD.2.10 Directors participate in selecting outside sources for needed services.

Note: *Directors of medical staff departments fulfill the responsibilities described in the "Medical Staff" chapter.*

Intent of LD.2.1 Through LD.2.10
Each department's leader is responsible for seeing that the department consistently functions well, and for the continuous improvement of the department's performance. In addition to their responsibilities for the department's internal functioning, department leaders integrate their department's activities with the rest of the hospital's primary functions, particularly the hospital's overall plan for care delivery.

Department leaders may delegate some responsibilities to others in the department or within the hospital. Responsibilities that may be delegated include
- developing and implementing policies and procedures that guide and support the department's provision of services;
- gathering and analyzing data associated with the continuous improvement of care and service quality; and
- maintaining quality control programs.

Although it may be appropriate for a director to delegate work to a qualified individual, the director is ultimately responsible for all the activities listed in LD.2.1. through LD.2.10.

The leaders of each department make their human resources and other resource requirements known to the hospital. This helps to ensure adequate staff, space, equipment, and other resources are available to meet patients' needs at all times. Patient care activities that require the use of special equipment, personnel, facilities, or services are performed only when appropriate resources are available. Equipment and supplies reflect the needs of the patient population served.

Standards

LD.2.11 Departments that are not medical staff services that provide patient care are directed by one or more qualified professionals.

LD.2.11.1 Responsibility for administrative direction and clinical direction is defined in writing.

LD.2.11.2 A qualified professional with appropriate clinical training and experience is responsible for the clinical direction of patient care.

LD.2.11.3 When a department has more than one director, the responsibilities of each are clearly defined in writing.

Intent of LD.2.11 Through LD.2.11.3
Departments providing patient care (for example, dietetic, nursing, respiratory care, physical rehabilitation) may be directed by a qualified professional with appropriate training and experience or by a qualified licensed independent practitioner who possesses appropriate clinical privileges. When a department includes one or more licensed independent practitioners, it is directed by a qualified member of the

medical staff with appropriate clinical privileges. In nonmedical staff departments, medical staff members who participate in clinical care are qualified licensed independent practitioners who are both trained and experienced in the clinical care provided.

Consistent with the intents of LD.2, LD.2.1, LD.2.5, LD.2.8, and LD.2.8.1 in the *1998–99 Comprehensive Accreditation Manual for Pathology and Clinical Laboratory Services*, clinical laboratory services may be directed by a qualified doctoral scientist. However, when the director of clinical laboratory services provides clinical consultation and medical opinions, the director is a physician, preferably a pathologist.

A physician member of the medical staff directs the emergency department.

When a clinical department has more than one director, the responsibilities of each are clearly defined in writing. This makes it easier to collaborate,cooperate, and avoid conflicts.

Standards and Intent Statements for Integrating and Coordinating Services

Standard
LD.3 Patient care services are integrated throughout the hospital.

Intent of LD.3
The leaders are responsible for appropriate integration of each patient care service into the overall functioning of the hospital. Integration enables specific services (for example, radiology services or laboratory services) to coordinate processes with those of other services, and participate in concerted efforts to improve the hospital's overall performance.

Standard
LD.3.1 The hospital's plan for the provision of patient care services describes the organization and functional relationships of departments.

Intent of LD.3.1
Forethought and careful planning are needed to integrate services with one another and with the hospital's overall daily functioning. The hospital's plan for the provision of patient care demonstrates this forethought. A planned approach to integrating patient care allows departments to understand the role and purpose of other services and how they may complement each other. The result is coordinated patient care across departments that is virtually seamless from the patient's perspective.

Standard
LD.3.2 The leaders foster communication and coordination among individuals and departments.

Intent of LD.3.2
To coordinate and integrate patient care, the leaders develop a culture that emphasizes cooperation and communication. An open communication system facilitates an interdisciplinary approach to

providing patient care. The leaders develop methods for promoting communication among services, individual staff members, and less formal structures such as quality action teams, performance-improvement teams, or members of standing committees.

This leadership role is commonly referred to as coaching.

Standard

LD.3.3 The leaders communicate with the leaders of health care delivery organizations corporately or functionally related to the hospital.

Intent of LD.3.3

Effective external communications are as important as internal communications. Because the provision of patient care does not occur in a vacuum, the hospital's leaders communicate effectively with the leaders of health care delivery organizations that are corporately and functionally related to the hospital. Leaders communicate both jointly and individually. Effective communication is necessary for hospital leaders to coordinate planning for patient care services with corporately or functionally related organizations.

Standard

LD.3.4 All departments develop policies and procedures in collaboration with associated departments.

Intent of LD.3.4

Written policies and procedures standardize practice for all staff and describe accepted methods for carrying out activities. It is important to collaboratively develop policies and procedures for those functions or processes that involve and invariably affect more than one department. Collaboration helps minimize conflicting practices and understandings. It also identifies functions or processes that might be more easily accomplished by cooperative effort. Finally, collaboration on policies and procedures creates opportunities to determine the best practice for the hospital.

It is similarly important for the hospital's administration and medical staff to approve all such policies and procedures, as appropriate to the nature of the policy or procedure, to ensure consistency throughout the hospital.

To ensure consistency throughout the hospital, the medical staff and administration approve all collaboratively developed department policies and procedures, as described at LD.1.7.

Standards and Intent Statements for Role in Improving Performance

Standard

LD.4 The hospital's leaders set expectations, develop plans, and manage processes to measure, assess, and improve the quality of the hospital's governance, management, clinical, and support activities.

Intent of LD.4

LD.4 through LD.4.5 describe the role the leaders play in supporting hospitalwide efforts to improve the performance of governance, management, clinical and patient care services, and support activities. The leaders' role in these efforts is critical to their success. LD.4 spells out *what* leaders do to ensure continuous improvement in the hospital's processes and functions. Succeeding standards (LD.4.1 through LD.4.5) detail the essential activities associated with carrying out these responsibilities—in other words, *how* leaders improve hospital performance.

These standards are based on the following principles:
- A hospital can take actions that result in desired, measurable change in processes that most affect patient outcomes.
- Processes are carried out by medical, nursing, and other clinicians; governing body members; managers; and support personnel. Many are carried out jointly.
- Processes are coordinated and integrated, which requires the attention of managerial and clinical leaders.
- Governance, managerial, medical, nursing, and other clinical and support staff are motivated and competent to perform processes well. Opportunities to improve processes—and patient outcomes—arise more frequently than errors and mistakes. The hospital's principal goal is to help everyone improve work processes without shirking the responsibility to address serious problems involving deficits in knowledge or skill.

Standard

LD.4.1 The leaders understand the approaches to and methods of performance improvement.

Intent of LD.4.1

The leaders need education about performance-improvement principles and methods to understand and implement performance-improvement initiatives. Education may include planned reading, discussions, visits to hospitals conducting performance-improvement efforts, use of consultants, and formal training programs. All leaders—administrative, governing body, clinical, and nonclinical—need to be educated.

Standard

LD.4.2 The leaders adopt an approach to performance improvement.

Intent of LD.4.2

Leaders select a hospitalwide approach to performance improvement and clearly define how all levels of the hospital will address improvement issues. There are many valid performance-improvement methodologies; the approach selected reflects the hospital's leadership style. The hospital documents performance-improvement activities at every level. The approach the leaders select provides for the following essential activities:
- Planning the process of improvement;
- Setting priorities for the scope and focus of measurement;
- Systematically measuring and assessing performance;
- Setting priories for improvement;
- Implementing improvement activities based on assessment conclusions; and
- Maintaining achieved improvements.

Standard

LD.4.3 Leaders ensure that important processes and activities are measured, assessed, and improved systematically throughout the hospital.

Intent of LD.4.3

Leaders prioritize the activities to be measured, assessed, and improved. Priorities relate to hospital-wide activities and patient health outcomes. Important internal processes and activities are those that affect patient outcomes most significantly. Leaders take steps to improve performance of these processes and activities throughout the hospital. To achieve this goal, each department collaborates as necessary with other departments in hospitalwide performance-improvement activities described in the "Improving Organization Performance" chapter of this book. Leaders ensure that data and other information necessary to improve performance are consistently identified, gathered, and assessed, both by each department internally and in collaboration with other departments as needed.

Standard

LD.4.3.1 All leaders participate in interdisciplinary, interdepartmental performance-improvement activities.

Intent of LD.4.3.1

Leading by example is important. Leaders set the tone for participation in interdisciplinary performance-improvement activities by participating in such activities themselves. Because performance improvement is not a process that can be delegated to nonmanagement staff alone, all leaders are responsible for team building. Interdepartmental performance-improvement activities are less effective when only nonmanagement staff are involved.

Standard

LD.4.3.2 Relevant information is forwarded to leaders and coordinators of hospitalwide performance-improvement activities.

Intent of LD.4.3.2

A successful, coordinated performance-improvement process depends on communication of its conclusions and recommendations to individuals responsible for implementing and coordinating improvements. Accountability is established for specific improvements to motivate their implementation. To do this, leaders also need relevant information from performance-improvement activities.

Standard

LD.4.3.3 Responsibility for acting on recommendations generated through performance-improvement activities is assigned and defined in writing.

Intent of LD.4.3.3

For process and procedure improvements to be implemented successfully, accountabilities must be defined and follow-up action taken. Follow-up action begins with a document that assigns responsibility for acting on performance-improvement recommendations to individuals, departments, or other hospital components (for example, committees). The document clearly describes the action to be taken, time frames, and other assignment parameters.

Leadership

Standard

LD.4.3.4 Leaders ensure that the processes for identifying and managing sentinel events are defined and implemented.*

Intent of LD.4.3.4

When a sentinel event occurs in a health care organization, it is necessary that appropriate individuals within the organization be aware of the event; investigate and understand the causes that underlie the event; and make changes in the organization's systems and processes to reduce the probability of such an event in the future. The leaders are responsible for establishing processes for the identification, reporting, analysis, and prevention of sentinel events and for ensuring the consistent and effective implementation of a mechanism to accomplish these activities including

- determination of a definition of *sentinel event*, that is approved by the leaders and communicated throughout the organization;
- communication of a process for reporting of sentinel events through established channels within the organization and, as appropriate, to external agencies in accordance with law and regulation;
- creation of a process for conducting thorough root cause analyses that focus on process and system factors; and
- determination of a risk reduction strategy and action plan that includes measurement of the effectiveness of process and system improvements to reduce risk.

Standards

LD.4.4 *The leaders allocate adequate resources for measuring, assessing, and improving the hospital's performance.*

LD.4.4.1 The leaders assign personnel needed to participate in performance-improvement activities.

LD.4.4.2 The leaders provide adequate time for personnel to participate in performance-improvement activities.

LD.4.4.3 The leaders provide information systems and data management processes for ongoing performance improvement.

LD.4.4.4 The leaders provide for staff training in the basic approaches to and methods of performance improvement.

Intent of LD.4.4 Through LD.4.4.4

Hospital leaders provide adequate human resources for this activity and give them sufficient time and support to be effective. Appropriate staff members are assigned in sufficient numbers to ensure progress in the pursuit of improvement priorities. Leaders allow enough time for performance-improvement activities and provide needed information and technical assistance. Each department determines what resources are sufficient for its improvement efforts.

---

* Effective January 1, 1999.

Standard

LD.4.5 The leaders measure and assess the effectiveness of their contributions to improving performance.

Intent of LD.4.5

The performance-improvement framework in the "Improving Organization Performance" chapter is used to design, measure, assess, and improve the leaders' performance and contribution to performance improvement.

The leaders
- set measurable objectives for improving hospital performance;
- gather information to assess their effectiveness in improving hospital performance;
- use pre-established, objective process criteria to assess their effectiveness in improving hospital performance;
- draw conclusions based on their findings and develop and implement improvement in their activities; and
- evaluate their performance to support sustained improvement.

Management of the Environment of Care

Overview

The **goal** of this function* is to provide a safe, functional, and effective environment for patients, staff members, and other individuals in the hospital. This is crucial to providing patient care and achieving good outcomes. Achieving this goal depends on performing the following processes:
- Planning by hospital leaders for the space, equipment, and resources needed to safely and effectively support the services provided. Planning and designing is consistent with the hospital's mission and vision.
- Educating staff about the role of the environment in safely and effectively supporting patient care. The hospital educates staff about the physical characteristics and the processes for monitoring and reporting on the health care environment.
- Developing standards to measure staff and hospital performance in managing and improving the environment of care.
- Implementing plans to create and manage the hospital's environment of care. An Information Collection and Evaluation System (ICES) is developed and used to continuously measure, assess, and improve the status of the environment of care.

"Environment of care" refers to a variety of sites where patients are treated. These include both inpatient settings (such as acute care hospitals, psychiatric hospitals, hospice facilities, subacute care facilities, or nursing homes) as well as outpatient settings (such as clinics, counseling centers, preadmission testing offices, infirmaries, same-day surgery centers, dialysis centers, or imaging centers). Such environments are made up of three basic components: building(s), equipment, and people. Effective management of the environment of care includes using processes and activities to
- reduce and control environmental hazards and risks;
- prevent accidents and injuries; and
- maintain safe conditions for patients, visitors, and staff.

The standards in this chapter focus on how everyone in the hospital participates in the processes and activities that make the care environment safe and effective. They also address department leaders' responsibility for identifying and communicating the care environment needs to the hospital and allocating appropriate space, equipment, and resources to safely and effectively support the hospital's services.

Note: *The standards in this chapter do not prescribe any particular structure (such as a safety committee), individual (such as one employee hired to be a safety officer), or format for the required designs and planning activities. The hospital needs to know the structural features of its own building(s) or its space within another building. The standards do not require the Statement of Conditions™ compliance document to be completed by anyone other than an employee of the hospital. This statement is the basis for corrective actions needed to make the environment of care as safe and useful as possible for patients and staff.*

---

* **function** A goal-directed, interrelated series of processes, such as continuum of care or management of information.

Standards

The following is a list of all standards for this function. If you have a questions about a term used here, please check the Glossary, pages 281 through 307. Terms that are critical to the understanding of the standard are defined in the footnotes of the next section of this chapter.

EC.1 *The organization designs a safe, accessible, effective, and efficient environment of care consistent with its mission, services, and law and regulation.*

EC.1.1 Newly constructed and existing environments of care are designed and maintained to comply with the *Life Safety Code.*®

EC.1.2 When designing the environment of care, the organization uses design criteria referenced by the health care community.

EC.1.3 A management plan addresses safety.

EC.1.4 A management plan addresses security.

EC.1.5 A management plan addresses control of hazardous materials and waste.

EC.1.6 A management plan addresses emergency preparedness.

EC.1.7 A management plan addresses life safety.

EC.1.8 A management plan addresses medical equipment.

EC.1.9 A management plan addresses utility systems.

EC.2 *The organization provides a safe, accessible, effective, and efficient environment of care consistent with its mission, services, and law and regulation.*

EC.2.1 Staff members have been oriented to and educated about the environment of care, and possess the knowledge and skills to perform their responsibilities under the environment of care management plans.

EC.2.2 The safety management plan is implemented.

EC.2.3 The security management plan is implemented.

EC.2.4 The hazardous materials and waste management plan is implemented.

EC.2.5 The emergency preparedness management plan is implemented.

EC.2.6 The life safety management plan is implemented.

Management of the Environment of Care

EC.2.7 The medical equipment management plan is implemented.

EC.2.8 The utility systems management plan is implemented.

EC.2.9 Drills are regularly conducted to test emergency preparedness.

EC.2.10 Fire drills are conducted regularly.

EC.2.11 Safety elements of the environment of care are maintained, tested, and inspected.

EC.2.12 Life safety elements in the environment of care are maintained, tested, and inspected.

EC.2.13 Medical equipment is maintained, tested, and inspected.

EC.2.14 Utility systems are maintained, tested, and inspected.

EC.3 *An organizationwide Information Collection and Evaluation System (ICES) is developed and used to evaluate and improve conditions in the environment of care.*

EC.3.1 The organization appoints an individual to direct an ongoing, organizationwide process to collect information about deficiencies and opportunities for improvement in environment of care management programs.

EC.3.2 The organization analyzes identified environment of care management issues and develops or approves recommendations for resolving them.

EC.3.3 The individual directing the safety program works with appropriate staff to implement recommendations and monitor their effectiveness.

EC.4 *The hospital provides a care environment that supports its mission and services.*

EC.4.1 Appropriate space to support patient services is provided.

EC.4.2 An environment that fosters a positive self-image for the patient and preserves his or her human dignity is provided.

EC.4.3 The built environment provides appropriate privacy to patients.

EC.4.4 The built environment supports the development and maintenance of the patient's interests, skills, and opportunities for personal growth when required.

EC.5 A nonsmoking policy is communicated and enforced throughout all buildings.

EC.5.1 Any exceptions to the prohibition are authorized for a patient by a licensed independent practitioner's written authorization, based on criteria that are defined by the medical staff.

Standards and Intent Statements for Design

Standard

EC.1 *The organization designs a safe, accessible, effective, and efficient environment of care consistent with its mission, services, and law and regulation.*

Intent of EC.1
The intent of this standard is self-evident.

Design of Buildings

Standard

EC.1.1 Newly constructed and existing environments of care are designed and maintained to comply with the *Life Safety Code*®*

Note: *This standard does not apply to environments of care classified as a business occupancy by the Life Safety Code® (LSC®) that occur as a freestanding building.*

Intent of EC.1.1
- A current, organizationwide Statement of Conditions™ compliance document[†] (SOC) has been prepared.
- Each building in which patients are housed or receive treatment
  - complies with the *Life Safety Code*® (*LSC*®), NFPA 101,® 1997;
    OR
  - does not comply with the *LSC*® but the resolution of all deficiencies is evidenced through
    - an equivalency approved by the Joint Commission or
    - continued progress in completing an acceptable Plan For Improvement. (SOC™—Part 4)

Standard

EC.1.2 When designing the environment of care, the organization uses design criteria referenced by the health care community.

Intent of EC.1.2
When planning for the size, configuration, and equipping the space of renovated, altered, or new construction, the organization uses

---

* *Life Safety Code*® and NFPA 101® are registered trademarks of the National Fire Protection Association, Inc, Quincy, Massachusetts. Effective January 1, 1998, the Joint Commission began referencing the *NFPA 101*,® *1997, Life Safety Code*® (*LSC*®), of the National Fire Protection Association. All facilities being surveyed will be evaluated using the 1997 edition of the *LSC*.® Buildings for which plans were approved after January 1, 1998, will be evaluated as "new construction" under the applicable occupancy chapters of the 1997 edition of the *LSC*.®

[†] **Statement of Conditions™ (SOC) compliance document** A proactive document that helps an organization to do a critical self-assessment of its current level of compliance and describe how to resolve any *Life Safety Code*® (*LSC*®) deficiencies. The SOC™ was created to be a "living, ongoing" management tool that should be used in a management process that continually identifies, assesses, and resolves *LSC*® deficiencies.

- *Guidelines for Design and Construction of Hospitals and Health Care Facilities,* 1996 edition, published by the American Institute of Architects; or
- applicable state rules and regulations; or
- similar standards or guidelines.

When site conditions or specific clinical needs require deviation from the referenced guidelines or standards, the organization identifies, when appropriate, the need for specialized staff training to effectively use the space and equipment provided.

Design of Management Plans

Standard

EC.1.3 A management plan addresses safety.

Intent of EC.1.3

The safety management plan describes how the organization will provide a physical environment free of hazards and manage staff activities to reduce the risk of injuries. The plan provides processes for
a. maintaining and supervising all grounds and equipment;
b. conducting risk assessment that proactively evaluates the impact of buildings, grounds, equipment, occupants, and internal physical systems on patient and public safety;
c. examining safety issues by appropriate representatives from administration, clinical services, and support services;
d. reporting and investigating all incidents of property damage, occupational illness, and patient, personnel, or visitor injury; and
e. ongoing hazard surveillance, including response to product safety recalls.

In addition, the plan establishes
f. a qualified individual(s) to oversee development, implementation, and monitoring of safety management;
g. an individual(s) to intervene whenever conditions pose an immediate threat to life or health or threaten damage to equipment or buildings;
h. an orientation and education program that addresses
  1. general safety processes,
  2. area-specific safety,
  3. specific job-related hazards, and
  4. provision of safety-related information through new employee orientation and continuing education;
i. ongoing monitoring of performance regarding actual or potential risk related to one or more of the following:
  - Staff knowledge and skills;
  - Level of staff participation;
  - Monitoring and inspection activities;
  - Emergency and incident reporting; or
  - Inspection, preventive maintenance, and testing of equipment;
j. safety policies and procedures are distributed, practiced, enforced, and reviewed as frequently as necessary, but at least every three years; and
k. how an annual evaluation of the safety management plan's objectives, scope, performance, and effectiveness will occur.

Standard

EC.1.4 A management plan addresses security.

Intent of EC.1.4

A security management plan describes how the organization will establish and maintain a security management program to protect staff, patients, and visitors from harm. The plan provides processes for
a. leadership's designation of personnel responsible for developing, implementing, and monitoring the security management plan;
b. addressing security issues concerning patients, visitors, personnel, and property;
c. reporting and investigating all security incidents involving patients, visitors, personnel, or property;
d. providing identification, as appropriate, for all patients, visitors, and staff;
e. controlling access to and egress from sensitive areas, as determined by the organization; and
f. providing vehicular access to urgent care areas.

In addition, the plan establishes
g. a security orientation and education program that addresses:
   1. processes for minimizing security risks for personnel in security sensitive areas;
   2. emergency procedures followed during security incidents; and
   3. processes for reporting security incidents involving patients, visitors, personnel, and property;
h. ongoing monitoring of performance regarding actual or potential risk related to one or more of the following:
   - Staff knowledge and skills;
   - Level of staff participation;
   - Monitoring and inspection activities;
   - Emergency and incident reporting; or
   - Inspection, preventive maintenance, and testing of equipment;
i. emergency security procedures that address
   1. actions taken in the event of a security incident or failure,
   2. handling of civil disturbances,
   3. handling of situations involving VIPs or the media, and
   4. provision of additional staff to control human and vehicle traffic in and around the environment of care during disasters; and
j. how an annual evaluation of the security management plan's objectives, scope, performance, and effectiveness will occur.

Standard

EC.1.5 A management plan addresses control of hazardous materials and waste.*

Intent of EC.1.5

A hazardous materials and waste management plan describes how the organization will establish and maintain a program to safely control hazardous materials and waste. The plan provides processes for

---

* **hazardous materials and waste** Materials, whose handling, use, and storage are guided or defined by local, state, or federal regulation (for example, the Occupational Safety and Health Administration's Regulations for Bloodborne Pathogens regarding the disposal of blood and blood-soaked items; Nuclear Regulatory Commission's regulations for the handling and disposal of radioactive waste), hazardous vapors (for example glutaraldehyde, ethylene oxide, nitrous oxide), and hazardous energy sources (for example, ionizing or nonionizing radiation, lasers, microwave, ultrasound). Though the Joint Commission considers infectious waste as falling into this category, federal regulations do not define infectious waste or medical waste as hazardous waste.

Management of the Environment of Care

a. selecting, handling, storing, using, and disposing of hazardous materials and waste from receipt or generation through use or final disposal;
b. establishing written criteria consistent with applicable law and regulation, to identify, evaluate, and inventory hazardous materials and waste used or generated;
c. managing chemical waste, chemotherapeutic waste, radioactive waste, and regulated medical or infectious waste, including sharps;
d. monitoring and disposing of hazardous gases and vapors;
e. providing adequate and appropriate space and equipment for safe handling and storage of hazardous materials and waste; and
f. reporting and investigating all hazardous materials or waste spills, exposures, and other incidents.
   In addition, the plan establishes
g. an orientation and education program for personnel who manage or have contact with hazardous materials and waste that addresses
   1. precautions for selecting, handling, storing, using, and disposing of hazardous materials and waste;
   2. emergency procedures for hazardous material and waste spills or exposure;
   3. health hazards of mishandling hazardous materials; and
   4. for all appropriate personnel, orientation and education about reporting procedures for hazardous materials and waste incidents, including spills or exposures;
h. ongoing monitoring of performance regarding actual or potential risk related to one or more of the following:
   - Staff knowledge and skills;
   - Level of staff participation;
   - Monitoring and inspection activities;
   - Emergency and incident reporting; or
   - Inspection, preventive maintenance, and testing of equipment;
i. emergency procedures describe the specific precautions, procedures, and protective equipment used during hazardous material and waste spills or exposures; and
j. how an annual evaluation of the hazardous materials and waste-management plan's objectives, scope, performance, and effectiveness will occur.

Standard

EC.1.6 A management plan addresses emergency preparedness.

Intent of EC.1.6

The emergency preparedness management plan describes how the organization will establish and maintain a program to ensure effective response to disasters* or emergencies affecting the environment of care. The plan provides processes for

a. implementing specific procedures in response to a variety of disasters;
b. defining and, when appropriate, integrating the organization's role with communitywide emergency preparedness efforts;
c. notifying external authorities of emergencies;

---

* **disaster** A natural or man-made event that significantly disrupts the environment of care, such as damage to the organization's building(s) and grounds due to severe wind storms, tornadoes, hurricanes, or earthquakes. Also, an event that disrupts care and treatment, such as loss of utilities (power, water, telephones) due to floods, riots, accidents, or emergencies within the organization or in the surrounding community.

1999 Hospital Accreditation Standards

    d. notifying personnel when emergency response measures are initiated;
    e. assigning available personnel in emergencies to cover all necessary staff positions;
    f. managing space, supplies, and security;
    g. evacuating the facility when the environment cannot support adequate patient care and treatment;
    h. establishing an alternative care site when the environment cannot support adequate patient care; and
    i. managing patients during emergencies, including scheduling, modification, or discontinuation of services, control of patient information, and patient transportation.

The plan identifies
    j. an alternative source of essential utilities;
    k. a backup communication system in the event of failure during disasters and emergencies;
    l. facilities for radioactive or chemical isolation and decontamination;
    m. alternate roles and responsibilities of personnel during emergencies; and

The plan establishes
    n. an orientation and education program for personnel who participate in implementing the emergency preparedness plan. Education addresses
        1. specific roles and responsibilities during emergencies,
        2. the information and skills required to perform duties during emergencies,
        3. the backup communication system used during disasters and emergencies, and
        4. how supplies and equipment are obtained during disasters or emergencies;
    o. ongoing monitoring of performance regarding actual or potential risk related to one or more of the following:
- Staff knowledge and skills;
- Level of staff participation;
- Monitoring and inspection activities;
- Emergency and incident reporting; or
- Inspection, preventive maintenance, and testing of equipment; and

    p. how an annual evaluation of the emergency preparedness safety management plan's objectives, scope, performance, and effectiveness will occur.

Standard

EC.1.7 A management plan addresses life safety.

Intent of EC.1.7

A life safety management plan describes how the organization will establish and maintain a life safety management program* to provide a fire-safe environment of care. The plan provides processes for
    a. protecting patients, personnel, visitors, and property from fire, smoke, and other products of combustion;
    b. inspection, testing, and maintaining fire protection and life safety systems, equipment, and components on a regular basis in accordance with standard EC.2.12;
    c. reviewing proposed acquisitions of bedding, window draperies, and other curtains, furnishings, decorations, wastebaskets, and other equipment for fire safety; and

---

* **life safety management program or process** An organization's documented management plan describing the processes for protecting patients, staff members, visitors, and property from fire and the product of combustion (smoke).

Management of the Environment of Care

   d. reporting and investigating fire protection deficiencies, failures, and user errors.

In addition, the plan establishes

   e. a life safety orientation and education program that addresses
      1. specific roles and responsibilities of personnel, physicians, and other licensed independent practitioners at a fire's point of origin,
      2. specific roles and responsibilities of personnel, physicians, and other licensed independent practitioners away from a fire's point of origin,
      3. specific roles and responsibilities of other personnel who must participate in the fire plan, such as volunteers, students, and physicians,
      4. use and functioning of fire alarm systems,
      5. specific roles and responsibilities in preparing for building evacuation,
      6. location and proper use of equipment for evacuating or transporting patients to areas of refuge, and
      7. building compartmentalization procedures for containing smoke and fire;
   f. ongoing monitoring of performance regarding actual or potential risk related to one or more of the following:
      - Staff knowledge and skills;
      - Level of staff participation;
      - Monitoring and inspection activities;
      - Emergency and incident reporting; or
      - Inspection, preventive maintenance, and testing of equipment;
   g. emergency procedures that address
      1. facilitywide fire-response needs,
      2. area-specific needs and fire evacuation routes,
      3. specific roles and responsibilities of personnel at a fire's point of origin,
      4. specific roles and responsibilities of personnel away from a fire's point of origin,
      5. specific roles and responsibilities of personnel in preparing for building evacuation; and
   h. how an annual evaluation of the life safety management plan's objectives, scope, performance, and effectiveness will occur.

Standard

EC.1.8 A management plan addresses medical equipment.

Intent of EC.1.8

A management plan describes how the organization will establish and maintain a medical equipment management program to promote safe and effective use of medical equipment. The plan provides processes for

   a. selecting and acquiring medical equipment;
   b. establishing criteria for identifying, evaluating, and taking inventory of medical equipment to be included in the management program before the equipment is used. These criteria address
      1. equipment function (diagnosis, care, treatment, and monitoring);
      2. physical risks associated with use;
      3. maintenance requirements; and
      4. equipment incident history;

      Note: *All medical equipment may be included in the program rather than a limited selection based on risk criteria.*

c. assessing and minimizing clinical and physical risks of equipment use through inspection, testing, and maintenance;
d. monitoring and acting on equipment hazard notices and recalls;
e. monitoring and reporting incidents in which a medical device is connected to the death, serious injury, or serious illness of any individual, as required by the Safe Medical Devices Act of 1990;
f. reporting and investigating equipment management problems, failures, and user errors.

In addition, the plan establishes
g. a medical equipment orientation and education program that addresses
   1. capabilities, limitations, and special applications of equipment;
   2. basic operating and safety procedures for equipment use;
   3. emergency procedures in the event of equipment failure;
   4. information and skills necessary to perform assigned maintenance responsibilities; and
   5. processes for reporting medical equipment management problems, failures, and user errors;
h. ongoing monitoring of performance regarding actual or potential risk related to one or more of the following:
   - Staff knowledge and skills;
   - Level of staff participation;
   - Monitoring and inspection activities;
   - Emergency and incident reporting; or
   - Inspection, preventive maintenance, and testing of equipment;
i. emergency procedures that address
   1. specific procedures in the event of equipment failure;
   2. when and how to perform emergency clinical interventions when medical equipment fails;
   3. availability of backup equipment; and
   4. how to obtain repair services; and
j. how an annual evaluation of the medical equipment management plan's objectives, scope, performance, and effectiveness will occur.

Standard

EC.1.9 A management plan addresses utility systems.*

Intent of EC.1.9

A management plan describes how the organization will establish and maintain a utility systems management program to
a. promote a safe, controlled, comfortable environment of care;
b. assess and minimize risks of utility failures; and
c. ensure operational reliability of utility systems;

The plan provides processes for
d. establishing criteria for identifying, evaluating, and taking inventory of critical operating components of systems to be included in the utility management program. These criteria address the impact of utility systems on
   1. life support systems,
   2. infection control systems,

---

* **utility systems** Organization systems for life support, surveillance, prevention, and control of infection; environment support; and equipment support. May include electrical distribution; emergency power; vertical and horizontal transport; heating, ventilating, and air conditioning; plumbing, boiler, and steam; piped gases; vacuum systems; or communication systems including data exchange systems.

Management of the Environment of Care

   3. environmental support systems,
   4. equipment-support systems, and
   5. communication systems;

Note: *All utility systems, rather than a limited selection of elements based on risk criteria, may be included in the management program.*
  e. inspecting, testing, and maintaining critical operating components;
  f. developing and maintaining current utility system operational plans to help ensure reliability, minimize risks, and reduce failures;
  g. mapping the distribution of utility systems and labeling controls for a partial or complete emergency shutdown; and
  h. investigating utility systems management problems, failures, or user errors and reporting incidents and corrective actions.

In addition, the plan establishes
  i. an orientation and education program that addresses
     1. utility systems' capabilities, limitations, and special applications,
     2. emergency procedures in the event of system failure,
     3. information and skills necessary to perform assigned maintenance responsibilities,
     4. location and instructions for use of emergency shutoff controls, and
     5. processes for reporting utility system management problems, failures, and user errors;
  j. ongoing monitoring of performance regarding actual or potential risk related to one or more of the following:
     - Staff knowledge and skills;
     - Level of staff participation;
     - Monitoring and inspection activities;
     - Emergency and incident reporting; or
     - Inspection, preventive maintenance, and testing of equipment;
  k. emergency procedures for utility system disruptions or failures that address
     1. specific procedures in the event of utility systems malfunction;
     2. identification of an alternative source of essential utilities;
     3. shutoff of malfunctioning systems and notification of staff in affected areas;
     4. obtaining repair services; and
     5. how and when to perform emergency clinical interventions when utility systems fail; and
  l. how an annual evaluation of the utility systems management plan's objectives, scope, performance, and effectiveness will occur.

Standards and Intent Statements for Implementation

Standard

EC.2 *The organization provides a safe, accessible, effective, and efficient environment of care consistent with its mission, services, and law and regulation.*

Intent of EC.2
The intent of this standard is self-evident.

Implementing Plans for Staff Orientation and Education
Standard
EC.2.1 Staff members have been oriented to and educated about the environment of care, and possess the knowledge and skills to perform their responsibilities under the environment of care management plans.*

Intent of EC.2.1
Personnel can describe or demonstrate
a. safety risks in the environment of care;
b. reporting procedures for incidents involving property, damage, occupational illness, and patient, personnel, or visitor injury;
c. actions to eliminate, minimize, or report safety risks;
d. facilitywide fire-response needs;
e. area-specific needs and fire evacuation routes;
f. their specific roles and responsibilities when at a fire's point of origin;
g. their specific roles and responsibilities when away from a fire's point of origin;
h. use and functioning of fire alarm systems;
i. their specific roles and responsibilities in preparing for building evacuation;
j. location and proper use of equipment for evacuating or transporting patients to refuge areas;
k. building compartmentalization procedures for containing smoke and fire.

Leaders can describe their role in developing safety policies and procedures and provide examples of safety management program goals and performance improvement standards.

    Personnel in security-sensitive areas of the environment of care can describe or demonstrate
l. processes for minimizing security risks;
m. emergency procedures for security incidents; and
n. reporting procedures for security incidents involving patients, visitors, personnel, and property.

Personnel who manage or have contact with hazardous materials and waste can describe or demonstrate
o. procedures and precautions for selecting, handling, storing, using, and disposing of hazardous materials and waste;
p. emergency procedures for handling hazardous material and waste spills or exposures;
q. health hazards of mishandling hazardous materials and waste; and
r. reporting procedures for hazardous materials and waste spills or exposures.

Personnel who implement the emergency preparedness plan can describe or demonstrate
s. their roles and responsibilities during emergencies;
t. their roles and past participation in organizationwide drills;
u. the backup communication system used during disasters and emergencies; and
v. how to obtain supplies and equipment during disasters or emergencies.

Medical equipment users can describe or demonstrate
w. capabilities, limitations, and special applications of equipment;
x. operating and safety procedures for equipment use;
y. emergency procedures in the event of equipment failure; and
z. processes for reporting equipment management problems, failures, and user errors.

---

* As described in EC.1.3 through EC.1.9, the organization has management plans for the following factors in the environment of care: safety, security, hazardous materials and waste, emergency preparedness, life safety, medical equipment, and utility systems.

Management of the Environment of Care

Medical equipment maintainers can demonstrate or describe
aa. knowledge and skills necessary to perform maintenance responsibilities; and
bb. processes for reporting equipment management problems, failures, and user errors.

Utility system users can describe or demonstrate
cc. utility system capabilities, limitations, and special applications;
dd. emergency procedures in the event of a system failure;
ee. processes for reporting utility system management problems, failures, and user errors;
ff. location and use of emergency shutoff controls; and
gg. whom to contact in emergencies.

Utility system maintainers can describe or demonstrate
hh. the knowledge and skills necessary to perform maintenance responsibilities;
ii. processes for reporting utility system management problems, failures, and user errors;
jj. location and use of emergency shutoff controls; and
kk. whom to contact in the event of an emergency.

Implementing Management Plans

Standard

EC.2.2 The safety management plan is implemented.

Intent of EC.2.2

The organization implements the safety management plan and performance improvement standards, including all features described in EC.1.3.

Standard

EC.2.3 The security management plan is implemented.

Intent of EC.2.3

The organization implements the security management plan and performance improvement standards, including all features described in EC.1.4.

Standard

EC.2.4 The hazardous materials and waste management plan is implemented.

Intent of EC.2.4

The organization implements the hazardous materials and waste management plan and performance improvement standards, including all features described in EC.1.5.

The organization also
a. maintains documentation, including required permits, licenses, and adherence to other regulations;
b. maintains manifests for handling of hazardous materials and waste;
c. properly labels hazardous materials and waste;
d. provides adequate, appropriate space and equipment for managing hazardous materials and waste; and
e. effectively separates hazardous materials and waste storage and processing areas from other areas of the facility.

Standard

EC.2.5 The emergency preparedness management plan is implemented.

Intent of EC.2.5

The organization implements the emergency preparedness management plan and performance improvement standards, including all features described in EC.1.6.

Standard

EC.2.6 The life safety management plan is implemented.

Intent of EC.2.6

The organization implements the life safety management plan and performance improvement standards, including all features described in EC.1.7.

The organization also
a. maintains current record drawings (or documents) addressing all structural features of fire protection;
b. develops a policy for use of interim life safety measures (ILSM*) that include written criteria to evaluate various $LSC^®$ deficiencies and construction hazards for determining when and to what extent one or more of the following are applicable;

The ILSM consist of the following actions:
1. Ensuring free and unobstructed exits. Personnel receive additional training when alternative exits are designated. Buildings or areas under construction must maintain escape routes for construction workers at all times. Means of exiting construction areas are inspected daily.
2. Ensuring free and unobstructed access to emergency services and for fire, police, and other emergency forces.
3. Ensuring fire alarm, detection, and suppression systems are in good working order. A temporary but equivalent system shall be provided when any fire system is impaired. Temporary systems must be inspected and tested monthly.

Note: *The* Life Safety Code, *NFPA 101, 1997 edition, requires that the municipal fire department (or applicable emergency forces group) is notified and a fire watch is provided whenever an approved fire alarm or automatic sprinkler system is out of service for more than four hours in a 24-hour period in an occupied building.*

4. Ensuring temporary construction partitions are smoke tight and built of noncombustible or limited combustible materials that will not contribute to the development or spread of fire.
5. Providing additional fire-fighting equipment and training personnel in its use.
6. Prohibiting smoking according to EC.5 throughout the organization's buildings, and in and adjacent to construction areas.
7. Developing and enforcing storage, housekeeping, and debris removal practices that reduce the building's flammable and combustible fire load to the lowest feasible level.

---

* **interim life safety measures (ILSM)** A series of 11 administrative actions required to temporarily compensate for the significant hazards posed by existing NFPA 101® 1997 *Life Safety Code®* ($LSC^®$)deficiencies or construction activities. ILSM apply to appropriate staff (including construction workers), must be implemented upon project development, and must be continuously enforced through project completion. Implementation of ILSM is required in or adjacent to all construction areas and throughout buildings with existing $LSC^®$ deficiencies. ILSM are intended to provide a level of life safety comparable to that described in Chapters 1–7, and the applicable occupancy chapters of the $LSC^®$. Each ILSM action must be documented through written policies and procedures. Frequencies for inspection, testing, training, and monitoring and evaluation must be established by the organization.

8. Conducting a minimum of two fire drills per shift per quarter.
9. Increasing hazard surveillance of buildings, grounds, and equipment, with special attention to excavations, construction areas, construction storage, and field offices.
10. Training personnel to compensate for impaired structural or compartmentalization features of fire safety.
11. Conducting organizationwide safety education programs to promote awareness of LSC® deficiencies, construction hazards, and ILSM.

c. implements, documents, and enforces appropriate interim life safety measures (ILSM) as determined by the organization.

Standard

EC.2.7 The medical equipment management plan is implemented.

Intent of EC.2.7

The organization implements the medical equipment management plan and performance improvement standards, including all features described in EC.1.8.

Standard

EC.2.8 The utility systems management plan is implemented.

Intent of EC.2.8

The organization implements the utility systems management plan and performance improvement standards, including all features described in EC.1.9.

 If applicable, the organization also

a. maintains a current, complete set of documents mapping the layout of each utility system and the location of controls for partial or complete shutdown;
b. properly installs an emergency power source that is adequately sized, designed, and fueled;
c. provides a reliable emergency power system, as required by occupancy classification, that supplies electricity to the following areas when normal electricity is interrupted:
   1. Alarm systems,
   2. Exit route illumination,
   3. Emergency communication systems, and
   4. Illumination of exit signs;
d. provides a reliable emergency power system, as required by the services provided, that supplies electricity to the following areas when normal electricity is interrupted:
   1. Blood, bone, and tissue storage units,
   2. Emergency/Urgent care areas,
   3. Elevators (at least one),
   4. Medical air compressors,
   5. Medical and surgical vacuum systems,
   6. Operating rooms,
   7. Postoperative recovery rooms,
   8. Special care units,
   9. Obstetrical delivery rooms; and
   10. Newborn nurseries.

Implementing Emergency Drills

Standard

EC.2.9 Drills are regularly conducted to test emergency preparedness.

Intent of EC.2.9

The emergency preparedness plan is executed twice a year, either in response to an emergency or in planned drills. Organizations that offer emergency services or are designated as disaster receiving stations perform at least one exercise yearly that includes an influx of volunteer or simulated patients. Exercises are conducted at least four months apart and no more than eight months apart.

Notes: 1. *Drills that involve packages of information that simulate patients, their family, and visitors are acceptable.*
2. *Tabletop exercises, though useful in planning or training, are **not** acceptable substitutes for a drill.*

Standard

EC.2.10 Fire drills are conducted regularly.

Intent of EC.2.10

Quarterly fire drills exercise all primary elements of the fire plan*† listed below. All personnel of all shifts in every building where patients are housed or treated participate in drills. Performance of all areas during fire drills is evaluated.

Note 1: *Staff in each free-standing building classified as a business occupancy, as defined by the Life Safety Code,® need only participate in one fire drill per shift annually. Staff in areas of the building that the organization occupies must participate in such drills.*

Note 2: *In lieu of observing all areas of the building for evaluation of staff performance, an organization may randomly observes different locations within the facility, provided the following are included:*
- *The smoke compartment from which the fire drill was initiated;*
- *Another smoke compartment on the same floor level and immediately adjacent to the fire drill location (if one exists);*
- *Another smoke compartment on a different floor level that is either immediately above or below the fire drill location (if one exists); and*
- *An additional number of smoke compartments, chosen randomly throughout the facility, that is equal to 20% of the total number of occupied smoke compartments in the building; or, when satisfactory fire drill experience and safety committee approval are evident, 10%, instead of 20%, of the total number of occupied smoke compartments in the building may be used.*

Fire drills test staff knowledge of
a. use and functioning of fire alarm systems (where such systems are available);
b. transmission of alarms (where such alarms are available);
c. containment of smoke and fire;
d. transfer to areas of refuge;
e. fire extinguishment;

---

* Effective January 1, 1999.

† Actual patient transfer or transport and building evacuation are not required. Properly documented actual or false alarms may be used for 50% of required drills for each shift, if all elements of the fire plan were implemented.

Management of the Environment of Care

f. specific fire-response duties; and
g. preparation for building evacuation.

Implementing Maintenance, Testing, and Inspection of the Operational Components of Plans

Standard

EC.2.11 Safety elements of the environment of care are maintained, tested, and inspected.

Intent of EC.2.11

Hazard surveillance surveys are performed in all patient care areas at least every six months and in non-patient care areas at least annually to identify environmental deficiencies, hazards, and unsafe practices.

Standard

EC.2.12 Life safety elements in the environment of care are maintained, tested, and inspected.

Intent of EC.2.12

The organization demonstrates and documents that fire alarm and detection equipment is tested as follows:*

a. Initiating devices
   1. all supervisory signal devices (except valve tamper switches) are tested at least quarterly,
   2. all valve tamper switches and water flow devices are tested at least semiannually, and
   3. all duct detectors, electromechanical releasing devices, heat detectors, manual fire alarm boxes, smoke detectors are tested at least annually;
b. Occupant Alarm Notification devices including all audible devices, speakers, and visible devices are tested at least annually; and
c. Off-premises Emergency Forces Notification transmission equipment is tested at least quarterly.
   The organization demonstrates and documents that automatic extinguishing equipment is inspected and tested as follows:
d. Water based automatic fire extinguishing systems†
   1. all fire pumps are tested at least weekly under no flow condition,
   2. all fire pumps are tested at least annually under flow,
   3. all water storage tank high and low water level alarms are tested at least semiannually,
   4. all water storage tank low water temperature alarms (during cold weather only) are tested at least monthly,
   5. main drain tests are conducted at least annually at all system risers, and
   6. all fire department connections are inspected quarterly.
e. Kitchen automatic fire extinguishing systems are inspected for proper operation at least semiannually (actual discharge of the fire extinguishing system is not required);
f. Carbon dioxide and other gaseous automatic fire extinguishing systems are tested for proper operation at least annually (actual discharge of the fire extinguishing system is not required);

---

* For additional guidance, see NFPA 72-1996 edition (Table 7-3.2).

† For additional guidance, see NFPA 25-1998 edition.

The organization demonstrates and documents that all portable fire extinguishers and standpipe systems are inspected, tested, and maintained as follows:

g. All portable fire extinguishers are*
   1. clearly identified,
   2. inspected at least monthly, and
   3. maintained at least annually;
h. All standpipe
   1. occupant hoses are hydrostatically tested five years after installation and at least every three years thereafter,[†] and
   2. systems receive water flow tests at least every five years;[‡]

The organization demonstrates and documents that building fire protection equipment is maintained as follows:

i. All fire and smoke dampers are operated (with fusible links removed where applicable) to verify they fully close at least every four years;[§]
j. All automatic smoke detection shutdown devices for air handling equipment are tested at least annually;[**] and
k. All horizontal and vertical sliding and rolling fire doors are tested for proper operation and full closure at least annually.[††]

Standard

EC.2.13 Medical equipment is maintained, tested, and inspected.

Intent of EC.2.13

The organization maintains documentation of

a. a current, accurate, and separate inventory of all equipment in the medical equipment management program, regardless of ownership;
b. performance and safety testing of all equipment in the management program prior to initial use and at least annually thereafter;
   Note: *An equipment time frame longer than 12 months may be justified based on previous experience and safety committee approval. The specification of an annual testing interval is not intended to be a single standard of testing needs. It is expected that organizations will apply professional judgment in establishing intervals so that risks and hazards are adequately managed.*
c. preventive maintenance and inspection of medical equipment according to a schedule based on current organizational experience and ongoing monitoring and evaluation;
d. annual chemical testing and monthly biological testing of water used in chronic renal dialysis; and
e. performance testing of all sterilizers used.

---

* For additional guidance, see NFPA 10-1994 edition (sections 1-6, 4-3, and 4-4).

[†] For additional guidance, see NFPA 1962-1993 edition (section 2-3).

[‡] For additional guidance, see NFPA 25-1998 edition.

[§] For additional guidance, see NFPA 90A-1996 edition (section 3-4.7).

[**] For additional guidance, see NFPA 90A-1996 edition (section 4-4.1).

[††] For additional guidance, see NFPA 80-1995 edition (section 15-2.4).

Management of the Environment of Care

Standard

EC.2.14 Utility systems are maintained, tested, and inspected.

Intent of EC.2.14

The organization maintains, tests, and inspects critical operating components of utility systems and maintains documentation of

a. a current, accurate, and separate inventory of all utility components in the utility management program;
b. performance and safety testing of each critical component in the program prior to initial use and at least annually thereafter;

   Note: *An equipment time frame longer than 12 months may be justified based on previous experience and safety committee approval. The specification of an annual testing interval is not intended to be a single standard of testing needs. It is expected that organizations will apply professional judgment in establishing intervals so that risks and hazards are adequately managed.*
c. preventive maintenance and inspection of utility systems according to a schedule based on current organizational experience and ongoing monitoring and evaluation; and
d. demonstration of the emergency power system's reliability by conducting
   1. monthly testing of each generator for at least 30 minutes under a dynamic load that is equal to or greater than the higher of the following load values:
      - 30% of the nameplate rating of the generator, after applying any applicable rating factors for site conditions or
      - 50% of either the calculated or greatest known load on the Emergency Power Supply System (EPSS); and

   Note: *Organizations may choose to test to less than 30% of the emergency generator's nameplate or 50% of the total emergency power supply system (EPSS) load. However, these organizations shall (in addition to performing a monthly test for 30 minutes under operating temperature) revise their existing documented management plan to conform to current NFPA 99® and NFPA 110® testing and maintenance activities. These activities shall include inspection procedures for assessing the evidence of wet stacking.**

   If diesel-powered generators show evidence of wet stacking, as determined from these inspection procedures, a resistive load bank or additional load test shall be conducted within twelve months (or more frequently if recommended by the generator's manufacturer). The following are the requirements for this test:
      - Duration—until the exhaust is clear of black smoke, but not less than 2 hours, and
      - Load—greater than or equal to 80% of nameplate.
   2. monthly testing of all automatic transfer switches.

---

* As per NFPA 110®, section 6–4.2 (1996 edition), wet stacking is a field term indicating the presence of unburned fuel or carbon in the exhaust system. Its presence is readily indicated by the presence of black smoke during engine-run operation.

Standards and Intent Statements for Measuring Outcomes of Implementation

Standard

EC.3 An organizationwide Information Collection and Evaluation System (ICES) is developed and used to evaluate and improve conditions in the environment of care.

Intent of EC.3

The ICES aggregates information from all major components of the environment of care. Data are collected about all management programs described in EC.1.3 through EC.1.9.

Standard

EC.3.1 The organization appoints an individual to direct an ongoing, organizationwide process to collect information about deficiencies and opportunities for improvement in environment of care management programs.

Intent of EC.3.1

The individual appointed to direct the safety program, sometimes referred to as a safety officer or director,
a. directs ongoing, organizationwide collection of information about deficiencies and opportunities for improvement in the environment of care;
b. reviews summaries of deficiencies, problems, failures, and user errors related to managing
 1. safety;
 2. security;
 3. hazardous materials and waste;
 4. emergency preparedness;
 5. life safety;
 6. medical equipment; and
 7. utility systems;
c. draws on other sources of information, such as published hazard or recall reports;
d. reports on findings, recommendations, actions taken, and results of measurement;
e. regularly participates in hazard surveillance and incident reporting; and
f. participates in the development of safety policies and procedures.

This individual reports on findings, recommendations, actions taken, and results of measurement.

Notes: 1. Patient incidents may be reported to staff in quality assessment, improvement, or other functions. However, at least a summary of incidents is shared with the safety officer.
2. The review of incident reports often requires that various legal processes be followed to preserve the confidentiality of information documented in the reports. Opportunities to improve care or to prevent future similar incidents are not lost as a result of the legal process followed.

Standard

EC.3.2 The organization analyzes identified environment of care management issues and develops or approves recommendations for resolving them.

Intent of EC.3.2

The organization has a multidisciplinary group (often known as the safety committee) composed of representation from administration, clinical services, and support services to carry out analysis of and seek resolution of safety management issues. Clinical service representatives may include physicians, nurses, pharmacists, laboratorians, or others appropriate to the hospital's mix of patient care providers. The committee meets at regular intervals to address issues related to managing the environment of care.

Safety issues are analyzed in a timely manner. Recommendations are developed and approved. Safety issues are communicated to the governing body, chief executive officer, directors of services, and individuals responsible for performance-improvement activities. Based on the ongoing monitoring of performance in each of the seven management areas, recommendations for one or more performance improvement activities are communicated at least annually to the organization's leaders.

An organization applies reasonable and prudent professional judgment when establishing meeting frequency so that risks, hazards, problems, failures, accidents, and incidents are minimized and resolved in a timely manner. (Meetings held more or less frequently than bimonthly are acceptable when supported by current organization experience and safety committee approval. Ongoing justification of meeting frequency is dependent on a satisfactory annual evaluation of performance as required by EC.1.3.)

Notes: 1. *The organization may communicate through a single source all safety related reports to the persons and organization components listed above. When indicated, specific information regarding improvement activities may be distributed to the department involved in addressing the identified issues.*
2. *Governing body issues may be communicated through a governing body liaison.*

Standard

EC.3.3 The individual directing the safety program works with appropriate staff to implement recommendations and monitor their effectiveness.

Intent of EC.3.3

Staff members with relevant expertise and job responsibilities implement and monitor safety improvements in the environment of care. The safety committee, department leader, or the safety officer establishes measurement guidelines. Measurement results are reported to the safety committee. The safety committee routes their actions and recommendations to applicable departments. Department leaders are aware of relevant safety committee action items.

Standards and Intent Statements for Other Environmental Considerations*

Standard

EC.4 *The hospital provides a care environment that supports its mission and services.*

Intent of EC.4

The care environment supports the care process and the needs of the population served.

---

* Formerly Social Environment.

Standard

EC.4.1 Appropriate space to support patient services is provided.

Intent of EC.4.1

a. The hospital provides appropriate interior space. The space is designed, equipped, and maintained to be comfortable, safe, clean, and attractive.
b. The hospital provides appropriate exterior space when required by the services provided. For example, when certain patient groups (such as pediatric, long-term care) experience long lengths of stay (for example, 30 days or more), the hospital provides access to the outdoors through appropriate use of hospital grounds, nearby parks and playgrounds, and adjacent countryside.
c. Lighting is suitable for the health care and patient specific activities being conducted.
d. Ventilation allows for acceptable levels of temperature, humidity, and elimination of odors. Ventilation is sufficient to remove odors and provide fresh air to each patient's room.
e. Closet and drawer space are provided for storing personal property and other items provided for use by patients. Lockers, drawers, or closet space is provided for patients who are in charge of their own personal grooming and wear street clothes (such as psychiatric patients who wear street clothes and are expected to meet their personal grooming needs).

Standard

EC.4.2 An environment that fosters a positive self-image for the patient and preserves his or her human dignity is provided.

Intent of EC.4.2

a. The environment of care enhances the positive self-image of patients and preserves their human dignity. Because a hospital program or unit at times becomes the patient's "home," the hospital provides an atmosphere that supports the patient's dignity. For example, in a long term care unit, a patient has space to display greeting cards, calendars, and other personal items important to his or her orientation and well being.
b. Door locks and other structural restraints used are consistent with the individual patient's needs, program policy, law, and regulation. All locking devices used are consistent with the requirements of the *Life Safety Code*® (*LSC*®), NFPA 101, 1997 edition. Emergency access provision is provided to all locked occupied spaces. Based on the patient population served, locking may include an entire patient unit or an individual bedroom or bathroom. For example,
   - locking a forensic patient sleeping room for security purposes;
   - locking a psychiatric seclusion room for patient observation purposes;
   - locking a psychiatric unit to limit patient egress;
   - locking a nursery and pediatric units to limit access;
   - locking a dementia unit to prevent resident elopement; or
   - providing locking devices for privacy needs during bathing and changing of clothes.
c. The hospital provides adequate storage space for permitting patients to wear their own clothing when appropriate. Hospitalized patients wear clothing suitable to their clinical condition. For example, hospital gowns provide easy emergency access to the anatomy of a patient in the ICU, whereas street clothes assist in the rehabilitation process of a patient in a substance use program.
d. The hospital provides adequate space for storing and makes available articles for grooming and personal hygiene appropriate to the patient's clinical status, developmental level, and age. Patients' feelings about themselves are influenced by how they are groomed. For example, when staff are

teaching activities of daily living skills to residents in a long term care unit, articles for grooming are important in redeveloping independent living skills. Access to items that may pose a danger, such as razor blades, may be restricted.

Standard

EC.4.3 The built environment provides appropriate privacy to patients.

Intent of EC.4.3

a. Where appropriate, space or equipment are arranged to ensure auditory and visual privacy. In rooms containing more than one patient, privacy may be provided by curtains, partitioning, or furniture placement.
b. Patients who desire private telephone conversations have access to space and phones appropriate to their clinical condition. Physically challenged individuals have similar access.
c. Each patient has a right to privacy in his or her sleeping room unless clinically contraindicated. For example, privacy may not be appropriate for some patients undergoing visual monitoring (such as for fall prevention).
d. The number of patients in a room is appropriate to the hospital's goals and the patients' ages, development levels, clinical conditions or diagnosis needs. Except when clinically justified in writing based on the program requirements, no more than eight patients sleep in a room. Sleeping rooms are assigned based on the patients' need for privacy, group support, independence, or safety. Private sleeping rooms are assigned to patients presenting a risk of predatory or violent behavior to other patients.

Standard

EC.4.4 The built environment supports the development and maintenance of the patient's interests, skills, and opportunities for personal growth when required.

Intent of EC.4.4

a. When appropriate, the environment of care allows for social interaction among patients through recreational interchange. The hospital makes adequate arrangements for patients' leisure-time activities which consider and respond to their needs. For example, depending upon an individual unit's or program's goals, facilities are available for providing patient snacks and for preparing meals. Thus, in a pediatric or adolescent service, recreational activities may include providing snacks and permitting patient participation in the selection of snacks.
b. Furnishings and equipment reflect patient characteristics related to age, level of disability, and therapeutic needs. For example, the environment accommodates equipment, such as wheelchairs, that are necessary for activities of daily living. The furniture and equipment chosen help to normalize the patient's living environment. Furnishings and equipment are suitable to the patients' ages (for example, pediatric, geriatric), maintained to be safe, and are in good repair.

Standards

EC.5 A nonsmoking policy is communicated and enforced throughout all buildings.

EC.5.1 Any exceptions to the prohibition are authorized for a patient by a licensed independent practitioner's written authorization, based on criteria that are defined by the medical staff.

Intent of EC.5 and EC.5.1

Patients, visitors, and staff are prohibited from smoking in any of the organization's buildings. These standards are intended to restrict smoking to a minimum and
- reduce risks to patients who smoke, including possible adverse effects on treatment;
- reduce risks of passive smoking for others; and
- reduce the risk of fire.

However, there may be medical reasons to permit some patients to smoke while in the hospital (for example, if sudden withdrawal may interfere with the patient's treatment). The smoking policy provides for such exceptions when authorized by a licensed independent practitioner.

Also, settings that provide longer-term care may have a policy that allows patients to smoke without a licensed independent practitioner's written authorization. In these instances, smoking occurs in designated locations that are environmentally separate from all patient care areas. Settings that provide longer-term care (that is, more than 30 days) for the following patient populations are included under this provision:
- Chronically mentally ill patients;
- Long-term or intermediate care and skilled nursing patients;
- Forensic psychiatry patients; and
- Postacute head trauma (social rehabilitation) patients.

When the hospital allows certain patients to smoke by either LIP order or long-term care exception,
- smoking may occur within the organization's building(s);
- the hospital acts to minimize the smoke to the greatest extent possible;
- the hospital discourages all such smoking; and
- the hospital provides education and options for smoking cessation activities.

These standards do not require that a designated smoking area for these patient population exceptions be a specific distance from patient care areas. A separate, well-ventilated room (such as a designated smoking lounge for authorized patient smoking) is an acceptable smoking area.

The hospital prohibits smoking (no medical exceptions allowed) for all hospital-based ambulatory care patients and for all child or adolescent patients. Visitors and staff within the hospital's building(s) may not smoke.

Management of Human Resources

Overview

The **goal** of the management of human resources function* is to identify and provide the right number of competent staff to meet the needs of patients served by the hospital.

A hospital needs an appropriate number of qualified people to fulfill its mission and meet the needs of the patients it serves.

The hospital's leaders† carry out the following processes and their related activities:

- *Planning*
  The leaders' planning process defines the qualifications, competencies, and staffing necessary to fulfill the hospital's mission.
- *Providing competent staff*
  The leaders provide for competent staff either through traditional employer-employee arrangements or contractual arrangements with other entities. An initial assessment reviews applicants' credentials and qualifications. Experience, education, and abilities are confirmed during orientation.
- *Assessing, maintaining, and improving staff competence*
  Ongoing, periodic competence assessment evaluates staff members' continuing abilities to perform throughout their association with the hospital.
- *Promoting self-development and learning*
  The leaders create a culture that fosters staff self-development and continued learning. Staff members in a hospital are encouraged to provide feedback about the work environment to leaders.

Note: *The standards in this chapter address these processes and their related activities, but do not apply solely to a human resources department. All hospital leaders perform the processes and activities in the Management of Human Resources function.*

---

* **function** A goal-directed, interrelated series of processes, such as continuum of care or management information.

† **leaders** The leaders described in the leadership function include at least the leaders of the governing body; the chief executive officer and other senior managers; department leaders; the elected and the appointed leaders of the medical staff and the clinical departments and other medical staff members in organizational administrative positions; and the nurse executive and other senior nursing leaders.

Standards

The following is a list of all standards for this function. If you have a questions about a term used here, please check the Glossary, pages 281 through 307. Terms that are critical to the understanding of the standard are defined in the footnotes of the next section of this chapter.

HR.1 The hospital's leaders define the qualifications and performance expectations for all staff positions.

HR.2 The hospital provides an adequate number of staff members whose qualifications are consistent with job responsibilities.

HR.3 *The leaders ensure that the competence of all staff members is assessed, maintained, demonstrated, and improved continually.*

HR.3.1 The hospital encourages and supports self-development and learning for all staff.

HR.4 An orientation process provides initial job training and information and assesses the staff's ability to fulfill specified responsibilities.

HR.4.1 The hospital orients and educates forensic staff about their responsibilities related to patient care.

HR.4.2 Ongoing in-service and other education and training maintain and improve staff competence.

HR.4.3 The hospital regularly collects aggregate data on competence patterns and trends to identify and respond to the staff's learning needs.

HR.5 The hospital assesses each staff member's ability to meet the performance expectations stated in his or her job description.

HR.6 The hospital addresses a staff member's request not to participate in any aspect of patient care.

HR.6.1 The hospital ensures that a patient's care will not be negatively affected if the hospital grants a staff member's request not to participate in an aspect of patient care.

HR.6.2 Policies and procedures specify those aspects of patient care that might conflict with staff members' cultural values or religious beliefs.

Standards and Intent Statements for Human Resources Planning

Standard

HR.1 The hospital's leaders define the qualifications and performance expectations for all staff positions.

Intent of HR.1

A hospital's ability to fulfill its mission and provide for its patients' needs is directly related to its ability to provide qualified, competent staff. The leaders track projected staffing needs against qualifications and competencies of current staff to identify any deficiencies to improve staffing levels. Leaders consider the following factors to project staffing needs:
- The hospital's mission;
- The case mix of patients served by the hospital or department, and the degree and complexity of care required by patients and their significant others;
- The care provided by the hospital, including treatment;
- The technology used in patient care; and
- The expectations of the hospital, its patients, and other customers.

The leaders provide a job description for each position that defines the qualifications and performance expectations in measurable terms.

Standard

HR.2 The hospital provides an adequate number of staff members whose qualifications are consistent with job responsibilities.

Intent of HR.2

Departments provide an adequate number of staff members with the experience and training needed to serve and fulfill the department's part of the hospital's mission. Department leaders compare projected needs to data and information on current staff numbers and qualifications. This analysis can support, if necessary, proposed modifications to each department's staff allocation. For each employee or contracted personnel, the department verifies the following elements, a through c, where relevant:
a. Education and training are consistent with applicable legal and regulatory requirements and hospital policy;
b. The individual is licensed, certified, or registered;
c. The individual's knowledge and experience are appropriate for his or her assigned responsibilities.
Evidence of these elements is present for each employee or contracted personnel.

Standard

HR.3 *The leaders ensure that the competence of all staff members is assessed, maintained, demonstrated, and improved continually.*

Intent of HR.3

The hospital assesses staff development needs on a hospitalwide, departmental, and individual level, and uses these assessments to plan continuing staff education. For example, when the hospital adopts new criteria for identifying possible victims of abuse, it educates emergency and other relevant staff members accordingly. Policies and procedures (and sometimes job descriptions) define performance expectations for each position in objective, measurable terms. The hospital measures performance regularly and expects each employee to perform competently.

Department leaders instill in staff a sense of ownership of their work processes—that is, they encourage staff members to act with appropriate authority and to take responsibility for their work. In addition, department leaders encourage staff to improve their performance continually, thereby improving the hospital's overall performance.

Supervisors contribute to a culture that values employees' human needs for self-respect and growth. Whenever feasible or possible, supervisors provide the staff with the support and encouragement needed to participate in professional associations and continuing education activities within or outside the hospital. Through formal and informal interaction with peers and colleagues from other hospitals and settings, staff competence improves.

A hospital can assess competence objectively in many ways. The hospital decides how to structure its assessment, evaluation, or appraisal process. If the hospital constructs its own competence-assessment process, it meets the following criteria:

- The hospital uses a combination of ongoing competence assessment and educational activities to maintain staff competence and
- An objective, measurable system is used periodically to evaluate job performance, current competencies, and skills.

For personnel provided through contractual arrangements, the hospital maintains a written job description and a completed competence assessment, evaluation, or appraisal tool for each individual.

Standard

HR.3.1 The hospital encourages and supports self-development and learning for all staff.

Intent of HR.3.1

Job performance is the result of both individual competence and the work environment. Besides assessing staff competence, the leaders create a work environment that helps staff members discover what they need to learn and acquire new knowledge and skills. Regular feedback from the staff helps the leaders create this kind of work environment.

Standards and Intent Statements for Orienting, Training, and Educating Staff

Standard

HR.4 An orientation process provides initial job training and information and assesses the staff's ability to fulfill specified responsibilities.

Intent of HR.4

The orientation process assesses each staff member's ability to fulfill specific responsibilities. The process familiarizes staff members with their jobs and with the work environment before the staff

Management of Human Resources

begins patient care or other activities. In this way, the process promotes safe and effective job performance. When the hospital uses volunteer services, volunteers are oriented to patient care, safety, infection control, and any other activities they are expected to perform competently.

Standard

HR.4.1 The hospital orients and educates forensic staff about their responsibilities related to patient care.

Intent of HR.4.1

In forensic services, staff members with no clinical training or experience (for example, correctional officers or guards) may become involved in activities that could support or hinder therapeutic goals for patients. The hospital trains these staff members in the following areas:
- How to interact with patients;
- Procedures for responding to unusual clinical events and incidents;
- The hospital's channels of clinical, security, and administrative communication; and
- The distinctions between administrative and clinical seclusion and restraint.

Standard

HR.4.2 Ongoing in-service and other education and training maintain and improve staff competence.

Intent of HR.4.2

The hospital ensures that each staff member participates in ongoing in-service education and other training to increase his or her knowledge of work-related issues. The hospital periodically reviews the staff's abilities to carry out job responsibilities, especially when introducing new procedures, techniques, technology, and equipment. Ongoing in-service and other education and training programs are appropriate to patient age groups served by the hospital.

Standard

HR.4.3 The hospital regularly collects aggregate data on competence patterns and trends to identify and respond to the staff's learning needs.

Intent of HR.4.3

The hospital regularly collects and analyzes aggregate data from a variety of sources to assess staff competence and pinpoint training needs. The hospital may extract data from performance evaluations and performance-improvement reports, it may survey the staff, or may conduct other needs assessment. The hospital analyzes patterns and trends, then responds by offering ongoing in-service education, training, and other teaching to meet identified needs. The hospital reports at least annually to the governing body on levels of competence, patterns and trends, and competence maintenance activities.

Standard and Intent Statement for Assessing Competence

Standard
HR.5 The hospital assesses each staff member's ability to meet the performance expectations stated in his or her job description.

Intent of HR.5
The hospital has a system to conduct periodic competence assessment and document findings for each staff member. When appropriate, the hospital considers special needs and behaviors of specific patient age groups in defining the qualifications, duties, and responsibilities of staff who do not have clinical privileges but who have regular clinical contact with patients (for example, radiology technologists and mental health technicians). Competency assessments of such individuals clearly address the ages of the patients they serve and the success with which employees produce the results expected from clinical interventions.

Standards and Intent Statements for Managing Staff Requests

Standards
HR.6 The hospital addresses a staff member's request not to participate in any aspect of patient care.

HR.6.1 The hospital ensures that a patient's care will not be negatively affected if the hospital grants a staff member's request not to participate in an aspect of patient care.

HR.6.2 Policies and procedures specify those aspects of patient care that might conflict with staff members' cultural values or religious beliefs.

Intent of HR.6 Through HR.6.2
The hospital respects its staff members' cultural values, ethics, and religious beliefs and the impact these may have on patient care. The hospital's process considers whether conflicting cultural values, ethics, or religious beliefs are sufficient grounds for granting requests not to participate in care. The hospital provides in writing the way such requests are managed, which is available for review by all staff members. To ensure that patient care and treatment will not suffer if the hospital excuses staff members from participating in an aspect of care, the hospital establishes alternative methods of care delivery for these situations.

Policy and procedures governing requests not to participate in an aspect of care, including treatment, address at least the following:
- How staff may request to be excused from participating in an aspect of patient care on grounds of conflicting cultural values, ethics, or religious beliefs; and
- How the hospital ensures that granting such a request will not negatively affect a patient's care or treatment.

Management of Information

Overview

The **goal** of the information-management function* is to obtain, manage, and use information to improve patient outcomes and individual and hospital performance in patient care, governance, management, and support processes.

Delivering health care to patients is a complex endeavor that is highly dependent on information.† Hospitals rely on information about the science of care, individual patients, care provided, results of care, as well as its performance to provide, coordinate, and integrate services. Like human, material, and financial resources, information is a resource that must be managed effectively by the hospital's leaders.

To achieve this goal, the following processes are performed well:
- Identifying information needs;
- Designing the structure of the information-management system;
- Defining and capturing‡ data§ and information;
- Analyzing data and transforming** it into information;
- Transmitting†† and reporting data and information; and
- Integrating and using information.

This chapter focuses on the performance of these processes in managing
- patient-specific data and information;
- aggregate data and information;
- expert knowledge-based information‡‡; and
- comparative performance data and information.

The standards in this chapter focus on organizationwide information planning and management processes to meet the organization's internal and external information needs. They describe a vision for effectively and continuously improving information management in health care organizations. Achieving this vision involves
- ensuring timely and easy access to complete information throughout the hospital;
- improving data accuracy;

---

* **function** A goal-directed, interrelated series of processes, such continuum of care or management of information.

† **information** Interpreted set(s) of data that can assist in decision making.

‡ **data capture** The acquisition or recording of data and information.

§ **data** Uninterpreted material, facts, or clinical observations.

** **data transformation** The process of changing the form of data representation, for example, changing data into information using decision-analysis tools.

†† **data transmission** The sending of data or information from one location to another.

‡‡ **knowledge-based information** A collection of stored facts, models, and information found in the clinical, scientific, and management literature that can be used for designing and redesigning processes and for problem solving.

- balancing requirements of security* and ease of access;
- using aggregate† and comparative data to pursue opportunities for improvement;
- redesigning information-related processes to improve efficiency; and
- increasing collaboration and information sharing to enhance patient care.

While efficiency may be improved by computerization and other technologies, the principles of good information management apply to all methods, whether paper-based or electronic. These standards are designed to be equally compatible with noncomputerized systems and future technologies.

---

* **data security** The protection of data from intentional or unintentional destruction, modification, or disclosure.

† **aggregate** To combine standardized data and information.

Management of Information

Standards

The following is a list of all standards for this function. If you have a questions about a term used here, please check the Glossary, pages 281 through 307. Terms that are critical to the understanding of the standard are defined in the footnotes of the next section of this chapter.

IM.1 The hospital plans and designs information-management processes to meet internal and external information needs.

IM.1.1 Internal and external information-management processes are appropriate for the hospital's size and the complexity of its services.

IM.1.1.1 The hospital bases management, staffing, and material resource allocations for information management on the scope and complexity of services provided.

IM.1.1.2 Appropriate clinical and administrative staff participate in assessing the hospital's information needs, and in selecting, integrating, and using information-management technology.

IM.2 *Confidentiality, security, and integrity of data and information are maintained.*

IM.2.1 The hospital determines appropriate levels of security and confidentiality for data and information.

IM.2.2 Collection, storage, and retrieval systems are designed to allow timely and easy use of data and information without compromising its security and confidentiality.

IM.2.3 Records and information are protected against loss, destruction, tampering, and unauthorized access or use.

IM.3 *Uniform data definitions and data capture methods are used whenever possible.*

IM.3.1 Minimum data sets, data definitions, codes, classifications, and terminology are standardized whenever possible.

IM.3.2 The hospital collects data in a timely, economic, and efficient manner and with the degree of accuracy, completeness, and discrimination necessary for their intended use.

IM.3.2.1 Medical records are reviewed on an ongoing basis for completeness and timeliness of information, and action is taken to improve the quality and timeliness of documentation that impacts patient care.

IM.3.2.1.1 A representative sample of records is included in the review process.

IM.4 Decision makers and other appropriate staff members are educated and trained in the principles of information management.

IM.5 Transmission of data and information is timely and accurate.

IM.5.1 The format and methods for disseminating data and information are standardized, whenever possible.

IM.6 Adequate integration and interpretation capabilities are provided.

IM.6.1 The hospital determines how long medical record information is retained, based on law and regulation and the information use for patient care, legal, research, and educational purposes.

IM.7 *The hospital defines, captures, analyzes, transforms, transmits, and reports patient-specific data and information related to care processes and outcomes.*

IM.7.1 The hospital initiates and maintains a medical record for every individual assessed or treated.

IM.7.1.1 Only authorized individuals make entries in medical records.

IM.7.2 The medical record contains sufficient information to identify the patient, support the diagnosis, justify the treatment, document the course and results, and promote continuity of care among health care providers.

IM.7.3 *The medical record thoroughly documents operative or other procedures and the use of anesthesia.*

IM.7.3.1 A preoperative diagnosis is recorded before surgery by the licensed independent practitioner responsible for the patient.

IM.7.3.2 Operative reports dictated or written immediately after surgery record the name of the primary surgeon and assistants, findings, technical procedures used, specimens removed, and postoperative diagnosis.

IM.7.3.2.1 The completed operative report is authenticated by the surgeon and filed in the medical record as soon as possible after surgery.

IM.7.3.2.2 When the operative report is not placed in the medical record immediately after surgery, a progress note is entered immediately.

IM.7.3.3 Postoperative documentation records the patient's vital signs and level of consciousness; medications (including intravenous fluids), blood, and blood components; any unusual events or postoperative complications; and management of such events.

IM.7.3.4 *Postoperative documentation records the patient's discharge from the postanesthesia care area by the responsible licensed independent practitioner or according to discharge criteria.*

IM.7.3.4.1 Compliance with discharge criteria is fully documented in the patient's medical record.

Management of Information

IM.7.3.5 Postoperative documentation records the name of the licensed independent practitioner responsible for discharge.

IM.7.4 For patients receiving continuing ambulatory care services, the medical record contains a summary list of known significant diagnoses, conditions, procedures, drug allergies, and medications.

IM.7.4.1 The list is initiated for each patient by the third visit and maintained thereafter.

IM.7.5 When emergency, urgent, or immediate care is provided, the time and means of arrival are also documented in the medical record.

IM.7.5.1 The medical record notes when a patient receiving emergency, urgent, or immediate care left against medical advice.

IM.7.5.2 The medical record of a patient receiving emergency, urgent, or immediate care notes the conclusions at termination of treatment, including final disposition, condition at discharge, and instructions for follow-up care.

IM.7.5.3 When authorized by the patient or a legally authorized representative, a copy of the emergency services provided is available to the practitioner or medical organization providing follow-up care.

IM.7.6 Medical record data and information are managed in a timely manner.

IM.7.7 Verbal orders of authorized individuals are accepted and transcribed by qualified personnel who are identified by title or category in the medical staff rules and regulations.

IM.7.8 Every medical record entry is dated, its author identified, and, when necessary, authenticated.

IM.7.9 The hospital can quickly assemble and have access to all relevant information from components of a patient's record, when the patient is admitted or is seen for ambulatory or emergency care.

IM.8 The hospital collects and analyzes aggregate data to support patient care and operations.

IM.9 The hospital provides systems, resources, and services to meet its needs for knowledge-based information in patient care, education, research, and management.

IM.9.1 The hospital's knowledge-based information resources are available, authoritative, and up to date.

IM.9.2 The hospital's services, resources, and systems for knowledge-based information are based on a needs assessment.

IM.10 *Comparative performance data and information are defined, collected, analyzed, transmitted, reported, and used consistent with national and state guidelines for data set parity and connectivity.*

IM.10.1 The hospital uses external reference databases for comparative purposes.

IM.10.2 The hospital contributes to external reference databases when required by law or regulation or when appropriate to the hospital.

IM.10.3 The security and confidentiality of data and information are maintained when contributing to or using external databases.

Management of Information

Standards and Intent Statements for Information Management Planning

Standard

IM.1 The hospital plans and designs information-management processes to meet internal and external information needs.

Intent of IM.1

A comprehensive needs assessment considers the following questions, as appropriate:
- What is the hospital's type, structure, size, and complexity?
- What are the needs of information users, including governance, leaders, clinical staff, inpatients, outpatients, patients' families, payers, purchasers, regulatory bodies, and accrediting bodies?
- What data and information does the hospital need to support planning?
- What data and information are needed for research and education?
- What are the relevant national and state guidelines for data set parity* and data connectivity† in interfacing information systems?
- What are the hospital's internal and external transmission requirements?
- What are the hospital's reporting needs over time (longitudinal reporting)?
- What data and information are needed for continuous performance improvement?
- What data and information does the hospital need to compare current performance with past performance? For benchmarking? For comparison with practice guidelines or parameters?
- What technology is appropriate?
- What technology is affordable?
- What does the hospital need to support customer and supplier relationships?
- What data and information does the hospital need to enhance cost-effectiveness (for example, to analyze resource use by patients with particular problems)?
- What data and information are needed to enhance work flow?
- What are the hospital's information requirements to support clinical and administrative decision making?
- Is the hospital planning to expand or redesign any services, such as library services, medical records, and computer services?
- What long-range plans are likely to affect the hospital's information needs?
    The organization identifies its needs based on its
- mission;
- goals;
- services;
- personnel;
- mode(s) of service delivery (for example, hospital, home care facility, ambulatory);
- resources; and
- access to affordable technology.

---

* **data parity** The degree to which data are equivalent.

† **data connectivity** The ability to link data from different sources or systems.

Standards

IM.1.1 Internal and external information-management processes are appropriate for the hospital's size and the complexity of its services.

IM.1.1.1 The hospital bases management, staffing, and material resource allocations for information management on the scope and complexity of services provided.

IM.1.1.2 Appropriate clinical and administrative staff participate in assessing the hospital's information needs, and in selecting, integrating, and using information-management technology.

Intent of IM.1.1 Through IM.1.1.2

Hospitals vary in size, complexity, governance, structure, decision-making processes, and resources. Information-management systems and processes vary accordingly. The hospital bases its information-management processes on a thorough analysis of internal and external information needs. The analysis considers what data and information are needed within and among departments, the medical staff, the administration, and the governing body, as well as information needed to support relationships with outside services, companies, and agencies. Leaders seek input from staff in a variety of areas and services. Appropriate individuals ensure that required data and information are provided efficiently for patient care, research, education, and management at every level.

Standards

IM.2 Confidentiality,* security, and integrity† of data and information are maintained.

IM.2.1 The hospital determines appropriate levels of security and confidentiality for data and information.

IM.2.2 Collection, storage, and retrieval systems are designed to allow timely and easy use of data and information without compromising its security and confidentiality.

IM.2.3 Records and information are protected against loss, destruction, tampering, and unauthorized access or use.

Intent of IM.2 Through IM.2.3

The hospital maintains the security and confidentiality of data and information, and is especially careful about preserving the confidentiality of sensitive data and information. The balance between data sharing and data confidentiality is addressed. The hospital determines the level of security and confidentiality maintained for different categories of information. Access to each category of information is based on need and defined by job title and function. An effective process defines
a. who has access to information;
b. the information to which an individual has access;
c. the user's obligation to keep information confidential;
d. when release of health information or removal of the medical record is permitted;

---

* **confidentiality** Restriction of access to data and information to individuals who have need, a reason, and permission for such access.

† **data integrity** The accuracy, consistency, and completeness of data.

e. how information is protected against unauthorized intrusion, corruption, or damage; and
f. the process followed when confidentiality and security are violated.

Hospital policy establishes that medical records may be removed from the hospital's jurisdiction and safekeeping only under a court order, subpoena, or statute.

The hospital addresses items a through f whenever it implements any new data and information collection, storage, and retrieval system(s).

Standards

IM.3 *Uniform data definitions* and data capture methods are used whenever possible.*

IM.3.1 Minimum data sets,[†] data definitions, codes, classifications, and terminology are standardized whenever possible.

IM.3.2 The hospital collects data in a timely, economic, and efficient manner and with the degree of accuracy, completeness, and discrimination necessary for their intended use.

Intent of IM.3 Through IM.3.2

Standardizing terminology, definitions, vocabulary, and nomenclature facilitates comparison of data and information within and among organizations. Abbreviations and symbols are also standardized. Uniformly applied and accepted definitions, codes, classifications, and terminology support data aggregation and analysis and provide criteria for decision analysis. Quality control systems are used to monitor data content and collection activities, and to ensure timely and economical data collection. Standardization is consistent with recognized state and federal standards. The hospital minimizes bias[‡] in the data and regularly assesses the data's reliability,[§] validity,** and accuracy.[††]

Standards

IM.3.2.1 Medical records are reviewed on an ongoing basis for completeness and timeliness of information, and action is taken to improve the quality and timeliness of documentation that impacts patient care.

IM.3.2.1.1 A representative sample of records is included in the review process.

Intent of IM.3.2.1 Through IM.3.2.1.1

The review of medical records addresses the presence, timeliness, legibility, and authentication of the following data and information, as appropriate to the organization's needs:

---

* **data definition** The identification of the data to be used in analysis.

[†] **minimum data set** An agreed-on and accepted set of terms and definitions constituting a core of data; a collection of related data items.

[‡] **bias** An influence on results that causes them to routinely depart from the true value.

[§] **data reliability** The stability, repeatability, or precision of the data.

** **data validity** Verification of correctness; reflects the true situation.

[††] **data accuracy** The extent to which data are free of errors.

- Identification data;
- Medical history, including the chief complaint; details of the present illness; relevant past, social, and family histories (appropriate to the patient's age); and an inventory by body system;
- A summary of the patient's psychosocial needs, as appropriate to the patient's age;
- A report of relevant physical examinations;
- A statement on the conclusions or impressions drawn from the admission history and physical examination;
- A statement on the course of action planned for the patient for this episode of care and of its periodic review, as appropriate;
- Diagnostic and therapeutic orders;
- Evidence of appropriate informed consent;
- Clinical observations, including the results of therapy;
- Progress notes made by the medical staff and other authorized staff;
- Consultation reports;
- Reports of operative and other invasive procedures, tests, and their results;
- Reports of any diagnostic and therapeutic procedures, such as pathology and clinical laboratory examinations and radiology and nuclear medicine examinations or treatment;
- Records of donation and receipt of transplants or implants;
- Final diagnosis(es);
- Conclusions at termination of hospitalization;
- Clinical resumés and discharge summaries;
- Discharge instructions to the patient or family; and
- When performed, results of autopsy.

    Medical record review is based on a representative sample (a sample representing the practitioners providing care and of the care provided). The review process is conducted by the medical staff, nursing, and other relevent clinical professionals. The focus of the review is on information available at the point of care.

    It is expected that findings from the medical record review, as well as medical record completion statistics, will be available for at least quarterly review and are evident in the reports of this review function (for example, medical record committee minutes or medical executive committee minutes).

Standard

IM.4 Decision makers and other appropriate staff members are educated and trained in the principles of information management.

Intent of IM.4

Individuals in the organization who generate, collect, analyze, and use data and information are educated and trained to effectively participate in managing information. This education and training enable these individuals to

- understand security and confidentiality of data and information;
- use measurement instruments, statistical tools, and data analysis methods for transforming data into relevant information;
- collect unbiased data, gathered with a control for confounding or corrected on the basis of acceptable methodologies;
- assist in interpreting data;
- use data and information to help in decision making;
- educate and support the participation of patients and family in care processes; and

- use indicators to assess and improve systems and processes over time.

Individuals are educated and trained as appropriate to their responsibilities, privileges, job descriptions, and data and information needs.

Standards

IM.5 Transmission of data and information is timely and accurate.

IM.5.1 The format and methods for disseminating data and information are standardized, whenever possible.

Intent of IM.5 and IM.5.1

Internally and externally generated data and information are accurately transmitted to users. The integrity of data and information is maintained, and there is adequate communication between data users and suppliers. The timing of transmission is appropriate to the data's intended use.

The format and methods of disseminating internal data and information are tailored to the needs of users and the hospital. Dissemination methods and formats provide for easy retrieval. The means by which data and information are exchanged is standardized whenever possible to facilitate interpretation.

Standards

IM.6 Adequate integration and interpretation capabilities are provided.

IM.6.1 The hospital determines how long medical record information is retained, based on law and regulation and the information use for patient care, legal, research, and educational purposes.

Intent of IM.6 and IM.6.1

The information-management process makes it possible to combine information from various sources and generate reports to support decision making. Specifically, the information-management process
a. coordinates collection of information;
b. makes information from one system available to another (for example, between clinical and organizational systems);
c. organizes data;
d. analyzes data;
e. interprets and clarifies data; and
f. generates and provides access to longitudinal data.

In addition, the information-management process provides the capability to link
g. patient care and nonpatient care data over time and among all care settings;
h. internal and external information sources;
i. patient care data and information from clinical literature; and
j. organizational data and management literature.

Data and information are retained for sufficient periods to comply with law and regulation and support patient care, management, legal documentation, research, and education.

Standards and Intent Statements for Patient-Specific Data and Information

Standards

IM.7 *The hospital defines, captures, analyzes, transforms, transmits, and reports patient-specific data and information related to care processes and outcomes.*

IM.7.1 The hospital initiates and maintains a medical record for every individual assessed or treated.

IM.7.1.1 Only authorized individuals make entries in medical records.

IM.7.2 The medical record contains sufficient information to identify the patient, support the diagnosis, justify the treatment, document the course and results, and promote continuity of care among health care providers.

Intent of IM.7 Through IM.7.2

Information-management processes provide for the use of patient-specific data and information to
- facilitate patient care;
- serve as a financial and legal record;
- aid in clinical research;
- support decision analysis; and
- guide professional and organizational performance improvement.

To facilitate consistency and continuity in patient care, specific data and information are required. Administrative and direct patient care providers produce and use this information for professional and organization improvement. Medical records contain sufficient information to
- identify the patient;
- support the diagnosis;
- justify the treatment;
- document the course and results; and
- facilitate continuity of care.

The environment in which patient-specific information is provided supports timely, accurate, secure, and confidential recording and use of patient-specific information. The system recalls historical patient data and is able to furnish data about current encounters. To facilitate consistency and continuity in patient care, the medical record contains very specific data and information, including

a. the patient's name, address, date of birth, and the name of any legally authorized representative;
b. the legal status of patients receiving mental health services;
c. emergency care provided to the patient prior to arrival, if any;
d. the record and findings of the patient's assessment*;
e. conclusions or impressions drawn from the medical history and physical examination;
f. the diagnosis or diagnostic impression;
g. the reasons for admission or treatment;
h. the goals of treatment and the treatment plan;

---

* See the "Assessment of Patients" chapter.

i. evidence of known advance directives;
j. evidence of informed consent, when required by hospital policy;
k. diagnostic and therapeutic orders, if any;
l. all diagnostic and therapeutic procedures and test results;
m. all operative and other invasive procedures performed, using acceptable disease and operative terminology that includes etiology, as appropriate;
n. progress notes made by the medical staff and other authorized individuals;
o. all reassessments and any revisions of the treatment plan;
p. clinical observations;
q. the patient's response to care;
r. consultation reports;
s. every medication ordered or prescribed for an inpatient;
t. every medication dispensed to an ambulatory patient or an inpatient on discharge;
u. every dose of medication administered and any adverse drug reaction;
v. all relevant diagnoses established during the course of care;
w. any referrals and communications made to external or internal care providers and to community agencies;
x. conclusions at termination of hospitalization;
y. discharge instructions to the patient and family; and
z. clinical resumes and discharge summaries, or a final progress note or transfer summary.

A concise clinical resume included in the medical record at discharge provides important information to other caregivers and facilitates continuity of care. For patients discharged to ambulatory (outpatient) care, the clinical resume summarizes previous levels of care. The discharge summary contains the following information:

- The reason for hospitalization;
- Significant findings;
- Procedures performed and treatment rendered;
- The patient's condition at discharge; and
- Instructions to the patient and family, if any.

For normal newborns with uncomplicated deliveries, or for patients hospitalized for less than 48 hours with only minor problems, a progress note may substitute for the clinical resume. The medical staff defines what problems and interventions may be considered minor. The progress note may be handwritten. It documents the patient's condition at discharge, discharge instructions, and follow-up care required.

When a patient is transferred within the same organization from one level of care to another (for example, from the hospital to residential care), and the caregivers change, a transfer summary may be substituted for the clinical resume. A transfer summary briefly describes the patient's condition at time of transfer, and the reason for the transfer. When the caregivers remain the same, a progress note may suffice.

Standards

IM.7.3 *The medical record thoroughly documents operative or other procedures* and the use of anesthesia.*

---

* **operative and other procedures** Includes operative, other invasive, and noninvasive procedures, such as radiotherapy, hyperbaric treatment, CAT scan, and MRI, that place the patient at risk. The focus is on procedures and is not meant to include medications that place the patient at risk.

IM.7.3.1 A preoperative diagnosis is recorded before surgery by the licensed independent practitioner responsible for the patient.

IM.7.3.2 Operative reports dictated or written immediately after surgery record the name of the primary surgeon and assistants, findings, technical procedures used, specimens removed, and postoperative diagnosis.

IM.7.3.2.1 The completed operative report is authenticated* by the surgeon and filed in the medical record as soon as possible after surgery.

IM.7.3.2.2 When the operative report is not placed in the medical record immediately after surgery, a progress note is entered immediately.

IM.7.3.3 Postoperative documentation records the patient's vital signs and level of consciousness; medications (including intravenous fluids), blood, and blood components; any unusual events or postoperative complications; and management of such events.

IM.7.3.4 *Postoperative documentation records the patient's discharge from the postanesthesia care area by the responsible licensed independent practitioner or according to discharge criteria.*

IM.7.3.4.1 Compliance with discharge criteria is fully documented in the patient's medical record.

IM.7.3.5 Postoperative documentation records the name of the licensed independent practitioner responsible for discharge.

Intent of IM.7.3 Through IM.7.3.5

In addition to the information required in all medical records,[†] the hospital documents all aspects of a surgical patient's preoperative, operative, and postoperative care. The record includes the preoperative diagnosis, a complete description of the surgical procedure and findings, the names of all practitioners involved in the patient's care, the postoperative course, evidence of the patient's readiness for discharge from postanesthesia care, and details of the discharge.

Operative reports are consistently placed in the medical record consistent with hospital policies and procedures and state laws. This requirement applies to outpatients as well as inpatients, including donors and recipients of organs and tissues. When the operative report is not placed in the medical record immediately—for example, when there is a transcription or filing delay—an operative progress note is entered in the medical record immediately after surgery to provide pertinent information for anyone required to attend to the patient.

Postoperative documentation includes at least the following records:
- Vital signs and level of consciousness;
- Medications (including intravenous fluids) and blood and blood components;
- Any unusual events or postoperative complications, including blood transfusion reactions, and the management of those events;

---

* **authenticate** To verify that an entry is complete, accurate, and final.

[†] See IM.7 through IM.7.2

- The names of providers of direct patient care nursing services, or the names of people who supervised that care if it was provided by someone other than a qualified registered nurse;
- The patient's discharge from the postanesthesia care, whether by a responsible licensed independent practitioner or by the use of relevant discharge criteria.

If discharge criteria are used, they are approved by the medical staff and rigorously applied to determine a patient's readiness for discharge. If the patient is discharged by a licensed independent practitioner, the practitioner's name is recorded in the postoperative documentation.

Standards

IM.7.4 For patients receiving continuing ambulatory care services, the medical record contains a summary list of known significant diagnoses, conditions, procedures, drug allergies, and medications.

IM.7.4.1 The list is initiated for each patient by the third visit and maintained thereafter.

Intent of IM.7.4 and IM.7.4.1

Patients sometimes receive ambulatory care services on a continuing basis, and often from more than one provider at the hospital. To promote continuity of care, both over time and among providers, the hospital maintains a record for any patient who is seen at three or more outpatient visits. The record, sometimes referred to as a "summary list," includes the following information:
- Known significant medical diagnoses and conditions;
- known significant operative and invasive procedures;
- known adverse and allergic drug reactions; and
- medications known to be prescribed for or used by the patient.

"Known" refers to information gathered as part of the ambulatory care assessment and treatment.

This information is in the same location in all records, so that providers can find it quickly. If more than one clinic in the hospital keeps a record of the patient, each record notes that there is additional information elsewhere (see IM.7.9).

Standards

IM.7.5 When emergency, urgent, or immediate care is provided, the time and means of arrival are also documented in the medical record.

IM.7.5.1 The medical record notes when a patient receiving emergency, urgent, or immediate care left against medical advice.

IM.7.5.2 The medical record of a patient receiving emergency, urgent, or immediate care notes the conclusions at termination of treatment, including final disposition, condition at discharge, and instructions for follow-up care.

IM.7.5.3 When authorized by the patient or a legally authorized representative, a copy of the emergency services provided is available to the practitioner or medical organization providing follow-up care.

Intent of IM.7.5 Through IM.7.5.3

The medical records of patients who have received emergency care contain not only the information required of all medical records, but additional information specific to the emergency visit. Such information is provided to the practitioner or organization responsible for follow-up care only when authorized by the patient or the legally authorized representative.

Standard

IM.7.6 Medical record data and information are managed in a timely manner.

Intent of IM.7.6

Timely entries are essential if a medical record is to be useful in a patient's care. A complete medical record is also important when a patient is discharged, since information in the record may be needed for clinical, legal, or performance-improvement purposes.

The hospital has a policy and procedures on the timely entry of all significant clinical information into the patient's medical record. Providers enter all such information accordingly.

Timely documentation of the patient's medical history, physical examination, and operative reports is especially important. A patient's medical record is complete when
- its contents reflect the patient's condition on arrival, diagnosis, test results, therapy, condition and in-hospital progress, and condition at discharge;
- its contents, including any required clinical resume or final progress notes, are assembled and authenticated; and
- all final diagnoses and complications are recorded without the use of symbols or abbreviations.

A medical record is considered delinquent when it has not been completed within a specific time following the patient's discharge. This time period is spelled out in the medical staff's rules and regulations and cannot exceed 30 days. The hospital measures medical record delinquency at regular intervals, no less frequently than every three months, and reports the data as part of medical record review function (IM.3.2).

Note: *If the average of the total number of records delinquent (for any reason) calculated from the last four quarterly measurements is equal to or exceeds twice the average monthly discharges, conditional accreditation will be recommended.*

Standard

IM.7.7 Verbal orders of authorized individuals are accepted and transcribed by qualified personnel who are identified by title or category in the medical staff rules and regulations.

Intent of IM.7.7

Practitioners often give orders verbally in the course of patient care. The quality of patient care may suffer if such orders are not received and recorded in a standard way. Each verbal order is dated and is identified by the names of the individuals who gave it and received it. And the record documents who implemented it. Individuals who receive verbal orders are qualified to do so and are authorized by the medical staff to do so as identified by title or category of personnel.

When required by state or federal law and regulation, verbal orders are authenticated within the specified time frame.

Standard

IM.7.8 Every medical record entry is dated, its author identified, and, when necessary, authenticated.

Management of Information

Intent of IM.7.8

The hospital has a system in place to
- assure that only authorized individuals make entries into medical records;
- identify the date and author of every entry in the medical record; and
- enable the author to authenticate an entry to verify it is complete, accurate, and final.

    The author authenticates those entries required by hospital policy. The hospital ensures that, at a minimum, entries of *histories and physical examinations, operative procedures, consultations*, and discharge summaries* are authenticated. Other entries are authenticated as specified by the hospital policy or medical staff bylaws or as required by state or federal law and regulation.

    Hospitals establish policies and mechanisms to assure that only an author can authenticate his or her own entry. Indications of authentication can include written signatures or initials, rubber-stamps, or computer "signatures" (or sequence of keys). The medical staff rules and regulations or policies define what entries, if any, by house staff or nonphysicians must be countersigned by supervising physicians.

Standard

IM.7.9 The hospital can quickly assemble and have access to all relevant information from components of a patient's record, when the patient is admitted or is seen for ambulatory or emergency care.

Intent of IM.7.9

Patients sometimes receive care in several areas of the hospital; as a result, records on the patient may exist in more than one location. To provide continuity of care, both over time and among providers, practitioners need ready access to all relevant information about the care a patient has received, regardless of where in the hospital that care was given.

    The hospital uses a patient-information system to integrate all relevant information from a patient's record from various locations or makes available a summary of information relevant for patient care when the patient is seen. This applies when a patient
- is admitted to the hospital;
- is seen for a prescheduled ambulatory care visit;
- is seen for an unscheduled outpatient visit; and
- comes in for emergency services.

The medical record, computer system, or organization policy indicates when part of the record has been filed elsewhere. The patient information is provided in a timely manner by hard copy or screen display.

Standards and Intent Statements for Aggregate Data and Information

Standard

IM.8 The hospital collects and analyzes aggregate data to support patient care and operations.

---

* The consultation report is a signed (authenticated) opinion of the consultant's findings for making a diagnosis for a specific patient or providing treatment advice on a specific patient. For the purpose of this standard, routine pathology and clinical laboratory reports and x-ray reports do not require authentication.

Intent of IM.8

The hospital aggregates and analyzes clinical and administrative data to support
- patient care;
- decision making;
- management and operations;
- analysis of trends over time;
- performance comparisons over time and with other organizations; and
- performance improvement.

The hospital is able to aggregate the following data and information:
a. Pharmacy transactions, as required by law and to control and account for all drugs;
b. Information about hazards and safety practices used to identify safety management issues to be addressed by the organization;
c. Records of radionuclides and radiopharmaceuticals, including the radionuclide's identity, the date received, method of receipt, activity, recipient's identity, date administered, and disposal;
d. Records of required reporting to authorities;
e. Performance measures of processes and outcomes;
f. Summaries of performance-improvement actions;
g. Practitioner-specific information*;
h. The ability to gather accurate, timely information for use in operational decision making and planning; and
i. Data and information to support clinical research.

Coding and retrieval systems are implemented for aggregating
j. medical record information about diagnoses and procedures;
k. patient demographic information; and
l. financial information.

Aggregate performance-improvement information includes information from risk management, utilization review, infection control, and safety management. Information about hazards and safety practices includes

m. summaries of the deficiencies, problems, failures, and user errors in safety management, life safety management, equipment management, and utilities management, as well as relevant published reports of hazards associated with any of these areas;
n. documented surveys, at least semiannually, of all areas of the facility to identify environmental hazards and unsafe practices; and
o. reports and investigations of all incidents involving property damage, occupational illness, or patient, personnel, or visitor injury.

A continuously maintained control register for emergency and outpatient services[†] includes at least the following information for every individual seeking care:
p. Identification, such as name, age, and gender;
q. Date, time, and means of arrival;
r. Nature of complaint;
s. Disposition; and
t. Time of departure.

---

* As defined in the "Medical Staff" chapter of this book.

[†] **outpatient services** Refers to a patient appointment system, and all the stated requirements do not apply.

Standards and Intent Statements for Knowledge-Based Information

Standard

IM.9 The hospital provides systems, resources, and services to meet its needs for knowledge-based information in patient care, education, research, and management.

Intent of IM.9

Knowledge-based information, often referred to as "literature," includes journal literature, reference information, and research data. It may be found in a variety of forms, including articles, abstracts, or indexes in print or electronic format; recent editions of texts, periodicals, and other professional resources; and patient education materials that meet individual and organizational needs. Knowledge-based information is authoritative and up to date. It supports clinical and management decision making, performance-improvement activities, patient and family education, continuing education of staff, and research.

This standard addresses the hospital's ability to provide knowledge-based information to those who need it. A hospital's need for knowledge-based information can be met in a variety of ways, including an on-site library department or unit, the services of a qualified medical librarian on site, or a variety of other cooperative arrangements for providing similar services to effectively meet the knowledge-based information needs of the institutions. These services may be shared with other hospitals or community resources, as long as needed information is easily accessible to hospital staff.

Appropriate knowledge-based information is acquired, assembled, and transmitted to users. Knowledge-based information management consists of systems, resources, and services to
- help health professionals acquire and maintain the knowledge and skills they need to care for patients;
- support clinical and management decision making;
- support performance improvement;
- satisfy research-related needs; and
- educate patients and families.

Standard

IM.9.1 The hospital's knowledge-based information resources are available, authoritative, and up to date.

Intent of IM.9.1

Knowledge-based resources are available and accessible to everyone in the hospital who needs them, including clinical and administrative staff, and patients and families when appropriate. These resources provide authoritative and up-to-date scientific, clinical, and managerial knowledge.

To be accessible, resources are in appropriate formats. For example, clinical and management literature may be available as paper or electronic journals, books, technical reports, and audiovisual media. Patient education material is often available in the form of brochures, articles, pamphlets, audiovisual materials, and models. Resources may also include externally produced databases and practice guidelines.

To select authoritative, up-to-date resources, the hospital may consult the
- *Selected List of Books and Journals for the Small Medical Library* (often called the Brandon-Hill list), published every other year by the Medical Library Association (MLA) in the *Bulletin of the MLA;*
- *Library for Internists,* published by the American College of Physicians every three years in the *Annals of Internal Medicine*;
- databases, publishing information, and reviews; and
- recommendations of resource users.

The hospital has a system for organizing knowledge-based information and providing it efficiently to users. Poison-control and formulary information is quickly and easily available when needed. A poison-control center hotline is usually the best source of up-to-date information on poisons.

Standard

IM.9.2 The hospital's services, resources, and systems for knowledge-based information are based on a needs assessment.

Intent of IM.9.2

When the hospital assesses its overall information needs, it looks at the need for knowledge-based information. The systems, resources, and services the hospital provides to meet these needs will depend on
- the services the hospital provides;
- the needs of those who will use the information.

Users include the medical and nursing staffs, administrators and managers, other health professional staff members, other hospital staff members, students, patients and their families, and researchers.

Specifically, the needs assessment addresses
- accessibility and timeliness;
- links with the hospital's internal information systems; and
- links with external databases and information networks.

Library and information services enable the hospital to
- respond to information requests from staff, patients, and families;
- anticipate information needs and systematically link literature to clinical and organizational processes; and
- provide relevant, current, and accurate information within appropriate time frames and in formats appropriate to users' needs.

Information is accessible in one or more of the following locations:
- At the work site;
- In a shared central collection at the hospital (for example, a professional library);
- From outside sources (such as vendors or other institutions), with acceptable time delays.

The quality of the information service can be judged by the following criteria:
- Accuracy;
- Currency;
- Relevance to the request;
- Speed of response;
- Format (ease of use); and
- Validity of the information.

Standards and Intent Statements for Comparative Data and Information

Standards

IM.10 *Comparative performance data and information are defined, collected, analyzed, transmitted, reported, and used consistent with national and state guidelines for data set parity and connectivity.*

IM.10.1 The hospital uses external reference databases for comparative purposes.

IM.10.2 The hospital contributes to external reference databases when required by law or regulation or when appropriate to the hospital.

IM.10.3 The security and confidentiality of data and information are maintained when contributing to or using external databases.

Intent of IM.10 Through IM.10.3

These standards address the hospital's ability to use and contribute to collections of performance data from multiple institutions. As part of its information-management activities, the hospital exchanges clinical and knowledge-based data and information with other health care organizations. These activities help the hospital develop its future capabilities and goals.

The hospital uses external data and information to identify areas in which its own performance deviates from expected patterns. The hospital also contributes its own information to external reference databases. To ensure that the data is comparable across institutions, the hospital follows national and state guidelines on form and content.

Surveillance, Prevention, and Control of Infection

Overview

The **goal** of the surveillance, prevention, and control of infection function* is to identify and reduce the risks of *acquiring* and *transmitting* infections among patients, employees, physicians and other licensed independent practitioners, contract service workers, volunteers, students, and visitors.

All hospitals run the risk of nosocomial infections—that is, infections *acquired* in the hospital—as well as infections *brought* into the hospital. These infections may be endemic† (common cause) or epidemic‡ (special cause), and they may affect patients, and health care workers and others who come into contact with patients.

Surveillance, prevention, and control of infection covers a broad range of processes and activities, both in direct patient care and in patient care support, that are coordinated and carried out by the hospital. This function also links with external organization support systems to reduce the risk of infection from the environment, including food and water sources.

---

* **function** A goal-directed, interrelated series of processes, such as continuum of care or management of information.

† **endemic infection** The habitual presence of an infection within a geographic area; may also refer to the usual prevalence of a given disease within such an area.

‡ **epidemic infection** An outbreak in a community or region of a group of infections of similar nature, clearly in excess of normal expectancy and derived from a common or propagated source.

Standards

The following is a list of all standards for this function. If you have a questions about a term used here, please check the Glossary, pages 281 through 307. Terms that are critical to the understanding of the standard are defined in the footnotes of the next section of this chapter.

IC.1 The organization uses a coordinated process to reduce the risks of endemic and epidemic nosocomial infections in patients and health care workers.

IC.1.1 The infection control process is managed by one or more qualified individuals.

IC.2 Case findings and identification of demographically important nosocomial infections provide surveillance data.

IC.3 The hospital reports, when appropriate, information about infections both internally and to public health agencies.

IC.4 The hospital takes action to prevent or reduce the risk of nosocomial infections in patients, employees, and visitors.

IC.5 The hospital takes action to control outbreaks of nosocomial infections when they are identified.

IC.6 The hospital's infection control process is designed to lower the risks and to improve the (proportional) rates or (numerical) trends of epidemiologically significant infections.

IC.6.1 Management systems support the infection control process.

IC.6.2 The infection control process includes at least one activity aimed at preventing the transmission of epidemiologically significant infections between patients and staff.

Standards and Intent Statements for Surveillance, Prevention, and Control of Infection

Standards

IC.1 The organization uses a coordinated process to reduce the risks of endemic and epidemic nosocomial infections in patients and health care workers.

IC.1.1 The infection control process is managed by one or more qualified individuals.

Intent of IC.1 and IC.1.1

The hospital's infection control process is based on sound epidemiologic principles and research on nosocomial infection. The specific program for controlling infection may differ from hospital to hospital, depending on factors such as the
- hospital's geographic location;
- patient volume;
- patient population served;
- hospital's clinical focus; and
- number of employees.

The hospital's infection control program addresses issues defined by that hospital to be epidemiologically important. Depending on the hospital, these may include
- device-related infections, especially those associated with intravascular devices, ventilators, and tube feeding;
- surgical site infections;
- nosocomial infections in special care units;
- infections caused by organisms that are antibiotic-resistant or in other ways epidemiologically important;
- nosocomial tuberculosis and other communicable diseases, especially vaccine-preventable infections; and
- infections in neonates.

The hospital connects its infection control program with the local health department to ensure appropriate *follow-up* and control of infection.

One or more qualified individuals oversee the infection control process. Their qualifications depend on the activities they will carry out, and may be met through
- education;
- training;
- experience; and
- certification or licensure. (Certification by the Certification Board for Infection Control [CBIC] is often a requirement for infection control practitioners.)

Standards

IC.2 Case findings and identification of demographically important nosocomial infections provide surveillance data.

IC.3 The hospital reports, when appropriate, information about infections both internally and to public health agencies.

IC.4 The hospital takes action to prevent or reduce the risk of nosocomial infections in patients, employees, and visitors.

IC.5 The hospital takes action to control outbreaks of nosocomial infections when they are identified.

Intent of IC.2 Through IC.5
The hospital's infection control process is comprehensive, encompassing both patient care and employee health services. The mechanisms that support this process are based on current scientific knowledge, accepted practice guidelines, and applicable law and regulation. They address the infection issues that are epidemiologically important to the hospital.

Standards
IC.6 The hospital's infection control process is designed to lower the risks and to improve the (proportional) rates or (numerical) trends of epidemiologically significant infections.

IC.6.1 Management systems support the infection control process.

IC.6.2 The infection control process includes at least one activity aimed at preventing the transmission of epidemiologically significant infections between patients and staff.

Intent of IC.6 Through IC.6.2
The infection control process is integrated with the hospital's overall process for assessing and improving organization performance. The hospital tracks risks, rates, and trends in nosocomial infections. It uses this information to improve its prevention and control activities and to reduce nosocomial infection rates to the lowest possible levels. The infection control program works with the employee health program to reduce the transmission of infections, including vaccine-preventable infections, from patients to staff and from staff to patients.

Management systems, including staff and data systems, help the hospital achieve these objectives. The specific role of management systems depends on the hospital's infection control process. Generally, they support activities such as data analysis, interpretation, and presentation of findings.

Governance

Overview

The governance of a hospital sets the organization policy that supports quality patient care. It does this by developing the mission, vision, policies, and bylaws that govern the hospital's operations. The "Leadership" chapter addresses how the activities of the hospital's leaders*—that is, the governing body or authority, management, and other leaders—are coordinated.

---

* **leaders** The leaders described in the leadership function include at least the leaders of the governing body; the chief executive officer and other senior managers; department leaders; the elected and the appointed leaders of the medical staff and the clinical departments and other medical staff members in organizational administrative positions; and the nurse executive and other senior nursing leaders.

Standards

The following is a list of all standards for this function. If you have a questions about a term used here, please check the Glossary, pages 281 through 307. Terms that are critical to the understanding of the standard are defined in the footnotes of the next section of this chapter.

GO.1 The hospital identifies how it is governed and the key individuals involved.

GO.2 *Those responsible for governance establish policy, promote performance improvement, and provide for organizational management and planning.*

GO.2.1 The hospital's governing body or authority adopts bylaws addressing its legal accountabilities and responsibility to the patient population served.

GO.2.2 The hospital's governing body or authority provides for appropriate medical staff participation in governance.

GO.2.2.1 The medical staff has the right to representation (through attendance and voice), by one or more medical staff members selected by the medical staff, at governing body meetings.

GO.2.2.2 Medical staff members are eligible for full membership in the hospital's governing body, unless legally prohibited.

GO.2.3 The hospital's governing body or authority establishes a criteria-based process for selecting a qualified and competent chief executive officer.

GO.2.4 The hospital's governing body or authority provides for compliance with applicable law and regulation.

GO.2.5 The hospital's governing body provides for the collaboration of leaders in developing, reviewing, and revising policies and procedures.

GO.2.6 The hospital's governing body or authority provides for conflict resolution.

Standards and Intent Statements for Governance

Standard

GO.1 The hospital identifies how it is governed and the key individuals involved.

Intent of GO.1

The hospital has a document that shows how it is governed. This document includes lines of authority relative to key planning, management, operations, and evaluation of responsibilities at each level of governance.

Standard

GO.2 *Those responsible for governance establish policy, promote performance improvement, and provide for organizational management and planning.*

Intent of GO.2

The hospital's governing body or authority ultimately is responsible for the quality of care the hospital provides. To carry out this responsibility, the governing body or authority provides for the effective functioning of activities related to
- delivering quality patient care;
- performance improvement;
- risk management;
- medical staff credentialing; and
- financial management.

Standard

GO.2.1 The hospital's governing body or authority adopts bylaws addressing its legal accountabilities and responsibility to the patient population served.

Intent of GO.2.1

The governing body or authority provides coordination and integration among the organization leaders to
- establish policy;
- maintain quality patient care;
- provide for necessary resources; and
- provide for organizational management and planning.
    At a minimum, the governing bylaws specify the
- organization's role and purpose;
- governing body's or authority's duties and responsibilities;
- process and criteria for selecting its members;
- governing body's or authority's organizational structure;
- relationship of responsibilities among those responsible for governing and any authority superior to the governing body or authority (if such exists), the chief executive officer, the medical staff, and other appropriate leaders;
- requirement for establishing a medical staff;
- requirement for establishing auxiliary organizations, if applicable; and
- definition of "conflict of interest."

Standards

GO.2.2 The hospital's governing body or authority provides for appropriate medical staff participation in governance.

GO.2.2.1 The medical staff has the right to representation (through attendance and voice), by one or more medical staff members selected by the medical staff, at governing body meetings.

GO.2.2.2 Medical staff members are eligible for full membership in the hospital's governing body, unless legally prohibited.

Intent of GO.2.2 Through GO.2.2.2

The medical staff contributes to the quality of care by coordinating their work with that of other leaders and those responsible for governing the organization. Through its participation in governance, the medical staff helps ensure that all medical staff members responsible for assessing, caring for, or treating patients are clinically competent and that clinical care rendered is appropriate. This participation also allows them the opportunity to contribute to the organization's planning, budgeting, safety management, and overall performance-improvement activities. The medical staff executive committee makes specific recommendations to the governing body for its approval (see MS.3.1.6 through MS.3.1.6.1.7 in the "Medical Staff" chapter). These recommendations relate to

- the medical staff's structure;
- the process designed for reviewing credentials and delineating individual clinical privileges;
- recommending individuals for medical staff membership;
- recommending delineated clinical privileges for each eligible individual;
- the organization of the medical staff's performance-improvement activities as well as the process designed for conducting, evaluating, and revising such activities;
- the process by which medical staff membership may be terminated; and
- the process designed for fair-hearing procedures.

Standard

GO.2.3 The hospital's governing body or authority establishes a criteria-based process for selecting a qualified and competent chief executive officer.

Intent of GO.2.3

The chief executive officer has the knowledge and skills necessary to perform the duties required of the hospital's senior leader. Among other criteria, education and relevant experience are important qualifications. The chief executive officer may be selected by the governing body. Or, the governing body may approve a chief executive officer selected by corporate management or another group.

Standard

GO.2.4 The hospital's governing body or authority provides for compliance with applicable law and regulation.

Intent of GO.2.4

The intent of this standard is self-evident.

Standard

GO.2.5 The hospital's governing body provides for the collaboration of leaders in developing, reviewing, and revising policies and procedures.

Intent of GO.2.5

Because most policies and procedures address cross-functional, interdisciplinary, multidepartmental activities, they need to be developed collaboratively to be effective. The governing body or authority and other leaders collaborate to develop, review, and revise key policies and procedures. Such policies and procedures are written and appear in bylaws, rules, regulations, protocols, or other documents. Those affected by policies and procedures are aware of their content.

Policies and procedures address key items regarding
- nursing care based on nursing standards of patient care and nursing practice standards (for example, critical care protocols, discharge planning) and
- the medical staff's responsibility for developing, adopting, and periodically reviewing its bylaws and rules and regulations consistent with organization policy and applicable law and other requirements (see MS.3 through MS.3.1 in the "Medical Staff" chapter).

Standard

GO.2.6 The hospital's governing body or authority provides for conflict resolution.

Intent of GO.2.6

The hospital has a system for resolving conflicts among leaders and the individuals under their leadership. Leaders regularly review the system's effectiveness, revising it as necessary.

Management

Overview

This chapter covers the responsibilities of the chief executive officer and executive management and the relationship between the governing body and the chief executive officer.

1999 Hospital Accreditation Standards

Standards

The following is a list of all standards for this function. If you have a questions about a term used here, please check the Glossary, pages 281 through 307. Terms that are critical to the understanding of the standard are defined in the footnotes of the next section of this chapter.

MA.1 The chief executive officer, selected by the governing body, is responsible for operating the hospital according to the authority conferred by the governing body.

MA.1.1 The chief executive officer has the education and experience necessary to carry out the responsibilities of the position.

MA.2 The chief executive officer provides for the hospital's compliance with applicable law and regulation and

MA.2.1 the chief executive officer reviews and promptly responds to reports and recommendations from planning, regulatory, and inspecting agencies, as outlined by the governing body.

MA.3 The chief executive officer, working with management, clinical, and administrative staff, provides for a well-managed hospital with clear lines of responsibility and accountability within departments and between departments and administration.

MA.4 The chief executive officer, working with management, clinical, and administrative staff, provides for internal controls protecting human, physical, financial, and information resources.

Management

Standards and Intent Statements for Management

Standards

MA.1 The chief executive officer,* selected by the governing body, is responsible for operating the hospital according to the authority conferred by the governing body.

MA.1.1 The chief executive officer has the education and experience necessary to carry out the responsibilities of the position.

Intent of MA.1 and MA.1.1

The governing body empowers a chief executive officer to be responsible for the hospital's management. Specific chief executive officer responsibilities include
- establishing effective operations;
- establishing information and support systems;
- recruiting and maintaining staff; and
- conserving physical and financial assets.

When chief executive officer responsibilities are performed by more than one individual, the governing body clearly defines each individual's responsibilities and the relationship between them. The chief executive officer is competent and has the education and experience required for the size, complexity, mission of the hospital, and the scope of services it provides.

Standards

MA.2 The chief executive officer provides for the hospital's compliance with applicable law and regulation and

MA.2.1 the chief executive officer reviews and promptly responds to reports and recommendations from planning, regulatory, and inspecting agencies, as outlined by the governing body.

Intent of MA.2 and MA.2.1

The hospital's chief executive officer provides for
- the hospital's compliance with applicable law and regulation and
- filing applicable legal documents and copies of the hospital's state licensure or certification.

The chief executive officer is responsible for implementing governing body policies. The governing body defines the chief executive officer's responsibility for acting on reports or recommendations from planning, regulatory, and inspecting agencies.

---

* Chief executive officer (CEO) is the term used in these standards for that position known to have other titles in different types of health care organizations, such as commanding officer in a military hospital, medical center director in a VA hospital, superintendent in a state psychiatric hospital, and so forth. A nonexhaustive list of those titles includes, but is not limited to: administrator, administrator and chief executive officer, administrator and chief operating officer, chief executive officer, commander, deputy commander for administration, director, executive director, executive vice president and director, president, president and chief executive officer, president and chief operating officer, vice president, vice president for operations, and vice president and chief executive officer.

Standards

MA.3 The chief executive officer, working with management, clinical, and administrative staff, provides for a well-managed hospital with clear lines of responsibility and accountability within departments and between departments and administration.

MA.4 The chief executive officer, working with management, clinical, and administrative staff, provides for internal controls protecting human, physical, financial, and information resources.

Intent of MA.3 and MA.4

The chief executive officer establishes lines of authority for planning, management, operations, and evaluation at each service level. The governing body provides the chief executive officer with policies to direct the hospital's operations. It also provides sufficient resources to realize the hospital's mission, goals, and objectives. The chief executive officer manages resources to meet the identified needs of the hospital and its patients.

The chief executive officer prepares reports for the governing body's review on
- short- and long-term plans;
- operations;
- program efficiency and effectiveness;
- the nature and extent of funding and other available resources;
- budgetary and financial performance; and
- capital and other resources.

Medical Staff

Overview

Medical staff members, in providing patient care and carrying out their other professional responsibilities in increasingly complex organizations, continue to actively participate and exercise professional leadership in measuring, assessing, and improving the performance of the organizations within which they practice. Medical staff leadership and participation in assessing and improving the quality of care delivered in health care organizations occur at the various levels within the organization:

- Interactions between individual staff members and patients;
- Their clinical departments; and
- Among the overall organization.

Several characteristics of the professional work of medical staff members contribute to the delivery of high-quality health care:

- Providing patient care within the parameters of their professional competence, as reflected in the scope of their clinical privileges;
- Practicing within the framework of (implicit or explicit) clinically relevant and scientifically valid standards, guidelines, and criteria;
- Participating in ongoing measurement, assessment, and improvement of both clinical and nonclinical processes and the resulting patient outcomes; and
- Leading the assessment and improvement of both clinical and nonclinical processes and the resulting patient outcomes primarily dependent on individuals with clinical privileges.

Standards

The following is a list of all standards for this function. If you have a questions about a term used here, please check the Glossary, pages 281 through 307. Terms that are critical to the understanding of the standard are defined in the footnotes of the next section of this chapter.

For the reader's convenience, MS.4.2.1.7 through MS.4.2.1.15 are included in this chapter. These standards have been adapted and their intent relocated to the "Leadership" chapter (pages 155 and 156). Their new standard numbers in the "Leadership" chapter are provided in parentheses after each standard.

Organization, Bylaws, Rules, and Regulations
The Organized Medical Staff

Individual members of the medical staff care for patients within an organization context. Within this context, members of the medical staff, as individuals and as a group, interface with, and actively participate in, important organization functions.

MS.1 One or more organized, self-governing medical staffs have overall responsibility for the quality of the professional services provided by individuals with clinical privileges,* as well as the responsibility of accounting therefore to the governing body.

MS.1.1 *Each medical staff has the following characteristics:*

MS.1.1.1 It includes fully licensed physicians and may include other licensed individuals permitted by law and by the hospital to provide patient care services independently in the hospital (both physicians and these other individuals are referred to as "licensed independent practitioners"†).

MS.1.1.2 *All medical staff members have delineated clinical privileges that define the scope of patient care services they may provide independently in the hospital.*

MS.1.1.3 All medical staff members and all others with delineated clinical privileges are subject to medical staff and departmental bylaws, rules and regulations, and policies and are subject to review as part of the organization's performance-improvement activities.

Documents Governing Activities of the Organized Medical Staff

Medical staff self-governance is delineated in documents that set out how the medical staff will organize and govern its affairs. Most typically it is delineated in bylaws, and essential components to be delineated are identified in these standards, including medical staff membership, the credentialing process, the role of the medical staff executive committee, and the structures necessary for ongoing

---

* **clinical privileges** Authorization granted by the appropriate authority (for example, a governing body) to a practitioner to provide specific care services in an organization within well-defined limits, based on the following factors, as applicable: license, education, training, experience, competence, health status, and judgment.

† **licensed independent practitioner** Any individual permitted by law and by the organization to provide care and services without direction or supervision, within the scope of the individual's license and consistent with individually granted clinical privileges.

activities of the medical staff. The medical staff bylaws, as adopted or amended by the medical staff and approved by the governing body, create a system of mutual rights and responsibilities between members of the medical staff and the hospital.

MS.2 *Each medical staff develops and adopts bylaws and rules and regulations to establish a framework for self-governance of medical staff activities and accountability to the governing body.*

MS.2.1 Medical staff bylaws and rules and regulations are adopted by the medical staff and approved by the governing body before becoming effective. Neither body may unilaterally amend the medical staff bylaws or rules and regulations.

MS.2.2 Medical staff bylaws and rules and regulations create a framework within which medical staff members can act with a reasonable degree of freedom and confidence.

MS.2.3 *Medical staff bylaws include provisions for at least the following:*

MS.2.3.1 *An executive committee of the medical staff;*

MS.2.3.2 Fair-hearing and appellate review mechanisms for medical staff members and other individuals holding clinical privileges;

MS.2.3.3 Mechanisms for corrective action, including indications and procedures for automatic and summary suspension of an individual's medical staff membership or clinical privileges;

MS.2.3.4 A description of the medical staff's organization, including categories of medical staff membership, when such exist, and appropriate officer positions, with the stipulation that each officer is a medical staff member;

MS.2.3.4.1 *The bylaws define*

MS.2.3.4.1.1 the method of selecting officers,

MS.2.3.4.1.2 the qualifications, responsibilities, and tenures of officers, and

MS.2.3.4.1.3 the conditions and mechanisms for removing officers from their positions;

MS.2.3.5 Requirements for frequency of meetings and for attendance;

MS.2.3.6 A mechanism designed to provide for effective communication among the medical staff, hospital administration, and governing body;

MS.2.3.6.1 *If there are multiple levels of governance, there is an established mechanism for the medical staff to communicate with all levels of governance involved in policy decisions affecting patient care services in the hospital.*

MS.2.3.7 A mechanism for adopting and amending the medical staff bylaws, rules and regulations, and policies; and

MS.2.3.8 Medical staff representation and participation in any hospital deliberation affecting the discharge of medical staff responsibilities.

MS.2.4 When necessary, the medical staff bylaws and rules and regulations are revised to reflect the hospital's current practices with respect to medical staff organization and functions.

MS.2.4.1 The medical staff bylaws, rules and regulations, and policies and the governing body's bylaws do not conflict.

MS.2.4.2 If significant changes are made in the medical staff bylaws, rules and regulations, or policies, medical staff members and other individuals who have delineated clinical privileges are provided with revised texts of the written materials.

MS.2.5 In hospitals participating in professional graduate education programs, the rules and regulations and policies specify the mechanisms by which house staff members are supervised by medical staff members in carrying out their patient care responsibilities.

Medical Staff Executive Function (Committee)

The medical staff executive committee has responsibilities, delegated by the medical staff, within the organization governance function. The medical staff executive committee carries out its work within the context of the organization functions of governance, leadership, and performance improvement. The medical staff executive committee is delegated the primary authority over activities related to the functions of self-governance of the medical staff and over activities related to the functions of performance improvement of the professional services provided by individuals with clinical privileges. The leadership of the hospital includes the medical staff leaders.*

MS.3 *The medical staff is organized to accomplish its functions.*

MS.3.1 There is an executive committee of the medical staff.

MS.3.1.1 The executive committee's function, size, and composition and the method of selecting its members are defined in the medical staff bylaws.

MS.3.1.2 The chief executive officer of the hospital or his or her designee attends each executive committee meeting on an ex-officio basis, with or without vote.

MS.3.1.3 No medical staff member actively practicing in the hospital is ineligible for membership on the executive committee solely because of his or her professional discipline or specialty.

MS.3.1.4 A majority of voting executive committee members are fully licensed physician members of the medical staff actively practicing in the hospital.

---

* **leaders** The leaders described in the leadership function include at least the leaders of the governing body; the chief executive officer and other senior managers; department leaders; the elected and the appointed leaders of the medical staff and the clinical departments and other medical staff members in organizational administrative positions; and the nurse executive and other senior nursing leaders.

Medical Staff

MS.3.1.5 The executive committee is empowered to act for the medical staff in the intervals between medical staff meetings.

MS.3.1.6 The executive committee is responsible for making medical staff recommendations directly to the governing body for its approval.

MS.3.1.6.1 Such recommendations pertain to at least the following:

MS.3.1.6.1.1 The medical staff's structure;

MS.3.1.6.1.2 The mechanism used to review credentials and to delineate individual clinical privileges;

MS.3.1.6.1.3 Recommendations of individuals for medical staff membership;

MS.3.1.6.1.4 Recommendations for delineated clinical privileges for each eligible individual;

MS.3.1.6.1.5 The participation of the medical staff in organization performance-improvement activities;

MS.3.1.6.1.6 The mechanism by which medical staff membership may be terminated; and

MS.3.1.6.1.7 The mechanism for fair-hearing procedures.

MS.3.1.7 The executive committee receives and acts on reports and recommendations from medical staff committees, clinical departments, and assigned activity groups.

Department Leadership

The leadership section outlines the role of medical staff department leaders. This responsibility is part of the organization leadership role of the medical staff, which is further explained in the "Leadership" chapter (pages 143 through 162).

MS.4 *When medical staff clinical departments exist:*

MS.4.1 Each department has effective leadership.

MS.4.1.1 The director of each department is certified by an appropriate specialty board, or affirmatively establishes comparable competence, through the credentialing process.
Note: *MS.4.1.1 applies only to those medical staff department directors who were appointed or reappointed after January 1, 1992. A medical staff department is currently defined as any structural unit of the medical staff (whether it is called a department, a service, a unit, a section, or something similar) in which the director is responsible for recommending privileges for individuals in the unit to the medical staff executive committee.*

MS.4.2 Medical staff department directors' responsibilities are specified in the medical staff bylaws and rules and regulations.

MS.4.2.1 Each department director is responsible for the following:

MS.4.2.1.1 All clinically related activities of the department;

MS.4.2.1.2 All administratively related activities of the department, unless otherwise provided for by the hospital;

MS.4.2.1.3 Continuing surveillance of the professional performance of all individuals in the department who have delineated clinical privileges;

MS.4.2.1.4 Recommending to the medical staff the criteria for clinical privileges that are relevant to the care provided in the department;

MS.4.2.1.5 *Recommending clinical privileges for each member of the department;*

MS.4.2.1.6 Assessing and recommending to the relevant hospital authority off-site sources for needed patient care services not provided by the department or the organization.

MS.4.2.1.7 *the integration of the department or service into the primary functions of the organization; (LD.2.1)*

MS.4.2.1.8 *the coordination and integration of interdepartmental and intradepartmental services; (LD.2.2)*

MS.4.2.1.9 *the development and implementation of policies and procedures that guide and support the provision of services; (LD.2.3)*

MS.4.2.1.10 *the recommendations for a sufficient number of qualified and competent persons to provide care or service; (LD.2.4)*

MS.4.2.1.11 *the determination of the qualifications and competence of department or service personnel who are not licensed independent practitioners and who provide patient care services; (LD.2.5)*

MS.4.2.1.12 *the continuous assessment and improvement of the quality of care and services provided; (LD.2.6)*

MS.4.2.1.13 *the maintenance of quality control programs, as appropriate; (LD.2.7)*

MS.4.2.1.14 *the orientation and continuing education of all persons in the department or service; and (LD.2.8)*

MS.4.2.1.15 *recommendations for space and other resources needed by the department or service. (LD.2.9)*

Medical Staff

MS.5.5.3 *involvement in a professional liability action under circumstances specified in the medical staff bylaws, rules and regulations, and policies.*

MS.5.5.3.1 At a minimum, final judgments or settlements involving the individual are reported.

MS.5.6 *Appointment or reappointment to the medical staff and the initial granting and renewal or revision of clinical privileges are also based on information regarding the applicant's competence.*

MS.5.7 Deliberations by the medical staff in developing recommendations for appointment to or termination from the medical staff and for the initial granting, revision, or revocation of clinical privileges include information provided by a peer(s) of the applicant.

MS.5.8 *A structured procedure, as defined by medical staff bylaws, rules and regulations, and medical staff policies, is used for the expeditious processing of complete applications for appointment, reappointment, and initial, renewed, or revised clinical privileges.*

MS.5.8.1 A separate record is maintained for each individual requesting medical staff membership or clinical privileges.

MS.5.8.2 Complete applications are acted on within a reasonable period of time, as specified in the medical staff bylaws.

MS.5.9 Gender, race, creed, or national origin are not used in making decisions regarding the granting or denying of medical staff membership or clinical privileges.

MS.5.10 *Each applicant*

MS.5.10.1 consents to the inspection of records and documents pertinent to his or her licensure, specific training, experience, current competence, and ability to perform the privileges requested, and, if requested, appears for an interview;

MS.5.10.1.1 The bylaws, rules and regulations, and policies of the medical staff indicate that the applicant for reappointment or renewal of clinical privileges is required to submit any reasonable evidence of current ability to perform privileges that may be requested.

MS.5.10.2 [Each applicant] pledges to provide for continuous care for his or her patients; and

MS.5.10.3 *[Each applicant] acknowledges any provisions in the medical staff bylaws for release and immunity from civil liability.*

MS.5.11 Appointment or reappointment to the medical staff and the granting, renewal, or revision of clinical privileges are made for a period of no more than two years.

MS.5.12 *Appraisal for reappointment to the medical staff or renewal or revision of clinical privileges is based on ongoing monitoring of information concerning the individual's*

MS.5.12.1 professional performance;

MS.5.12.2 judgment; and

MS.5.12.3 clinical or technical skills.

MS.5.13 Departmental or major clinical service recommendations are part of the basis for developing recommendations for continued membership on the medical staff or for delineating individual clinical privileges.

MS.5.14 All individuals who are permitted by law and by the hospital to provide patient care services independently in the hospital have delineated clinical privileges, whether or not they are medical staff members.

MS.5.14.1 The delineation of an individual's clinical privileges includes the limitations, if any, on an individual's privileges to admit and treat patients or direct the course of treatment for the conditions for which the patients were admitted.

MS.5.14.2 There is a mechanism designed to ensure that all individuals with clinical privileges only provide services within the scope of privileges granted.

MS.5.14.3 When physicians or other individuals eligible for delineated clinical privileges are engaged by the hospital to provide patient care services pursuant to a contract, their clinical privileges to admit or treat patients are defined through medical staff mechanisms.

MS.5.14.4 When appropriate, the chief executive officer or his or her designee may grant temporary clinical privileges for a limited period of time on the recommendation of the director of the applicable clinical department, when available, or the president of the medical staff in all other circumstances.

MS.5.15 Whatever mechanism for granting and renewal or revision of clinical privileges is used, evidence indicates that the clinical privileges are hospital specific and based on the individual's demonstrated current competence.

MS.5.15.1 *Privileges are related to*

MS.5.15.1.1 *an individual's documented experience in categories of treatment areas or procedures;*

MS.5.15.1.2 *the results of treatment; and*

MS.5.15.1.3 *the conclusions drawn from organization performance-improvement activities when available.*

MS.5.15.2 Board certification is an excellent benchmark and is considered when delineating clinical privileges.

MS.5.15.3 When privilege delineation is based primarily on experience, the individual's credentials record reflects the specific experience and successful results that form the basis for the granting of privileges.

Medical Staff

MS.5.15.4 When the medical staff uses a system involving classification or categorization of privileges, the scope of each level of privileges is well defined, and the standards to be met by the applicant are stated clearly for each category.

MS.5.15.5 When medical staff clinical departments exist, all licensed independent practitioners are assigned to at least one clinical department and are granted clinical privileges that are relevant to the care provided in that department.

MS.5.15.5.1 There is a satisfactory method to coordinate appraisal for granting or renewal or revision of clinical privileges when an individual currently holding clinical privileges or applying for clinical privileges requests privileges that are relevant to the care provided in more than one department or clinical specialty area.

MS.5.15.6 The exercise of clinical privileges within any department is subject to the rules and regulations of that department and to the authority of the department's director.*

MS.5.15.7 When there are no medical staff clinical departments, all individuals with clinical privileges have their privileges recommended and the quality of their care reviewed through designated medical staff mechanisms, described in the medical staff or governing body bylaws and rules and regulations.

Care of the Patient

Caring for patients continues to be the nucleus of activity around which all health care organization functions revolve. Members of the medical staff are intricately involved in carrying out, and in providing leadership in, all patient care functions conducted by individuals with clinical privileges.

MS.6 Individuals who admit patients are granted specific privileges to do so.

MS.6.1 Individuals are granted the privilege to admit patients to inpatient services in accordance with state law and criteria for standards of medical care established by the medical staff.

MS.6.2 A patient admitted for inpatient care has a medical history taken and an appropriate physical examination performed by a qualified physician.[†]

MS.6.2.1 Qualified oral and maxillofacial surgeons[‡] may perform the medical history and physical examination, if they have such privileges, in order to assess the medical, surgical, and anesthetic risks of the proposed operative and other procedure(s).

---

* **department director** (as related to the intent of this standard) Medical staff department director who has responsibility for clinical directorship of the department.

[†] **physician, qualified** A doctor of medicine or doctor of osteopathy who, by virtue of education, training, and demonstrated competence, is granted clinical privileges by the organization to perform specific diagnostic or therapeutic procedure(s) and who is fully licensed to practice medicine.

[‡] **oral and maxillofacial surgeon, qualified** An individual who has successfully completed a postgraduate program in oral and maxillofacial surgery accredited by a nationally recognized accrediting body approved by the U.S. Department of Education. As determined by the medical staff, the individual is also currently competent to perform a complete history and physical examination in order to assess the medical, surgical, and anesthetic risks of the proposed operative and other procedure(s).

MS.6.2.2 Other licensed independent practitioners who are permitted to provide patient care services independently may perform all or part of the medical history and physical examination, if granted such privileges.

MS.6.2.2.1 The findings, conclusions, and assessment of risk are confirmed or endorsed by a qualified physician prior to major high-risk (as defined by the medical staff) diagnostic or therapeutic interventions.

MS.6.2.2.2 Dentists are responsible for the part of their patients' history and physical examination that relates to dentistry.

MS.6.2.2.3 Podiatrists are responsible for the part of their patients' history and physical examination that relates to podiatry.

MS.6.3 The medical staff determines those noninpatient services (for example, ambulatory surgery), if any, for which a patient must have a medical history taken and appropriate physical examination performed by a qualified physician who has such privileges, except as provided for in MS.6.2.1 through MS.6.2.2.3.

MS.6.4 Individuals provide treatment and perform operative and other procedure(s) within those areas of competence indicated by the scope of their delineated clinical privileges.

MS.6.5 The management of each patient's care is the responsibility of a qualified licensed independent practitioner with appropriate clinical privileges.

MS.6.5.1 Management of a patient's general medical condition is the responsibility of a qualified physician member of the medical staff.

MS.6.5.2 The medical staff, through its designated mechanism, determines the circumstances under which consultation or management by a physician or other qualified licensed independent practitioner is required.

MS.6.6 When a hospital that provides psychiatric or substance-abuse services determines that multidisciplinary treatment plans are appropriate, written policies address multidisciplinary treatment plans.

MS.6.6.1 The written policies provide for appropriate physician involvement in and approval of the multidisciplinary treatment plan.

MS.6.7 In hospitals that do not primarily provide psychiatric or substance-abuse services, the medical staff's role in the care or appropriate referral of patients who are emotionally ill, who become emotionally ill while in the hospital, or who suffer the results of alcoholism or drug abuse is clearly defined in a written plan.

MS.6.8 *There is a mechanism designed to ensure that the same level of quality of patient care is provided by all individuals with delineated clinical privileges, within medical staff departments, across departments, and between members and nonmembers of the medical staff who have delineated clinical privileges.*

Continuing Medical Education

This section focuses on the importance of self-development and continuing medical education, as well as on activities related to improving organization performance.

MS.7 All individuals with delineated clinical privileges participate in continuing education.

MS.7.1 Hospital-sponsored educational activities are offered.

MS.7.1.1 *These activities relate, at least in part, to*

MS.7.1.1.1 the type and nature of care offered by the hospital; and

MS.7.1.1.2 the findings of performance-improvement activities.

MS.7.2 *Each individual's participation in continuing education is documented; and*

MS.7.2.1 considered in decisions about reappointment to the medical staff or renewal or revision of individual clinical privileges.

Medical Staff Role in Performance Improvement

The performance-improvement function defines the framework for the medical staff to improve clinical and nonclinical processes that require medical staff leadership or participation. Where a clinical process is the primary responsibility of physicians, physicians take the leadership role in improving the process.

MS.8 *The medical staff has a leadership role in organization performance-improvement activities designed to*

MS.8.1 ensure that when the performance of a process is dependent primarily on the activities of one or more individuals with clinical privileges (for example, on what surgeons as a component of the medical staff do), the medical staff provides leadership for the process measurement, assessment, and improvement. These processes include, though are not limited to, those within the:

MS.8.1.1 Medical assessment and treatment of patients;

MS.8.1.2 Use of medications; (PI.3.2.2)

MS.8.1.3 Use of blood and blood components; (PI.3.2.3)

MS.8.1.4 Use of operative and other procedure(s); (PI.3.2.1)

MS.8.1.5 Efficiency of clinical practice patterns; and

MS.8.1.6 Significant departures from established patterns of clinical practice.

MS.8.2 ensure that the medical staff participates in the measurement, assessment, and improvement of other patient care processes. The processes include, though are not limited to, those related to:

MS.8.2.1 Education of patients and families;

MS.8.2.2 Coordination of care with other practitioners and hospital personnel, as relevant to the care of an individual patient; and

MS.8.2.3 Accurate, timely, and legible completion of patients' medical records. (IM.3.2.1)

MS.8.3 ensure that when the findings of the assessment process are relevant to an individual's performance, the medical staff is responsible for determining their use in peer review or the ongoing evaluations of a licensed independent practitioner's competence, in accordance with the standards on renewing or revising clinical privileges delineated in this chapter;

MS.8.4 ensure that the findings, conclusions, recommendations, and actions taken to improve organization performance are communicated to appropriate medical staff members; and

MS.8.5 ensure that the medical staff, with other appropriate hospital staff, develops and uses criteria that identify deaths in which an autopsy should be performed.

MS.8.5.1 *The medical staff attempts to secure autopsies in all deaths that meet the criteria.*

MS.8.5.2 The mechanism for documenting permission to perform an autopsy is defined.

MS.8.5.3 There is a system for notifying the medical staff, and specifically the attending practitioner, when an autopsy is being performed.

Standards and Intent Statements for Organization, Bylaws, Rules, and Regulations

The Organized Medical Staff

Individual members of the medical staff care for patients within an organization context. Within this context, members of the medical staff, as individuals and as a group, interface with, and actively participate in, important organization functions.

Standards

MS.1 One or more organized, self-governing medical staffs have overall responsibility for the quality of the professional services provided by individuals with clinical privileges,* as well as the responsibility of accounting therefore to the governing body.

MS.1.1 *Each medical staff has the following characteristics:*

MS.1.1.1 *It includes fully licensed physicians and may include other licensed individuals permitted by law and by the hospital to provide patient care services independently in the hospital (both physicians and these other individuals are referred to as "licensed independent practitioners"[†]).*

MS.1.1.2 *All medical staff members have delineated clinical privileges that define the scope of patient care services they may provide independently in the hospital.*

MS.1.1.3 *All medical staff members and all others with delineated clinical privileges are subject to medical staff and departmental bylaws, rules and regulations, and policies and are subject to review as part of the organization's performance-improvement activities.*

Intent of MS.1 Through MS.1.1.3

A single, organized, self-governing medical staff provides clear responsibility and accountability for overseeing the quality of care being provided to a hospital's patient population. However, mergers and consolidations in the health care field have created a growing proliferation of new organization structures and relationships that can blur this traditional line of patient care accountability. This is particularly true when a single hospital serves different patient populations in geographically distant sites.

To accommodate these realities, it is important to acknowledge that within a single hospital organization, separate medical staffs—providing care to separate patient populations at *geographically distinct sites*—may comfortably co-exist and be capable of meeting the accountabilities envisioned within these standards.

To assure that these accountabilities are met, the following bases are to be used in determining whether a hospital may have more than one medical staff:

---

* **clinical privileges** Authorization granted by the appropriate authority (for example, a governing body) to a practitioner to provide specific care services in an organization within well-defined limits, based on the following factors, as applicable: license, education, training, experience, competence, health status, and judgment.

† **licensed independent practitioner** Any individual permitted by law and by the organization to provide care and services without direction or supervision, within the scope of the individual's license and consistent with individually granted clinical privileges.

- A hospital with a single governing body that has one inpatient care delivery site has a single, organized medical staff;
- A hospital with a single governing body that has multiple inpatient care delivery sites, all of which serve the same patient population and are geographically *proximate* to the other sites, has a single organized medical staff;
- A hospital with a single governing body that has multiple inpatient care delivery sites, some or all of which serve different patient populations, but are geographically *proximate* to the other sites, may have either a single organized medical staff for all sites or separate medical staffs at two or more sites; and
- A hospital with a single governing body that has multiple inpatient care delivery sites, each of which serves a *different* patient population and is geographically *distant* from the other site(s), may have a separate organized medical staff at each site.

A single group of physicians that constitute a medical staff may be accountable for services in more than one accredited hospital.

Note: *A hospital site is considered* proximate or distant *based on whether the patient population does or does not have access to and does or does not use the services provided at the other sites. The* patient population *consists of those individuals who choose the hospital as their primary source of inpatient care and for whom the hospital designs and delivers services consistent with its mission.*

Documents Governing Activities of the Organized Medical Staff

Medical staff self-governance is delineated in documents that set out how the medical staff will organize and govern its affairs. Most typically it is delineated in bylaws, and essential components to be delineated are identified in these standards, including medical staff membership, the credentialing process, the role of the medical staff executive committee, and the structures necessary for ongoing activities of the medical staff. The medical staff bylaws, as adopted or amended by the medical staff and approved by the governing body, create a system of mutual rights and responsibilities between members of the medical staff and the hospital.

Standard

MS.2 *Each medical staff develops and adopts bylaws and rules and regulations to establish a framework for self-governance of medical staff activities and accountability to the governing body.*

Intent of MS.2

This intent of this standard is self-evident.

Standards

MS.2.1 Medical staff bylaws and rules and regulations are adopted by the medical staff and approved by the governing body before becoming effective. Neither body may unilaterally amend the medical staff bylaws or rules and regulations.

MS.2.2 Medical staff bylaws and rules and regulations create a framework within which medical staff members can act with a reasonable degree of freedom and confidence.

MS.2.3 *Medical staff bylaws include provisions for at least the following:*

Medical Staff

MS.2.3.1 An executive committee of the medical staff;

MS.2.3.2 Fair-hearing and appellate review mechanisms for medical staff members and other individuals holding clinical privileges;

MS.2.3.3 Mechanisms for corrective action, including indications and procedures for automatic and summary suspension of an individual's medical staff membership or clinical privileges;

MS.2.3.4 A description of the medical staff's organization, including categories of medical staff membership, when such exist, and appropriate officer positions, with the stipulation that each officer is a medical staff member;

MS.2.3.4.1 The bylaws define

MS.2.3.4.1.1 the method of selecting officers,

MS.2.3.4.1.2 the qualifications, responsibilities, and tenures of officers, and

MS.2.3.4.1.3 the conditions and mechanisms for removing officers from their positions;

MS.2.3.5 Requirements for frequency of meetings and for attendance;

MS.2.3.6 A mechanism designed to provide for effective communication among the medical staff, hospital administration, and governing body;

MS.2.3.6.1 *If there are multiple levels of governance, there is an established mechanism for the medical staff to communicate with all levels of governance involved in policy decisions affecting patient care services in the hospital.*

MS.2.3.7 A mechanism for adopting and amending the medical staff bylaws, rules and regulations, and policies; and

MS.2.3.8 Medical staff representation and participation in any hospital deliberation affecting the discharge of medical staff responsibilities.

Intent of MS.2.1 Through MS.2.3.8
The intents of these standards are self-evident.

Standards
MS.2.4 When necessary, the medical staff bylaws and rules and regulations are revised to reflect the hospital's current practices with respect to medical staff organization and functions.

MS.2.4.1 The medical staff bylaws, rules and regulations, and policies and the governing body's bylaws do not conflict.

MS.2.4.2 If significant changes are made in the medical staff bylaws, rules and regulations, or policies, medical staff members and other individuals who have delineated clinical privileges are provided with revised texts of the written materials.

Intent of MS.2.4 Through MS.2.4.2
The intent of these standards are self-evident.

Standard
MS.2.5 In hospitals participating in professional graduate education programs, the rules and regulations and policies specify the mechanisms by which house staff members are supervised by medical staff members in carrying out their patient care responsibilities.

Intent of MS.2.5
Medical staff rules and regulations and policies define the mechanism(s) designed for supervising house staff. For example, the supervising medical staff member is often required to countersign the history and physical examination taken by a house staff member, or the supervising medical staff member may change a statement made in the record by the house staff member and initial the change. Such actions are consistent with the supervisory rules of most hospital teaching programs.

Privileging of the house staff is not required, but if house staff members are not privileged, they must have a job description. The job descriptions do not have to be for the individual, but for the level of care that person is allowed to provide. Medical staff rules and regulations and policies also delineate those house staff members who may write patient care orders and the circumstances under which they may do so, without prohibiting the medical staff from writing orders.

Medical Staff Executive Function (Committee)
The medical staff executive committee has responsibilities, delegated by the medical staff, within the organization governance function. The medical staff executive committee carries out its work within the context of the organization functions of governance, leadership, and performance improvement. The medical staff executive committee is delegated the primary authority over activities related to the functions of self-governance of the medical staff and over activities related to the functions of performance improvement of the professional services provided by individuals with clinical privileges. The leadership of the hospital includes the medical staff leaders.*

Standard
MS.3 *The medical staff is organized to accomplish its functions.*

Intent of MS.3
The intent of this standard is self-evident.

---

* **leader** An individual who sets expectations, develops plans, and implements procedures to assess and improve the quality of the organization's governance, management, clinical, and support functions and processes. Leaders include, when applicable to the organization's structure, the owners, members of the governing body, the chief executive officer and other senior managers, and the leaders of the licensed independent practitioners.

Medical Staff

Standards

MS.3.1 There is an executive committee of the medical staff.

MS.3.1.1 The executive committee's function, size, and composition and the method of selecting its members are defined in the medical staff bylaws.

MS.3.1.2 The chief executive officer of the hospital or his or her designee attends each executive committee meeting on an ex-officio basis, with or without vote.

MS.3.1.3 No medical staff member actively practicing in the hospital is ineligible for membership on the executive committee solely because of his or her professional discipline or specialty.

MS.3.1.4 A majority of voting executive committee members are fully licensed physician members of the medical staff actively practicing in the hospital.

MS.3.1.5 The executive committee is empowered to act for the medical staff in the intervals between medical staff meetings.

MS.3.1.6 The executive committee is responsible for making medical staff recommendations directly to the governing body for its approval.

MS.3.1.6.1 *Such recommendations pertain to at least the following:*

MS.3.1.6.1.1 The medical staff's structure;

MS.3.1.6.1.2 The mechanism used to review credentials and to delineate individual clinical privileges;

MS.3.1.6.1.3 Recommendations of individuals for medical staff membership;

MS.3.1.6.1.4 Recommendations for delineated clinical privileges for each eligible individual;

MS.3.1.6.1.5 The participation of the medical staff in organization performance-improvement activities;

MS.3.1.6.1.6 The mechanism by which medical staff membership may be terminated; and

MS.3.1.6.1.7 The mechanism for fair-hearing procedures.

MS.3.1.7 The executive committee receives and acts on reports and recommendations from medical staff committees, clinical departments, and assigned activity groups.

Intent of MS.3.1 Through MS.3.1.7

Medical staff bylaws define in detail the medical staff executive committee's function, size, composition, method of selecting committee members, and frequency of committee meetings. Minutes of all deliberations of this committee are available for review and indicate that the committee carries out its stated functions.

Medical staff executive committee functions include, but are not limited to,
- reviewing and acting on reports of medical staff committees, departments, and other assigned activity groups;
- reviewing the credentials of applicants for medical staff membership and delineated clinical privileges;
- making recommendations regarding the mechanism designed to review credentials and delineate individual clinical privileges to the governing body;
- making recommendations for medical staff membership and delineated clinical privileges to the governing body (subject to any applicable state law);
- organizing the medical staff's organization performance-improvement activities and establishing a mechanism designed to conduct, evaluate, and revise such activities;
- developing the mechanism by which medical staff membership may be terminated; and
- creating the mechanism designed for use in fair hearing procedures.

Documenting its conclusions, recommendations, and actions taken is an important function of the medical staff executive committee.

An appropriate committee structure is established to carry out the functions and activities of the medical staff executive committee. The medical staff as a whole may serve as the executive committee if it meets the requirements specified in MS.3.1 through MS.3.1.6.1.7. In smaller and less complex hospitals where the entire medical staff functions as the executive committee, it is often designated as a "committee of the whole." Other nonphysician medical staff executive committee members may include, but are not limited to, the chief executive officer or designee, the nurse executive, or a governing body member. The medical staff bylaws define the voting status of committee members who are not medical staff members.

Department Leadership

The leadership section outlines the role of medical staff department leaders. This responsibility is part of the organization leadership role of the medical staff, which is further explained in the "Leadership" chapter (pages 143 through 162).

Standards

MS.4 *When medical staff clinical departments exist:*

MS.4.1 *Each department has effective leadership.*

MS.4.1.1 The director of each department is certified by an appropriate specialty board, or affirmatively establishes comparable competence, through the credentialing process.

Note: *MS.4.1.1 applies only to those medical staff department directors who were appointed or reappointed after January 1, 1992. A medical staff department is currently defined as any structural unit of the medical staff (whether it is called a department, a service, a unit, a section, or something similar) in which the director is responsible for recommending privileges for individuals in the unit to the medical staff executive committee.*

Intent of MS.4 Through MS.4.1.1

The responsibilities of the medical staff department directors include
- establishing, together with medical staff and administration, the type and scope of services required to meet the needs of the patients and the hospital;

- developing and implementing policies and procedures that guide and support the provision of services in the department;
- recommending to the medical staff the criteria for clinical privileges in the department;
- recommending clinical privileges for each department member;
- continuing surveillance of the professional performance of all individuals with clinical privileges in the department; and
- assessing and improving the quality of care and services provided in the department.

Fulfilling these responsibilities requires knowledge about the care and services provided in the department. Board certification can be an excellent benchmark of the individual's capability to fulfill these responsibilities.

Therefore, the director of each medical staff department is certified by an appropriate specialty board, or the medical staff affirmatively determines, through the privilege delineation process, that he or she possesses comparable competence. An appropriate specialty board is one

- that certifies in a specialty relevant to the services provided in the department and
- whose certification can serve as a reliable benchmark. The certification process includes examination of credentials (including supervised training and experience in an appropriate educational program), knowledge of the applicant at the time of certification, and issuance of a certificate based on the adequacy of those credentials and knowledge.

The hospital and its medical staff determine whether the specialty is relevant to the services provided by the department. This determination is documented.

Note: *For some hospital departments, there may be only one or two relevant specialty boards. Examples of such situations include (1) the American Board of Radiology and the American Osteopathic Board of Radiology for diagnostic radiology services; (2) the American Board of Pathology and the American Osteopathic Board of Pathology for pathology services; and (3) the American Board of Nuclear Medicine and the American Board of Radiology (or American Osteopathic Board of Radiology) for nuclear medicine services.*

For other hospital departments, there may be a number of relevant specialty boards. Examples include (1) the American Board of Emergency Medicine, the American Board of Surgery, the American Board of Pediatrics, and the American Board of Internal Medicine for emergency services; and (2) the American Board of Internal Medicine, the American Board of Family Practice, and the American Board of Pediatrics for family medicine services.

To decide whether certification by a specific board is a reliable benchmark, the hospital and its medical staff determine both the relevance of the board certification to the individual's responsibilities and the credibility of the board providing this certification. In making the latter determination, the hospital and its medical staff can rely on the determination of an appropriate external agency, such as recognition by or membership in the American Board of Medical Specialties, the Council on Post-Secondary Accreditation (in dentistry), or the American Osteopathic Association. As an alternative, the hospital and its medical staff may conduct their own review of a board's criteria and processes for providing certification.

In the absence of board certification, the medical staff establishes, through the privilege delineation process, that a candidate for directorship possesses competence comparable to that of an individual with board certification. This can be accomplished by identifying the knowledge and skills expected of a board-certified individual and determining that the candidate has such knowledge and skills.

Standards

MS.4.2 Medical staff department directors' responsibilities are specified in the medical staff bylaws and rules and regulations.

MS.4.2.1 Each department director is responsible for the following:

MS.4.2.1.1 All clinically related activities of the department;

MS.4.2.1.2 All administratively related activities of the department, unless otherwise provided for by the hospital;

MS.4.2.1.3 Continuing surveillance of the professional performance of all individuals in the department who have delineated clinical privileges;

MS.4.2.1.4 Recommending to the medical staff the criteria for clinical privileges that are relevant to the care provided in the department;

MS.4.2.1.5 Recommending clinical privileges for each member of the department;

MS.4.2.1.6 Assessing and recommending to the relevant hospital authority off-site sources for needed patient care services not provided by the department or the organization.

MS.4.2.1.7 through MS.4.2.1.15 have been relocated to the "Leadership" chapter of this book. The standard numbers in parentheses indicate where these standards are now located in the "Leadership" chapter.

MS.4.2.1.7 *the integration of the department or service into the primary functions of the organization; (LD.2.1)*

MS.4.2.1.8 *the coordination and integration of interdepartmental and intradepartmental services; (LD.2.2)*

MS.4.2.1.9 *the development and implementation of policies and procedures that guide and support the provision of services; (LD.2.3)*

MS.4.2.1.10 *the recommendations for a sufficient number of qualified and competent persons to provide care or service; (LD.2.4)*

MS.4.2.1.11 *the determination of the qualifications and competence of department or service personnel who are not licensed independent practitioners and who provide patient care services; (LD.2.5)*

MS.4.2.1.12 *the continuous assessment and improvement of the quality of care and services provided; (LD.2.6)*

MS.4.2.1.13 *the maintenance of quality control programs, as appropriate; (LD.2.7)*

MS.4.2.1.14 *the orientation and continuing education of all persons in the department or service; and (LD.2.8)*

MS.4.2.1.15 *recommendations for space and other resources needed by the department or service. (LD.2.9)*

Intent of MS.4.2 Through MS.4.2.1.15

The medical staff director of each department is responsible for the ongoing, effective operation of the department and for assessing and improving its activities. Such responsibilities encompass not only the internal functioning, but also the integration of each department into the overall functioning of the organization.

Fulfilling these responsibilities enables the integration of the department into the overall functioning of the organization, the coordination of its services with those of other departments, and the improvement of the services it provides.

Standards and Intent Statements for Credentialing

The Credentialing Process*

The medical staff is responsible for a credentialing process. The credentialing process includes a series of activities designed to collect relevant data that will serve as the basis for decisions regarding appointments and reappointments to the medical staff, as well as delineation of clinical privileges for individual members of the medical staff. Although the specific information used to make decisions regarding appointments and reappointments is at the discretion of the individual organization, the range of information used should be explicit. In addition, within, and at the discretion of, an organization, the specific information required for appointment may differ from the information required for reappointment. The required information should include data on qualifications such as licensure and training or experience, and data on actual performance that is collected and assessed initially and in an ongoing process.

Standards

MS.5 The organization establishes mechanisms for hospital-specific appointment and reappointment of medical staff members and for granting and renewing or revising hospital-specific clinical privileges.

MS.5.1 The governing body appoints and reappoints to the medical staff and grants initial, renewed, or revised clinical privileges, based on medical staff recommendations, in accordance with the bylaws, rules and regulations, and policies of the medical staff and of the hospital.

MS.5.1.1 Each applicant for medical staff membership is oriented to these bylaws, rules and regulations, and policies and agrees in writing that his or her activities as a medical staff member will be bound by them.

---

* **credentialing** The process of obtaining, verifying, and assessing the qualifications of a health care practitioner to provide patient care services in or for a health care organization.

MS.5.1.2 Individuals in administrative positions who desire medical staff membership or clinical privileges are subject to the same procedures as all other applicants for membership or privileges.

Intent of MS.5 Through MS.5.1.2

The processes of appointment and reappointment to the medical staff and of granting and renewing or revising clinical privileges all involve using information about an applicant to decide whether the individual will be authorized to practice within the hospital and, if so, what the individual will be authorized to do within the hospital. Because these processes consider the specific hospital's characteristics, supportive resources, and staff, the processes are designed to yield hospital-specific decisions. Hospital-specific decisions mean that the privileges granted to an applicant are based not only on the applicant's qualifications, but also on consideration of the procedures and types of care or services that can be performed or provided within the hospital. If an applicant's training or experience is in a specific area(s), corresponding privileges can be granted only if the hospital has adequate facilities, equipment, number and types of qualified support personnel, and any necessary support services. Specialists whose services may be contracted, such as radiologists and emergency service physicians, are also granted hospital-specific privileges.

Because the decisions to be made, and the data on which these decisions rely, are quite similar for appointment and reappointment and for granting, renewing, and revising clinical privileges, the sequence of steps in the processes and the sources of data often overlap and may occur in unison. For this reason, these standards identify the common characteristics of all these processes and draw attention to the few differences.

MS.5.1 stipulates that applicable medical staff and hospital bylaws, rules and regulations, and policies specify that the governing body grants medical staff membership and clinical privileges. The governing body reviews recommendations made by the medical staff executive committee, the documentation on which recommendations are based, and records of any hearings or appeals addressing adverse decisions. The governing body's decision is based on the information submitted and is guided by legitimate patient care considerations, medical staff bylaws, and rules and regulations.

The governing body is not bound by the medical staff recommendations but has the ultimate authority to render a decision, adverse or not, as long as the decision is neither arbitrary, capricious, discriminatory, nor contrary to the bylaws.

The mechanisms used for appointment and reappointment to the medical staff and for granting, renewing, and revising clinical privileges are fully described in the bylaws, rules and regulations, and policies of the medical staff and the hospital, and yield hospital-specific decisions. The description of each mechanism is detailed enough to permit tracking of the procedural steps in an applicant's appointment or reappointment to the medical staff or in the initial granting, renewing, or revising of clinical privileges. Separate decisions are made regarding an application for medical staff membership or application for clinical privileges. To avoid unnecessary delay, time limits are specified for each step of each process.

Appointment or reappointment to the medical staff is not granted solely on the basis of an applicant's membership on the medical staff of another hospital. Individuals in administrative positions who are on the medical staff or who seek appointment to the medical staff are appointed or reappointed through the same procedure used for all other members of the medical staff. Likewise, individuals in administrative positions who have or who seek clinical privileges achieve and maintain their clinical privileges through the same procedure used for all other individuals with delineated clinical privileges. The applicant, medical staff, and governing body adhere to the mechanism designed for hospital-specific appointment and reappointment and for granting, renewing, and revising delineated clinical privileges.

An applicant for appointment or reappointment or clinical privileges is informed of existing bylaws, rules and regulations, and policies regarding the application process and agrees, in writing, that he or she will be bound by them. Medical staff members and other individuals who have delineated clinical privileges are informed of any changes in existing bylaws, rules and regulations, and policies of the medical staff and governing body.

Standards

MS.5.2 There are mechanisms, including a fair hearing and appeal process, for addressing adverse decisions for existing medical staff members and other individuals holding clinical privileges for renewal, revocation, or revision of clinical privileges.

MS.5.2.1 *These mechanisms may differ for medical staff members and other individuals holding clinical privileges.*

Intent of MS.5.2 Through MS.5.2.1

Mechanisms for fair hearing and appeal processes, in accordance with all applicable statutes, are designed to allow adverse decisions to be aired and understood. The hospital has a mechanism (as specified in the medical staff and governing body bylaws) designed to provide a fair hearing, which includes the scheduling of hearing requests, the procedures hearings are to follow, the composition of the hearing committee, and the agenda for the hearing. Similarly, the hospital has a mechanism (as specified in the medical staff and governing body bylaws) designed for appealing an adverse decision.

Standards

MS.5.3 *The mechanisms for appointment or reappointment and initial granting and renewal or revision of clinical privileges are*

MS.5.3.1 approved and implemented by the medical staff and governing body;

MS.5.3.2 fully documented in the medical staff bylaws, rules and regulations, and policies; and

MS.5.3.3 *described to each applicant.*

Intent of MS.5.3 Through MS.5.3.3

The mechanisms designed for appointment or reappointment and for granting, renewing, or revising clinical privileges are formally approved by the medical staff and governing body and are fully documented in the medical staff bylaws, rules and regulations, and policies. The description of each mechanism is detailed enough to permit tracking of the procedural steps taken when examining credentials files.

Standards

MS.5.4 The mechanisms provide for professional criteria that are specified in the medical staff bylaws and uniformly applied to all applicants for medical staff membership, medical staff members, or applicants for delineated clinical privileges. These criteria constitute the basis for granting initial or continuing medical staff membership and for granting initial, renewed, or revised clinical privileges.

MS.5.4.1 Each clinical department makes recommendations to the medical staff regarding professional criteria for clinical privileges.

MS.5.4.2 The professional criteria are designed to assure the medical staff and governing body that patients will receive quality care.

MS.5.4.3 The professional criteria at least pertain to evidence of current licensure, relevant training or experience, current competence, and ability to perform the privileges requested.*

Intent of MS.5.4 Through MS.5.4.3

The medical staff bylaws specify professional criteria for medical staff membership and for clinical privileges. These criteria are designed to help establish an applicant's background, current competence, and physical and mental ability to discharge patient care responsibilities. Moreover, they are designed to help assure the medical staff and governing body that patients will receive quality care. *Four core criteria* are essential to establishing and maintaining a qualified and competent medical staff:
- Current licensure;
- Relevant training or experience;
- Current competence; and
- Ability to perform the privileges requested.

Each credentials file indicates that these criteria are uniformly and individually applied.

Each clinical department develops its own criteria for determining an applicant's ability to provide patient care services within the scope of clinical privileges requested. These criteria are in addition to the medical staff criteria for medical staff membership and clinical privileges. For renewing or revising clinical privileges, these criteria could include procedures performed and their outcomes and could be based on pertinent results of review of operative and other procedure(s),† medication usage, blood usage, medical records, and other performance-improvement activities, as appropriate. Additional criteria may be based on mortality rates, utilization management, meeting and committee attendance, and risk-management data.

The hospital may elect to add other reasonable criteria, such as the ability to provide adequate facilities and support services for the applicant and the applicant's patients; patient care needs for additional staff members with the applicant's skill and training; current evidence of adequate professional liability insurance; and the applicant's geographic location. When medical staff bylaws specify additional criteria, their uniform application is documented in credentials files.

---

* The Americans with Disabilities Act (ADA) bars certain discrimination based on physical or mental impairment. Toward preventing such discrimination, the act prohibits or mandates various activities.

Hospitals need to determine the applicability of the ADA to their medical staff. If applicable, the hospital should examine its privileging or credentialing procedures as to how and when it ascertains and confirms the ability of an applicant to perform the privileges requested. For example, the act may prohibit inquiry as to the physical or mental health status of an applicant prior to making an offer of membership and privileges, but may not prohibit such inquiry after an offer is extended (contingent on the ascertainment of health status). The act does not appear to prohibit inquiry as to the ability of the applicant (without specific reference to health matters) to perform the specific privileges requested. Thus, this latter inquiry may be made and confirmed as a component of the application process.

The Joint Commission cannot provide legal advice to hospitals. However, the Joint Commission has and will absolutely construe MS.5.4 through MS.5.4.3, MS.5.10.1, and MS.5.10.1.1 in such a manner as not to be inconsistent with hospital efforts to comply with the ADA.

† **operative and other procedures** Includes operative, other invasive, and noninvasive procedures, such as radiotherapy, hyperbaric treatment, CAT scan, and MRI, that place the patient at risk. The focus is on procedures and is not meant to include medications that place the patient at risk.

Appropriate documentation for each of the *four core criteria* includes, but is not limited to, the following:

- **Current licensure.** Current licensure is verified at the time of appointment and initial granting of clinical privileges by a letter or computer printout obtained from the appropriate state licensing board or from any state licensing board if in a federal service. Verifying current licensure with the licensing board by telephone is also acceptable, if this verification is documented. There is a mechanism designed to ensure verification and documentation of current licensure for all practitioners.

   At the time of reappointment to the medical staff, and at the time of renewal or revision of clinical privileges, current licensure is confirmed with the primary source or by viewing the applicant's current license or registration.

- **Relevant training or experience.** At the time of appointment and initial granting of clinical privileges, the hospital obtains verification of relevant training or experience from the primary source(s), whenever feasible. This includes letters from professional schools (for example, medical and dental) or residency or postdoctoral programs. Information from credentials verification organizations (CVOs), such as the American Medical Association's Physician Masterfile, may also be used. (See the Example of Implementation for MS.5.4.3.2 for a list of principles that can be used to evaluate a CVO's services.)

   Information from secondary sources, including the Federation of State Medical Boards Action Data Bank, is considered supplementary and not sufficient, by itself, to meet this condition. For applicants who have just completed training in an approved residency or postdoctoral program, a letter from the program director is sufficient. Board certification in medical specialties is confirmed by the listings in the *Official ABMS Directory of Board Certified Medical Specialists*, published by the American Board of Medical Specialists (ABMS). If the applicant or hospital uses a phrase such as "board qualified," such qualification is confirmed by a letter from the relevant ABMS specialty board.

- **Current competence.** Current competence at the time of appointment and initial granting of clinical privileges cannot be determined on the basis of board certification or admissibility alone. Rather, it is verified in writing by individuals personally acquainted with the applicant's professional and clinical performance, either in teaching facilities or in other hospitals. The hospital has obtained information directly from the primary source(s) in the form of letters from authoritative sources, which contain informed opinions on each applicant's scope and level of performance. Letters that describe the applicant's actual clinical performance in general terms, the satisfactory discharge of his or her professional obligations as a medical staff member, and his or her ethical performance are acceptable. However, ideally, letters also address at least the following two specific aspects of current competence:
  - For applicants in fields doing operative and other procedure(s), the types of operative procedures performed as the surgeon of record; the handling of complicated deliveries; or the skill demonstrated in performing invasive procedures, including information on appropriateness and outcomes. In the case of applicants in nonsurgical fields, the types and outcomes of medical conditions managed by the applicant as the responsible physician should be addressed.
  - The applicant's clinical judgment and technical skills.

   At the time of reappointment, current competence is determined by the results of performance-improvement activities (see MS.5.12.3 and MS.5.15.1.3), peer recommendations (see MS.5.7), and departmental or major clinical service recommendations (see MS.5.13).

- **Ability to perform privileges requested.** The applicant's ability to perform privileges requested must be evaluated. This evaluation is documented in the individual's credentials file. Such documentation may include the applicant's statement that no health problems exist that could affect his or her practice; such a statement, however, must be confirmed. For an applicant for appointment or initial clinical privileges, the statement is confirmed by the director of a training program, by the chief of services or chief of staff at another hospital at which the applicant holds privileges, or by a currently licensed physician designated by the hospital. For an applicant for reappointment or renewal or revision of clinical privileges, the statement is confirmed by at least a countersignature on the applicant's statement by a department director in a departmentalized hospital or by the chief of staff in a nondepartmentalized hospital (see MS.5.10.1.1).

Standards

MS.5.4.3.1 For an applicant for initial appointment to the medical staff and for initial granting of clinical privileges, the hospital verifies information about the applicant's licensure, specific training, experience, and current competence provided by the applicant with information from the primary source(s) whenever feasible.

MS.5.4.3.1.1 Action on an individual's application for appointment or initial clinical privileges is withheld until the information is available and verified.

MS.5.4.3.2 *The hospital is also encouraged to consider additional information concerning the applicant from other sources, including the Federation of State Medical Boards Physician Disciplinary Data Bank. These databases and other sources may provide the hospital with information that is new or that may flag an inconsistency when compared with the individual's application.*

Intent of MS.5.4.3.1 Through MS.5.4.3.2

When hospitals evaluate an individual for clinical privileges, they verify the information in the application that relates to the individual's licensure, training, experience, and competence from primary sources (see Notes, pages 257 and 258), whenever possible. In addition, the standards recognize the value of obtaining information from other sources, such as the AMA Physician Masterfile.

Hospitals may use an external agency (for example, county medical society, hospital association, AMA Physician Masterfile) to collect information from primary sources provided that the agency also furnishes the hospital with any additional information from the primary source(s). The hospital then evaluates the individual's credentials by comparing the information in his or her application with the information provided by the primary source to the external agency. Additional information may be required to supplement the external agency information to fully evaluate each applicant.

The "Health Care Quality Improvement Act of 1986" (Title IV of Pub. L. 99-660, as amended) requires the establishment of the National Practitioner Data Bank (NPDB), to which the following information must be reported in a timely manner by the appropriate agencies:
- Medical malpractice payments;
- Licensure disciplinary actions;
- Adverse clinical privilege actions taken by a health care entity (for example, hospitals, health maintenance organizations, group practices); and
- Adverse actions affecting professional society membership.

Adverse professional review actions taken by health care entities against health care practitioners other than physicians and dentists may also be reported.

Under the act, hospitals must query the NPDB at the time of initial medical staff appointments and initial granting of clinical privileges, as well as at least every two years thereafter for information on physicians, dentists, and other health care practitioners granted clinical privileges. Such queries should be performed on a timely basis to ensure that all relevant information is received by an organization before finalizing appointments and the granting of privileges.

It may not always be feasible to obtain information from the primary source. In rare or occasional instances, a primary source, such as an educational institution or a hospital, no longer exists, or the applicant's records have been lost or destroyed. Applicants may have received education, training, and experience partially or wholly in a foreign country, and for political or other reasons, information regarding their professional background is not accessible. However, when undue delay occurs in deriving information from a primary source, medical staff appointment is withheld pending receipt of this information. Under these circumstances, the applicant may be given temporary privileges for a limited time in accordance with applicable medical staff bylaws, rules and regulations, and policies, as well as state and federal regulations. Designated equivalent sources or other reliable secondary sources may also be used if there has been a documented attempt to contact the primary source.

Notes:
1. *Designated equivalent sources are selected agencies that have been determined to maintain a specific item(s) of credential information that is identical to the information at the primary source. These designated equivalent sources are*
   - *the American Medical Association (AMA) Physician Masterfile for verification of a physician's medical school graduation and residency completion;*
   - *the American Board of Medical Specialties (ABMS) for verification of a physician's board certification;*
   - *the Education Commission for Foreign Medical Graduates (ECFMG) for verification of a physicians graduation from a foreign medical school.*

      These designated equivalent sources may be used by a hospital, a network, the network's components, or a credentials verification organization (CVO) that is used by the hospital, network or its components. Other designated equivalent sources may exist for certain applicants, such as for licensure verification of an applicant in the federal service. The hospital should communicate with the Joint Commission to determine whether a specific agency qualifies as a designated equivalent source under such special circumstances. The physician profiles from the AMA Physician Masterfile also include other primary source-reported information that is similar to primary source-verified information provided by a CVO. Use of this additional information is subject to the guidelines set forth in Note 2.

2. *Any hospital, network, or component thereof that bases its decisions in part on information obtained from a CVO should have confidence in the completeness, accuracy, and timeliness of that information. To achieve this level of confidence in the information, the hosopital, the network, or component should evaluate the agency providing the information initially and then periodically as appropriate. The principles that guide such an evaluation include the following:*
   - *The agency makes known to the user what data and information it can provide.*
   - *The agency provides documentation to the user describing how its data collection, information development, and verification process(es) are performed.*
   - *The user is provided with sufficient, clear information on database functions. This information includes any limitations of information available from the agency (for example, practitioners not included in the database); the time frame for agency responses to requests for information; and a summary overview of quality control processes relating to data integrity, security, transmission accuracy, and technical specifications.*
   - *The user and agency agree on the format for transmission of an individual's credentials information from the agency.*

- *The user can easily discern which information, transmitted by the agency, is from a primary source and which is not.*
- *When the agency transmits information that can become out of date (such as licensure, board certification), it provides the date on which the information was last updated from the primary source.*
- *The agency certifies that the information transmitted to the user accurately presents the information obtained by it.*
- *The user can discern whether the information transmitted by the agency from a primary source is* all *the primary source information in the agency's possession pertinent to a given item and, if not, where additional information can be obtained.*
- *When necessary, the user can engage the agency's quality control processes to resolve concerns about transmission errors, inconsistencies, or other data issues that may be identified from time to time.*

Standards

MS.5.4.4 Decisions on reappointments or on revocation, revision, or renewal of clinical privileges must consider criteria that are directly related to the quality of care.

MS.5.4.4.1 Such decisions are subject to a fair hearing and appeal process.

MS.5.4.5 Decisions on appointments or on granting of clinical privileges must consider criteria that are directly related to the quality of care.

Intent of MS.5.4.4 Through MS.5.4.5

The determination of initial appointment or reappointment or of granting, revocation, revision, or renewal of clinical privileges is based on a variety of criteria. If criteria are used that are unrelated to the quality of care or professional competency, evidence exists that the impact of resulting decisions on the quality of care is evaluated. For medical staff members and other individuals holding clinical privileges, the decisions about the impact on the quality of care is subject to a fair hearing and appeal process (as are credentialing decisions that are based on criteria directly related to the quality of care).

Standards

MS.5.5 *The medical staff bylaws, rules and regulations, or policies define the information to be provided by each applicant for appointment or reappointment to the medical staff and initial, renewed, or revised clinical privileges, including at least*

MS.5.5.1 previously successful or currently pending challenges to any licensure or registration (state or district, Drug Enforcement Administration) or the voluntary relinquishment of such licensure or registration;

MS.5.5.2 voluntary or involuntary termination of medical staff membership or voluntary or involuntary limitation, reduction, or loss of clinical privileges at another hospital; and

MS.5.5.3 *involvement in a professional liability action under circumstances specified in the medical staff bylaws, rules and regulations, and policies.*

MS.5.5.3.1 At a minimum, final judgments or settlements involving the individual are reported.

Intent of MS.5.5 Through MS.5.5.3.1
Each applicant for medical staff appointment or reappointment or for initial, renewed, or revised clinical privileges provides certain information defined in the medical staff bylaws, rules and regulations, or policies. This information is intended to supplement the core criteria (current licensure, relevant training or experience, current competence, and ability to perform privileges requested). Specifically, medical staff bylaws and rules and regulations require each applicant to provide information regarding the following, when applicable:
- Challenges to any licensure or registration, or voluntary or involuntary relinquishment of such licensure or registration; and
- Voluntary or involuntary termination of medical staff membership, or voluntary or involuntary limitation, reduction, or loss of clinical privileges.

Bylaws and rules and regulations also specify the circumstances under which an individual is to report involvement in a professional liability action. At a minimum, these circumstances include final judgments or settlements in which the medical staff member is involved.

Each credentials file for medical staff members and others with clinical privileges contains information relative to standards MS.5.5.1, MS.5.5.2, and MS.5.5.3.1.

Standard
MS.5.6 *Appointment or reappointment to the medical staff and the initial granting and renewal or revision of clinical privileges are also based on information regarding the applicant's competence.*

Intent of MS.5.6
The intent of this standard is self-evident.

Standard
MS.5.7 Deliberations by the medical staff in developing recommendations for appointment to or termination from the medical staff and for the initial granting, revision, or revocation of clinical privileges include information provided by a peer(s)* of the applicant.

Intent of MS.5.7
Recommendation(s) from peers (appropriate practitioners in the same professional discipline as the applicant—for example, physician, dentist, podiatrist—who have firsthand knowledge of the applicant) are in the credentials files and reflect part of the basis for recommending appointment or reappointment and granting, renewing, or revising clinical privileges. If there are no peers on the medical staff who are knowledgeable about the applicant, a peer recommendation is obtained from outside the hospital, such as the local county or regional medical society, or a practitioner in the community or on the medical staff of another hospital. It is advisable, when possible, to include recommendations from an individual(s) in the same specialty. The peer recommendations refer, as appropriate, to relevant training or experience; current competence; fulfillment of obligations as a medical staff member; and

---

* **peer** Individual from the same discipline (for example, physician and physician, dentist and dentist) and with essentially equal qualifications.

any effects of health status on the privileges being recommended. Sources for peer recommendations may include

- an organization performance-improvement committee, the majority of whose members are the applicant's peers;
- a reference letter(s) or documented telephone conversation(s) about the applicant from a peer(s) who is a member of the hospital's medical staff or who is from outside the hospital, but knowledgeable about the applicant's competence;
- a department or major clinical service chairperson who is a peer; or
- the medical staff executive committee, the majority of whose members are the applicant's peers.

Standards

MS.5.8 *A structured procedure, as defined by medical staff bylaws, rules and regulations, and medical staff policies, is used for the expeditious processing of complete applications for appointment, reappointment, and initial, renewed, or revised clinical privileges.*

MS.5.8.1 A separate record is maintained for each individual requesting medical staff membership or clinical privileges.

MS.5.8.2 Complete applications are acted on within a reasonable period of time, as specified in the medical staff bylaws.

Intent of MS.5.8 Through MS.5.8.2

As described in the intent of MS.5, medical staff bylaws clearly define the steps in processing applications for medical staff appointment or reappointment and initial, renewed, or revised clinical privileges. Unnecessary delay is avoided by establishing specific time frames (for example, 90 days) for expeditiously processing complete applications.

The complexity of, and myriad details involved in, the application process for appointment or reappointment to the medical staff and for granting, renewing, or revising clinical privileges require that individual records be maintained for each applicant.

Standard

MS.5.9 Gender, race, creed, or national origin are not used in making decisions regarding the granting or denying of medical staff membership or clinical privileges.

Intent of MS.5.9

Decisions regarding appointment, reappointment, and initial, renewed, or revised clinical privileges are rendered based on the merits of the applicant's credentials. Discriminatory practices based on gender, race, creed, or national origin are not part of the decision-making process.

Standards

MS.5.10 *Each applicant*

MS.5.10.1 consents to the inspection of records and documents pertinent to his or her licensure, specific training, experience, current competence, and ability to perform the privileges requested*, and, if requested, appears for an interview;

Intent of MS.5.10 and MS.5.10.1
There is a procedure for obtaining and documenting the consent of all applicants for medical staff membership and clinical privileges allowing the hospital to inspect all records and documents pertaining to the individual's licensure, specific training, experience, current competence, and ability to perform privileges requested. The applicant's consent extends to supplying information necessary for obtaining relevant records and documents and to appearing for an interview with the credentials committee, medical staff executive committee, or other representatives of the medical staff, hospital administration, or the governing board, if required or requested. The applicant's consent is documented.

Standard
MS.5.10.1.1 The bylaws, rules and regulations, and policies of the medical staff indicate that the applicant for reappointment or renewal of clinical privileges is required to submit any reasonable evidence of current ability to perform privileges that may be requested.

Intent of MS.5.10.1.1
Evidence of current ability to perform privileges requested may be required of applicants for reappointment or renewal of clinical privileges. In many cases, the applicant's department chairperson or chief of service will evaluate the individual's ability to perform privileges requested.

In instances in which there is doubt about an applicant's ability to perform privileges requested, an evaluation by someone other than the applicant's department chairperson or chief of service may be necessary to resolve the issue. The request for such an evaluation rests with the executive committee of the medical staff. Many federal facilities and some private hospitals require an annual physical examination at reappointment; such an examination meets the intent of this standard.

Standards
MS.5.10.2 [Each applicant] pledges to provide for continuous care for his or her patients; and

MS.5.10.3 *[Each applicant] acknowledges any provisions in the medical staff bylaws for release and immunity from civil liability.*

Intent of MS.5.10.2 and MS.5.10.3
Medical staff members are responsible for providing for continuous care for their patients. Hospital bylaws require applicants to acknowledge this responsibility and any provisions in the medical staff bylaws for release and immunity from civil liability.

Standard
MS.5.11 Appointment or reappointment to the medical staff and the granting, renewal, or revision of clinical privileges are made for a period of no more than two years.

---

* See footnote on **credentialing process** on page 235.

Intent of MS.5.11
A period of no more than two years is established between appointment and subsequent reappointments and between granting, renewing, or revising clinical privileges in order to review the performance of medical staff members and of other practitioners granted clinical privileges. This review can be done more often, if desired. Initial appointment is granted for a provisional period, which is specified in the medical staff bylaws and consistently applied to all applicants.

Standards

MS.5.12 *Appraisal for reappointment to the medical staff or renewal or revision of clinical privileges is based on ongoing monitoring of information concerning the individual's*

MS.5.12.1 professional performance;

MS.5.12.2 judgment; and

MS.5.12.3 clinical or technical skills.

Intent of MS.5.12 Through MS.5.12.3
A reappraisal is conducted at the time of reappointment or renewal or revision of clinical privileges. The reappraisal includes confirmation of adherence to medical staff membership requirements stated in medical staff bylaws, rules and regulations, and policies.

Relevant information from organization performance-improvement activities is considered when evaluating professional performance, judgment, and clinical or technical skills (see the "Improving Organization Performance" chapter, PI.4.2, and MS.8 through MS.8.4). Any results of peer review of the individual's clinical performance are also included.

Credentials files contain clear evidence (for example, a signed statement by the department chairperson or service chief recommending that privileges be granted) that the full range of privileges has been included in the reappraisal, particularly privileges for performing high-risk procedures and treating high-risk conditions, and that the information is substantive and practitioner specific.

The effectiveness of the reappraisal process may be measured by objective documentation in credentials files that, within the past few years, an individual's privileges were increased, reduced, or terminated because of
1. assessments of his or her documented performance;
2. nonuse of privileges for a high-risk procedure or treatment over a period of two years; or
3. emergence of new technologies.

Because hospital practices and clinical techniques change over time, it would be unusual if clinical privileges were not to change also.

Standard

MS.5.13 Departmental or major clinical service recommendations are part of the basis for developing recommendations for continued membership on the medical staff or for delineating individual clinical privileges.

Intent of MS.5.13
Credentials files used for reappointment to the medical staff or granting, renewing, or revising clinical privileges contain the recommendation of the department or major clinical service to which the individual

is applying. This recommendation comes through the department or major clinical service chairperson (see MS.5.12) or chief of staff in a nondepartmentalized hospital. Mechanisms designed for department or major clinical service recommendations may include:
- Concurrence (evidenced, at least, by the signature of the department or major clinical service chairperson) with the applicant-specific recommendations (including an applicant-specific statement of the basis thereof) of a departmental committee concerning the applicant's reappointment to the medical staff or initial granting, renewal, or revision of clinical privileges. One way to provide an applicant-specific statement is to write a narrative. Another way could consist of a document indicating that the department chairperson, chief of staff, or an appropriate committee has reviewed every item required by the Joint Commission and the hospital's medical staff bylaws, rules and regulations, and policies and made an applicant-specific judgment about each required item or
- An applicant-specific statement (including the basis thereof) by the chairperson of the department or major clinical service noting that the individual is recommended for reappointment to the medical staff or to be granted or have renewed the requested privileges. If the chairperson of the department or major clinical service is the applicant's peer, this recommendation can also fulfill the requirement for MS.5.7.

In either case, the department or major clinical service recommendation is based on evidence of relevant training and experience; current competence (including any available relevant results of ongoing appraisals of clinical performance and practice); any effects of health status on the privileges to be recommended; and, if the level or scope of privileges was previously increased, evidence of satisfactory performance in accordance with those privileges.

Standard

MS.5.14 All individuals who are permitted by law and by the hospital to provide patient care services independently in the hospital have delineated clinical privileges, whether or not they are medical staff members.

Intent of MS.5.14

MS.5.14 applies to all individuals permitted by law and by the hospital to provide patient care services independently without supervision or direction. These individuals have delineated clinical privileges, whether or not they are medical staff members. "Delineated," when used in the context of clinical privileges, means an accurate, detailed, and specific description of the clinical privileges granted. Granting "general" privileges in any specialty does not meet the intent of these standards because the limits and specifics of the privileges granted are not defined.

The clinical qualifications of medical staff members are relevant to their responsibilities within the organization structure. Some individuals who may be permitted by law and by the hospital to provide patient care independently in the hospital, such as clinical psychologists, might not be members of the hospital's medical staff either because of limitations on medical staff membership under applicable law or regulation or because of hospital choice. Such individuals, if providing patient care without supervision or direction, must have delineated clinical privileges. A supervised clinical practitioner may have a job description rather than delineated clinical privileges.

Clinical privileges may be defined several ways. For example, they may be categorized by
- practitioner specialty;
- level of training and experience;
- patient risk categories;
- lists of procedures or treatments; or

- any combination of the methods listed above—particularly a combination of patient risk categories and lists of procedures.

An acceptable model might combine patient risk categories with specific clinical areas (for example, cardiovascular diseases, endocrinology), invasive procedures (for example, cardiac catheterization, Swan-Ganz catheterization), biopsies, and interpretation of special noninvasive procedures (for example, echocardiograms). This approach to categorizing and listing procedures for recommending clinical privileges can be applied to all specialties.

Standard
MS.5.14.1 The delineation of an individual's clinical privileges includes the limitations, if any, on an individual's privileges to admit and treat patients or direct the course of treatment for the conditions for which the patients were admitted.

Intent of MS.5.14.1
Regardless of the method used to delineate an individual's clinical privileges, the limitations on the individual's privileges to admit and treat patients or direct the course of treatment for the conditions for which the patients were admitted are specified. For example, it may be that a surgeon with privileges to perform cardiovascular procedures, including arterial grafts, is not privileged to resect abdominal aortic aneurysms until he or she has been observed while operating under supervision by an experienced cardiovascular surgeon. Likewise, it may be that a family practitioner is privileged to admit a suspected myocardial infarction case to the coronary care unit but is not privileged to manage that patient.

Standard
MS.5.14.2 There is a mechanism designed to ensure that all individuals with clinical privileges only provide services within the scope of privileges granted.

Intent of MS.5.14.2
The medical staff or hospital uses an effective mechanism(s) designed for assessing whether individuals with clinical privileges provide services within the scope of privileges granted. For example, the operating room staff compares the surgical procedures to be performed against a current list of the practitioners' privileges; the special care unit staff screen admission requests and orders for special procedures against a current list of the practitioners' privileges in the special care unit; a pharmacist or other designated individual(s) verifies prescribing or ordering privileges by nonmembers of the medical staff or limitations on prescribing or ordering for certain medical staff members. These lists are updated as changes in clinical privileges for each practitioner are made.

Standard
MS.5.14.3 When physicians or other individuals eligible for delineated clinical privileges are engaged by the hospital to provide patient care services pursuant to a contract, their clinical privileges to admit or treat patients are defined through medical staff mechanisms.

Intent of MS.5.14.3
The hospital often contracts with physicians or other individuals eligible for clinical privileges to perform patient care services. A specified medical staff mechanism(s) defines the clinical privileges of

Medical Staff

these individuals to admit or treat patients. This mechanism(s) is defined in the medical staff bylaws, rules and regulations, and policies and includes the criteria for granting clinical privileges.

Standard

MS.5.14.4 When appropriate, the chief executive officer or his or her designee may grant temporary clinical privileges for a limited period of time on the recommendation of the director of the applicable clinical department, when available, or the president of the medical staff in all other circumstances.

Intent of MS.5.14.4

Issuing temporary clinical privileges can fulfill an important patient care need. For example, if the only physician privileged to perform a highly specialized service becomes ill, disabled, or is otherwise unable to perform this service, a qualified physician may be brought in and given temporary privileges to provide this service while his or her credentials are being reviewed for medical staff membership and delineated clinical privileges. In another example, a recently recruited applicant whose specialized training is needed to perform necessary procedures may be given temporary privileges while his or her credentials are being processed. In both examples, however, the applicant would have to possess a current license and registration and demonstrate current competence.

Medical staff bylaws, rules and regulations, or policies stipulate that all temporary privileges granted must be time limited. The chief executive officer (CEO) is authorized to grant such privileges on the recommendation of either the applicable clinical department chairperson or the president of the medical staff, and a provision for a designee(s) to act in the absence of the CEO, when necessary (for example, in an emergency), is specified in the bylaws, rules and regulations, or policies of the medical staff or hospital.

Medical staff bylaws, rules and regulations, or policies describe the mechanism used for granting temporary clinical privileges and stipulate that, in an emergency, any medical staff member who has clinical privileges is permitted to provide any type of patient care necessary as a life-saving measure or to prevent serious harm—regardless of his or her medical staff status or clinical privileges—provided that the care provided is within the scope of the individual's license.

In facilities with approved graduate medical education programs, such emergency care may be provided by properly supervised members of the house staff.

Primary source verification (a documented phone call is acceptable) of licensure and current competence is required prior to the granting of temporary privileges.

Standards

MS.5.15 Whatever mechanism for granting and renewal or revision of clinical privileges is used, evidence indicates that the clinical privileges are hospital specific and based on the individual's demonstrated current competence.

MS.5.15.1 *Privileges are related to*

MS.5.15.1.1 *an individual's documented experience in categories of treatment areas or procedures;*

MS.5.15.1.2 *the results of treatment; and*

MS.5.15.1.3 the conclusions drawn from organization performance-improvement activities when available.

MS.5.15.2 Board certification is an excellent benchmark and is considered when delineating clinical privileges.

MS.5.15.3 When privilege delineation is based primarily on experience, the individual's credentials record reflects the specific experience and successful results that form the basis for the granting of privileges.

Intent of MS.5.15 Through MS.5.15.3
Regardless of the mechanisms used to grant, renew, or revise clinical privileges, the privileges granted are hospital specific—that is, they are based not only on the applicant's qualifications, but also on a consideration of the procedures and types of care or services that can be performed or provided within a specific hospital. If an applicant's training or experience is in a specific area(s), corresponding privileges can be granted only if the hospital has adequate facilities, equipment, number and types of qualified support personnel, and any necessary support services. When services of a specialist, such as a radiologist or an emergency service physician, are contracted, the specialist is granted hospital-specific privileges.

Granting, renewal, or revision of clinical privileges is also based on the individual's demonstrated current competence. For renewal or revision of privileges, this may be determined, in part, by a review of relevant results of medical staff performance improvement activities. Specific instances of treatment outcomes and the results of other assessment and improvement activities may also be included. An evaluation of the applicant's clinical judgment and technical skills in performing procedures and in patient treatment and management is also included in an evaluation of current competence.

Note: *Current competence is addressed in MS.5.4.3 and MS.5.12 through MS.5.12.3.*

Standard
MS.5.15.4 When the medical staff uses a system involving classification or categorization of privileges, the scope of each level of privileges is well defined, and the standards to be met by the applicant are stated clearly for each category.

Intent of MS.5.15.4
The intent of this standard is self-evident.

Standard
MS.5.15.5 When medical staff clinical departments exist, all licensed independent practitioners are assigned to at least one clinical department and are granted clinical privileges that are relevant to the care provided in that department.

Intent of MS.5.15.5
The intent of this standard is self-evident.

Standard

MS.5.15.5.1 *There is a satisfactory method to coordinate appraisal for granting or renewal or revision of clinical privileges when an individual currently holding clinical privileges or applying for clinical privileges requests privileges that are relevant to the care provided in more than one department or clinical specialty area.*

Intent of MS.5.15.5.1
The intent of this standard is self-evident.

Standard

MS.5.15.6 *The exercise of clinical privileges within any department is subject to the rules and regulations of that department and to the authority of the department's director.**

Intent of MS.5.15.6
The intent of this standard is self-evident.

Standard

MS.5.15.7 *When there are no medical staff clinical departments, all individuals with clinical privileges have their privileges recommended and the quality of their care reviewed through designated medical staff mechanisms, described in the medical staff or governing body bylaws and rules and regulations.*

Intent of MS.5.15.7
The intent of this standard is self-evident.

Care of the Patient
Caring for patients continues to be the nucleus of activity around which all health care organization functions revolve. Members of the medical staff are intricately involved in carrying out, and in providing leadership in, all patient care functions conducted by individuals with clinical privileges.

Standards

MS.6 *Individuals who admit patients are granted specific privileges to do so.*

MS.6.1 Individuals are granted the privilege to admit patients to inpatient services in accordance with state law and criteria for standards of medical care established by the medical staff.

MS.6.2 A patient admitted for inpatient care has a medical history taken and an appropriate physical examination performed by a qualified physician.†

---

* **department director** (as related to the intent of this standard) Medical staff department director who has responsibility for clinical directorship of the department.

† **physician, qualified** A doctor of medicine or doctor of osteopathy who, by virtue of education, training, and demonstrated competence, is granted clinical privileges by the organization to perform specific diagnostic or therapeutic procedure(s) and who is fully licensed to practice medicine.

MS.6.2.1 Qualified oral and maxillofacial surgeons* may perform the medical history and physical examination, if they have such privileges, in order to assess the medical, surgical, and anesthetic risks of the proposed operative and other procedure(s).

MS.6.2.2 Other licensed independent practitioners who are permitted to provide patient care services independently may perform all or part of the medical history and physical examination, if granted such privileges.

MS.6.2.2.1 The findings, conclusions, and assessment of risk are confirmed or endorsed by a qualified physician prior to major high-risk (as defined by the medical staff) diagnostic or therapeutic interventions.

MS.6.2.2.2 Dentists are responsible for the part of their patients' history and physical examination that relates to dentistry.

MS.6.2.2.3 Podiatrists are responsible for the part of their patients' history and physical examination that relates to podiatry.

MS.6.3 The medical staff determines those noninpatient services (for example, ambulatory surgery), if any, for which a patient must have a medical history taken and appropriate physical examination performed by a qualified physician who has such privileges, except as provided for in MS.6.2.1 through MS.6.2.2.3.

MS.6.4 Individuals provide treatment and perform operative and other procedure(s) within those areas of competence indicated by the scope of their delineated clinical privileges.

MS.6.5 The management of each patient's care is the responsibility of a qualified licensed independent practitioner with appropriate clinical privileges.

MS.6.5.1 Management of a patient's general medical condition is the responsibility of a qualified physician member of the medical staff.

MS.6.5.2 The medical staff, through its designated mechanism, determines the circumstances under which consultation or management by a physician or other qualified licensed independent practitioner is required.

Intent of MS.6 Through MS.6.5.2

Only individuals granted specific privileges in accordance with state law and criteria for standards of medical care established by the medical staff may admit patients to inpatient services. Regardless of the method used to delineate an individual's clinical privileges, the limitations on the individual's privileges to admit and treat patients or direct the course of treatment for the conditions, which the patients were admitted are specified. However, the medical staff may choose to also recommend that a

---

* **oral and maxillofacial surgeon, qualified** An individual who has successfully completed a postgraduate program in oral and maxillofacial surgery accredited by a nationally recognized accrediting body approved by the U.S. Department of Education. As determined by the medical staff, the individual is also currently competent to perform a complete history and physical examination in order to assess the medical, surgical, and anesthetic risks of the proposed operative and other procedure(s).

licensed independent practitioner be granted temporary appointment as defined by organization or medical staff policy. A qualified physician is responsible for the inpatient's history and appropriate physical examination, but nonphysicians, such as dentists and podiatrists, may be responsible for patient histories and physical findings respective to their areas of expertise.

Medical staff bylaws may specify that oral and maxillofacial surgeons be granted privileges to admit patients to inpatient services for oral and maxillofacial surgery; to perform and record the history and physical examination; and to assess the medical, surgical, and anesthetic risk of an operative and other procedure(s).

Other nonphysician, licensed independent practitioners (for example, depending on state law and the hospital's decision, nurse anesthetists, nurse practitioners, physician assistants, and midwives) may be granted privileges to perform all or part of a history and physical examination. Under these circumstances, the medical staff determines which diagnostic and therapeutic interventions are high risk; before these interventions are performed, a physician must confirm or endorse the findings, conclusions, and assessment of risk.

MS.6.3 introduces the same principles for a medical history and physical examination for ambulatory situations as required for inpatients. MS.6.5 through MS.6.5.2 address responsibilities for the management of care.

Standards

MS.6.6 When a hospital that provides psychiatric or substance-abuse services determines that multidisciplinary treatment plans are appropriate, written policies address multidisciplinary treatment plans.

MS.6.6.1 The written policies provide for appropriate physician involvement in and approval of the multidisciplinary treatment plan.

Intent of MS.6.6 and MS.6.6.1

The intents of these standards are self-evident.

Standard

MS.6.7 In hospitals that do not primarily provide psychiatric or substance-abuse services, the medical staff's role in the care or appropriate referral of patients who are emotionally ill, who become emotionally ill while in the hospital, or who suffer the results of alcoholism or drug abuse is clearly defined in a written plan.

Intent of MS.6.7

The intent of this standard is self-evident.

Standard

MS.6.8 *There is a mechanism designed to ensure that the same level of quality of patient care is provided by all individuals with delineated clinical privileges, within medical staff departments, across departments, and between members and nonmembers of the medical staff who have delineated clinical privileges.*

Intent of MS.6.8
Patients are entitled to receive a comparable level of care for the same condition, regardless of which department provides the care (for example, internal medicine, pediatrics), the discipline of the practitioner (for example, surgeon, podiatrist), or the setting (for example, ambulatory clinic, inpatient department). This comparability is evaluated through performance-improvement activities (for example, by using similar indicators) and by the clinical privileging process (for example, by establishing similar criteria for similar privileges).

Continuing Medical Education
This section focuses on the importance of self-development and continuing medical education, as well as on activities related to improving organization performance.

Standards

MS.7 All individuals with delineated clinical privileges participate in continuing education.

MS.7.1 Hospital-sponsored educational activities are offered.

MS.7.1.1 *These activities relate, at least in part, to*

MS.7.1.1.1 the type and nature of care offered by the hospital; and

MS.7.1.1.2 the findings of performance-improvement activities.

MS.7.2 *Each individual's participation in continuing education is documented; and*

MS.7.2.1 considered in decisions about reappointment to the medical staff or renewal or revision of individual clinical privileges.

Intent of MS.7 Through MS.7.2.1
Continuing education is an adjunct to maintaining clinical skills and current competence. Many state departments of licensure and registration require a specified number of hours of continuing education to maintain licensure. These same hours may be used to satisfy hospital requirements, provided that the education programs are acceptable to the hospital. Educational activities relate, at least in part, to the privileges granted.

A hospital of sufficient size and resources is the ideal site to sponsor educational activities that are consonant with the hospital's mission, the population served, and the patient care services provided. Results of organization performance-improvement activities can augment the source material and database for hospital-sponsored educational activities. Documentation of each individual's participation in such educational activities is required.

Medical Staff Role in Performance Improvement
The performance-improvement function defines the framework for the medical staff to improve clinical and nonclinical processes that require medical staff leadership or participation. Where a clinical process is the primary responsibility of physicians, physicians take the leadership role in improving the process.

Standards

MS.8 *The medical staff has a leadership role in organization performance-improvement activities designed to*

MS.8.1 ensure that when the performance of a process is dependent primarily on the activities of one or more individuals with clinical privileges (for example, on what surgeons as a component of the medical staff do), the medical staff provides leadership for the process measurement, assessment, and improvement. These processes include, though are not limited to, those within the:

MS.8.1.1 Medical assessment and treatment of patients;

MS.8.1.2 Use of medications; (PI.3.1.1)

MS.8.1.3 Use of blood and blood components; (PI.3.1.1)

MS.8.1.4 Use of operative and other procedure(s); (PI.3.1.1)

MS.8.1.5 Efficiency* of clinical practice patterns; and

MS.8.1.6 Significant departures from established patterns of clinical practice.

MS.8.2 *ensure that the medical staff participates in the measurement, assessment, and improvement of other patient care processes. The processes include, though are not limited to, those related to:*

MS.8.2.1 Education of patients and families;

MS.8.2.2 Coordination of care with other practitioners and hospital personnel, as relevant to the care of an individual patient; and

MS.8.2.3 Accurate, timely, and legible completion of patients' medical records. (IM.3.2.1)

MS.8.3 ensure that when the findings of the assessment process are relevant to an individual's performance, the medical staff is responsible for determining their use in peer review or the ongoing evaluations of a licensed independent practitioner's competence, in accordance with the standards on renewing or revising clinical privileges delineated in this chapter;

MS.8.4 ensure that the findings, conclusions, recommendations, and actions taken to improve organization performance are communicated to appropriate medical staff members; and

Intent of MS.8 Through MS.8.4

Members of the medical staff are involved in activities to measure, assess, and improve performance on an organizationwide basis. They are involved in

---

* **efficiency** The relationship between the outcomes (results of care) and the resources used to deliver care.

- the measurement of outcomes and of processes, as defined in the "Improving Organization Performance" chapter, and in the assessment of performance in relation to the design of processes and their expected or intended outcomes, in order to identify opportunities for improvement;
- evaluation of individuals with clinical privileges whose performance is questioned as a result of the measurement and assessment activities;
- communication to appropriate medical staff members of the findings, conclusions, recommendations, and actions taken to improve organization performance; and
- implementation of changes to improve performance.

The medical staff should assure a leadership role in the improvement of clinical processes that are dependent primarily on individuals with clinical privileges, such as surgery, physical examinations, and prescribing of medication.

Standards

MS.8.5 ensure that the medical staff, with other appropriate hospital staff, develops and uses criteria that identify deaths in which an autopsy should be performed.

MS.8.5.1 *The medical staff attempts to secure autopsies in all deaths that meet the criteria.*

MS.8.5.2 The mechanism for documenting permission to perform an autopsy is defined.

MS.8.5.3 There is a system for notifying the medical staff, and specifically the attending practitioner, when an autopsy is being performed.

Intent of MS.8.5 Through MS.8.5.3

The intent of these standards are self-evident.

Medical Staff

Selected Medical Staff Standards Pertinent to Admission, Performing a History and Physical Examination, and Treatment by Physicians and Other Licensed Independent Practitioners

1. All licensed independent practitioners have delineated privileges.

MS.5.14 All individuals who are permitted by law and by the hospital to provide patient care services independently in the hospital have delineated clinical privileges, whether or not they are medical staff members.

MS.5.14.1 The delineation of an individual's clinical privileges includes the limitations, if any, on an individual's privileges to admit and treat patients or direct the course of treatment for the conditions for which the patients were admitted.

MS.5.14.2 There is a mechanism designed to ensure that all individuals with clinical privileges only provide services within the scope of privileges granted.

2. All licensed independent practitioners are assigned to a medical staff department.

MS.5.15.5 *When medical staff clinical departments exist, all licensed independent practitioners are assigned to at least one clinical department and are granted clinical privileges that are relevant to the care provided in that department.*

3. Admission is by a licensed independent practitioner with privileges.

MS.6 *Individuals who admit patients are granted specific privileges to do so.*

MS.6.1 Individuals are granted the privilege to admit patients to inpatient services in accordance with state law and criteria for standards of medical care established by the medical staff.

4. A history and physical exam is performed by a physician.

MS.6.2 A patient admitted for inpatient care has a medical history taken and an appropriate physical examination performed by a qualified physician.*

4(a) Exceptions

MS.6.2.1 Qualified oral and maxillofacial surgeons[†] may perform the medical history and physical examination, if they have such privileges, in order to assess the medical, surgical, and anesthetic risks of the proposed operative and other procedure(s).

---

* **physician, qualified** A doctor of medicine or doctor of osteopathy who, by virtue of education, training, and demonstrated competence, is granted clinical privileges by the organization to perform specific diagnostic or therapeutic procedure(s) and who is fully licensed to practice medicine.

† **oral and maxillofacial surgeon, qualified** An individual who has successfully completed a postgraduate program in oral and maxillofacial surgery accredited by a nationally recognized accrediting body approved by the U.S. Department of Education. As determined by the medical staff, the individual is also currently competent to perform a complete history and physical examination in order to assess the medical, surgical, and anesthetic risks of the proposed operative and other procedure(s).

MS.6.2.2 Other licensed independent practitioners who are permitted to provide patient care services independently may perform all or part of the medical history and physical examination, if granted such privileges.

MS.6.2.2.1 The findings, conclusions, and assessment of risk are confirmed or endorsed by a qualified physician prior to major high-risk (as defined by the medical staff) diagnostic or therapeutic interventions.

MS.6.2.2.2 Dentists are responsible for the part of their patients' history and physical examination that relates to dentistry.

MS.6.2.2.3 Podiatrists are responsible for the part of their patients' history and physical examination that relates to podiatry.

MS.6.3 The medical staff determines those noninpatient services (for example, ambulatory surgery), if any, for which a patient must have a medical history taken and appropriate physical examination performed by a qualified physician who has such privileges, except as provided for in MS.6.2.1 through MS.6.2.2.3.

5. Treatment is managed by a licensed independent practitioner with privileges.

MS.6.5 The management of each patient's care is the responsibility of a qualified licensed independent practitioner with appropriate clinical privileges.

MS.6.5.1 Management of a patient's general medical condition is the responsibility of a qualified physician member of the medical staff.

MS.6.5.2 The medical staff, through its designated mechanism, determines the circumstances under which consultation or management by a physician or other qualified licensed independent practitioner is required.

Nursing

Overview

The nurse executive
- ensures the continuous and timely availability of nursing services to patients;
- ensures that nursing standards of patient care and standards of nursing practice are consistent with current nursing research findings and nationally recognized professional standards;
- implements the findings of current research from nursing and other literature into the policies and procedures governing the provision of nursing care;
- ensures that nursing service staff carry out applicable processes in the patient care and organizationwide functions described in this book;
- assigns responsibility to individuals or groups of nursing staff members to act on improving the nursing service's performance;
- actively participates in the hospital's leadership functions;
- collaborates with other hospital leaders in designing and providing patient care and services;
- participates with hospital leaders in providing for a sufficient number of appropriately qualified nursing staff members to care for patients; and
- develops, presents, and manages the nursing services' portion of the hospital's budget.

To promote quality patient care, nursing services, including nursing care, are provided on a continuous basis, 24 hours a day, 7 days a week, to those patients requiring such care and service. Nursing monitors each patient's status and coordinates the provision of nursing care while assisting other professionals in implementing their plans of care. To accomplish this goal, the hospital provides a sufficient number of qualified nursing staff members to
- assess the patient's nursing care needs;
- plan and provide nursing care interventions;
- prevent complications and promote improvement in the patient's comfort and wellness; and
- alert other care professionals to the patient's condition, as appropriate.

Standards

The following is a list of all standards for this function. If you have a questions about a term used here, please check the Glossary, pages 281 through 307. Terms that are critical to the understanding of the standard are defined in the footnotes of the next section of this chapter.

NR.1 Nursing services are directed by a nurse executive who is a registered nurse qualified by advanced education and management experience.

NR.2 The nurse executive has the authority and responsibility for establishing standards of nursing practice.

NR.3 Nursing policies and procedures, nursing standards of patient care, and standards of nursing practice are approved by the nurse executive or a designee(s).

NR.4 *The nurse executive and other nursing leaders participate with leaders from the governing body, management, medical staff, and clinical areas in planning, promoting, and conducting organizationwide performance-improvement activities.*

Nursing

Standards and Intent Statements for Nursing

Standard
NR.1 Nursing services are directed by a nurse executive who is a registered nurse qualified by advanced education and management experience.

Intent of NR.1
The nurse executive directs the nursing service. "Directs" does not mean that the nurse executive has to have line authority over those who provide nursing care. In most situations such authority and responsibility involve some degree of line authority, with several nurse-employees who report to an executive other than the nurse executive.

Even when the organization's structure is decentralized, an identified nurse leader at the executive level coordinates and provides authority and accountability for the nurse executive functions listed in the following paragraphs.

This applies to organizations that decentralize nursing as a part of an overall decentralized organization structure (for example, patient-focused models, decentralization by service units or product-line or service-line management), rather than organizations in which *only* nursing is decentralized. In a decentralized organization, a nurse leader is identified to function at the executive level to provide effective and coordinated leadership to deliver nursing care. In those organizations, the identified nurse leader may be the elected chair of a nursing council or nursing executive committee, or designated by some other means. Identified nurse leaders functioning in the executive role do so for at least one year or more.

Organizations that result from mergers and consolidations often serve different patient populations in *geographically distant sites*. To accommodate these realities, it is important to acknowledge that organization designs can be flexible yet capable of meeting the accountabilities envisioned within this standard and its intent.

Regardless of the organization's structure or scope of the nurse executive's line authority, one nurse executive or nurse leader at the executive level, qualified by advanced education and management experience, has the authority and responsibility to address the following four functions:
1. Developing organizationwide patient care programs, policies, and procedures that describe how patients' nursing care needs or patient populations receiving nursing care are assessed, evaluated, and met;
2. Developing and implementing the organization's plans for providing nursing care to those patients requiring nursing care;
3. Participating with governing body, management, medical staff, and clinical leaders in the organization's decision-making structures and processes; and
4. Implementing an effective, ongoing program to measure, assess, and improve the quality of nursing care delivered to patients.

The nurse executive is currently licensed as a registered professional nurse in the state, commonwealth, or territory as required by law. The nurse executive's education and experience are directly related to the hospital's stated mission and also to the nursing care needs of the patient population(s) served. When the nurse executive is appointed, his or her education and experience, with respect to the following six factors, are considered in making the appointment decision:
1. The education requirements for the position. The registered nurse executive possesses the knowledge and skills associated with a master's degree in nursing or related field or another appropriate

postgraduate degree, or there is evidence of a plan to obtain these qualifications. It is *not* the master's degree that is required but the knowledge and skills associated with graduate-level education. When this is not the case, there is a written plan to obtain this level of knowledge and skill. Specifically, knowledge of the following is sought:
   a. Current theoretical approaches to delivering nursing care and strategies for examining and applying relevant concepts and
   b. Current leadership, management, and performance-improvement concepts and the ability to participate in developing and implementing strategies to address opportunities for improving the nursing care delivered to patients;
2. The organization's scope and complexity and the position's authority and responsibility;
3. The scope and complexity of the nursing care needs of the major patient population(s) served;
4. The education and experience required for leadership peers. For example, in an organization that expects its chief financial officer and other corporate officers to possess at least a master's degree in their appropriate professional discipline, it's reasonable for the organization to expect the nurse executive to possess a master's degree. When leadership peers are expected to have a doctoral degree or appropriate professional certification, the nurse executive possesses similar qualifications;
5. The availability of nursing support staff and services to help the nurse executive address the responsibilities required in this chapter; and
6. Applicable federal, state, and local law and regulation that affect the nurse executive's education or experience.

Decentralized organization structures with geographically distant sites also have a process for selecting, electing, or appointing one appropriately prepared, identified nurse as its nurse executive. This individual
- participates in defined and established meetings of the organization's corporate leaders (when such leaders exist), with other clinical and managerial leaders and
- has the authority to speak on behalf of nursing to the same extent that other organization leaders speak for their respective disciplines or departments. The identified nurse executive possesses the requisite knowledge and skills associated with graduate-level education.

Note: *A hospital site is considered proximate or distant based on whether the patient population does or does not have access to and does or does not use the services provided at the other sites. The patient population consists of those individuals who choose the hospital as their primary source of inpatient care and for whom the hospital designs and delivers services consistent with its mission.*

Standards

NR.2 The nurse executive has the authority and responsibility for establishing standards of nursing practice.

NR.3 Nursing policies and procedures, nursing standards of patient care, and standards of nursing practice are approved by the nurse executive or a designee(s).

NR.4 *The nurse executive and other nursing leaders participate with leaders from the governing body, management, medical staff, and clinical areas in planning, promoting, and conducting organizationwide performance-improvement activities.*

Intent of NR.2 Through NR.4

The nurse executive, registered nurses, and other designated nursing staff members write
- nursing policies and procedures;
- nursing standards of patient care;
- standards of nursing practice; and
- standards to measure, assess, and improve patient outcomes.

The nurse executive's authority and responsibility for these activities is defined in a contract, written agreement, letter, memorandum, job or position description, or other document. Regardless of how nursing policies, procedures, and nursing standards are developed, the nurse executive, or a designee(s), exercises final authority over those associated with providing nursing care. This authority may be delegated. Nonetheless, the nurse executive is responsible for ensuring that nursing policies, procedures, and standards describe and guide how the nursing staff provides the nursing care required by all patients and patient populations served by the hospital and as defined in the hospital's plan(s) for providing nursing care.

All nursing policies, procedures, and standards are defined, documented, and accessible to the nursing staff in written or electronic format. Regardless of how it is documented, each element is approved by the nurse executive, or designee(s), before it is implemented.

The nurse executive and other nursing staff members collaborate with appropriate governing body, management, medical staff, and other clinical and managerial leaders in developing, implementing, reviewing, revising, and monitoring organizationwide performance-improvement activities.

Glossary

abuse   Intentional maltreatment of an individual which may cause injury, either physical or psychological. *See also* neglect.

  mental abuse   Includes humiliation, harassment, and threats of punishment or deprivation.

  physical abuse   Includes hitting, slapping, pinching, or kicking. Also includes controlling behavior through corporal punishment.

  sexual abuse   Includes sexual harassment, sexual coercion, and sexual assault.

accreditation   A determination by an accrediting body that an eligible health care organization complies with applicable Joint Commission standards. *See also* accreditation decision.

accreditation appeal   The process through which an organization that has been preliminarily denied Joint Commission accreditation exercises its right to a hearing by an Appeals Hearing Panel, followed by a review of the Panel's report and recommendation by the Joint Commission's Board of Commissioners.

Accreditation Committee   The committee of the Joint Commission's Board of Commissioners responsible for oversight of its accreditation process.

accreditation cycle   The three-year term at the conclusion of which accreditation expires unless a full survey is performed.

accreditation decision   The conclusion regarding an organization's status after evaluation of the results of a Joint Commission on-site survey; recommendations of the surveyor(s); and any other relevant information, such as documentation of compliance with standards, documentation of plans to correct deficiencies, or evidence of recent improvements. The decision may be accreditation with commendation, accreditation (with or without type I recommendations), provisional accreditation, conditional accreditation, preliminary nonaccreditation, or not accredited.

  accreditation with commendation   The highest accreditation decision awarded by the Joint Commission to an organization that has demonstrated exemplary performance.

  accreditation (with or without type I recommendations)   A determination by an accrediting body that an eligible health care organization complies with applicable Joint Commission standards.

  provisional accreditation   An accreditation decision that results when an organization has demonstrated substantial compliance with the selected structural standards used in the first of two surveys conducted under the Joint Commission's Early Survey Policy, Option One. The second survey is conducted approximately six months after the first to allow the organization sufficient time to demonstrate a track record of performance. Provisional accreditation status continues until the organization completes a full survey.

  conditional accreditation   An accreditation decision that results when an organization is not in substantial compliance with Joint Commission standards but is believed to be capable of achieving acceptable compliance within a stipulated time period. Evidence of correction must be found through a short-term follow-up survey for the organization to be considered for full accreditation status.

preliminary nonaccreditation An accreditation decision that is assigned to an organization when it is found to be in significant noncompliance with Joint Commission standards or when its accreditation is preliminarily withdrawn by the Joint Commission for other reasons (for example, falsification of documents) *prior* to the determination of the final accreditation decision (for example, not accredited). Preliminary nonaccreditation is an appealable accreditation decision.

not accredited An accreditation decision that results when an organization has been denied accreditation, when its accreditation is withdrawn by the Joint Commission, or when it withdraws from the accreditation process. This designation also describes any organization that has never applied for accreditation.

accreditation decision grid A single-page display of the performance areas that summarizes the standards in each Joint Commission accreditation manual. The grid format allows for the presentation of a numerical summary of aggregated compliance scores for a number of related Joint Commission standards. Each score on the grid reflects an organization's assigned level of compliance for standards relating to a key performance area. *See also* summary grid score.

accreditation decision rules Rules based on grid element scores and specific standards compliance issues that determine the accreditation decision, as well as the scope (which and how many elements require monitoring) and type (focused surveys or written progress reports) of follow-up monitoring required for compliance deficiencies.

accreditation duration The three-year time period during which an organization, found to be in compliance with Joint Commission standards, is awarded accreditation.

accreditation history An account of past Joint Commission accreditation decisions for an organization. The Joint Commission may publicly disclose the accreditation history on request.

accreditation manuals The ten Joint Commission books delineating current standards for specified types of health care organizations, networks, or services. The books are designed for use in organization or network self-assessment. The ten manuals are *Accreditation Manual for Preferred Provider Organizations; Comprehensive Accreditation Manual for Ambulatory Care; Comprehensive Accreditation Manual for Behavioral Health Care; Comprehensive Accreditation Manual for Health Care Networks; Comprehensive Accreditation Manual for Home Care; Comprehensive Accreditation Manual for Hospitals; Comprehensive Accreditation Manual for Long Term Care; Comprehensive Accreditation Manual for Long Term Care Pharmacies; Comprehensive Accreditation Manual for Managed Behavioral Health Care;* and *Comprehensive Accreditation Manual for Pathology and Clinical Laboratory Services.*

accreditation survey An evaluation of an organization to assess its level of compliance with applicable Joint Commission standards and to make determinations regarding its accreditation status. The survey includes evaluation of documentation of compliance provided by organization staff; verbal information concerning the implementation of standards or examples of their implementation that will enable a determination of compliance to be made; on-site observations by surveyors; and an opportunity for education and consultation regarding standards compliance and performance improvement.

Glossary

Accreditation Watch An attribute of an organization's Joint Commission accreditation status. A health care organization is placed on Accreditation Watch when a sentinel event has occurred and a thorough and credible root cause analysis of the sentinel event has not been completed within a specified time frame. Although Accreditation Watch status is not an official accreditation category, it can be publicly disclosed by the Joint Commission.

accreditation with commendation *See* accreditation decision.

activities coordinator, qualified An individual who is licensed or registered, if applicable, in the state in which he or she practices as a therapeutic recreation therapist or as an activities professional and is eligible for certification as such by a recognized accrediting body; or an individual who has had at least two years of experience in a social or recreational program within the past five years, one year of which was full time in a patient activities program in a health care setting; or an individual who is a qualified occupational therapist or occupational therapy assistant; or an individual who has the documented equivalent education, training, or experience.

activity services Structured activities designed to help an individual develop or maintain creative, physical, and social skills through participation in recreation, art, dance, drama, social, or other activities.

administration, administrative (*adj*) The fiscal and general management of an organization, as distinct from the direct provision of services.

admitting privileges Authority issued to admit individuals to a health care organization. Individuals with admitting privileges may practice only within the scope of the clinical privileges granted by the organization's governing body.

advance directive A document or documentation allowing a person to give directions about future medical care or to designate another person(s) to make medical decisions if the individual loses decision-making capacity. Advance directives may include living wills, durable powers of attorney, do-not-resuscitate (DNRs) orders, right to die, or similar documents expressing the individual's preferences as specified in the Patient Self-Determination Act.

advocate A person who represents the rights and interests of another individual as though they were the person's own, in order to realize the rights to which the individual is entitled, obtain needed services, and remove barriers to meeting the individual's needs.

aggregate To combine standardized data and information.

aggregate survey data Information on key organization performance areas and standards collected from organizations and networks surveyed by the Joint Commission. This is combined to produce a database of information concerning the performance of the organizations and networks during a specified time interval.

aggregation The process by which the scores of individual standards in a grid element are consolidated into a single grid element score. *See also* grid element score; recommendation, type I.

aggregation rules The specific rules, listed by grid element, used to incorporate all Joint Commission survey findings into 45 grid element scores. The format of the rules is commonly referred to as the algorithm. Aggregation rules are reviewed and approved by the Joint Commission Board of Commissioner's Accreditation Committee. *See also* Accreditation Committee; algorithm; grid element; grid element score.

algorithm A series of steps for determining grid element scores addressing a specific

issue. *See also* aggregation rules; grid element score.

ambulatory health care occupancy *See* occupancy.

anesthesia The administration to an individual, in any setting, for any purpose, by any route (general, spinal, or other), of major regional anesthesia or sedation (with or without analgesia) for which there is a reasonable expectation that, in the manner used, the analgesia or sedation will result in the loss of protective reflexes.

anesthetizing location Any area ordinarily used for the administration of anesthetic agents.

appropriateness The degree to which the care and services provided are relevant to an individual's clinical needs, given the current state of knowledge.

art therapy The use of art and artistic processes specifically selected and administered by a qualified art therapist to restore, maintain, or improve an individual's mental, emotional, or social functioning.

assess To transform data into information by analyzing it.

assessment
1. For purposes of performance improvement, the systematic collection and review of patient-specific data.
2. For purposes of patient assessment, the process established by an organization for obtaining appropriate and necessary information about each individual seeking entry into a health care setting or service. The information is used to match an individual's need with the appropriate setting, care level, and intervention.

audiological assessment A process to delineate the site and degree of auditory dysfunction using audiological tests such as pure tone air-conduction thresholds, speech reception thresholds, speech discrimination measurements, impedance measurements, and others.

audiologist, qualified An individual who has a master's degree from an audiology program approved by a nationally recognized professional accrediting body; who has completed a supervised clinical fellowship year and passed a national examination in audiology or has the documented equivalent in education, training, or experience; and who meets any current legal requirements for licensure.

audiology services Services provided by a qualified audiologist, either directly or through written agreement with another organization or individual, to assist individuals in hearing and balance and their underlying processes.

audiometric screening A process to screen hearing that may include such tests as pure tone air-conduction thresholds, pure tone air-conduction suprathreshold screenings, impedance measurements, or observations of reactions to auditory stimuli.

authenticate To verify that an entry is complete, accurate, and final.

availability The degree to which appropriate care is available to meet an individual's needs.

behavior management The use of basic learning techniques, such as biofeedback, reinforcement, or aversion therapy, to manage and improve an individual's behavior.

behavioral health A broad array of mental health, chemical dependency, forensic, mental retardation, developmental disabilities, and cognitive rehabilitation services provided in settings such as acute, long term, and ambulatory.

bias An influence on results that causes them to routinely depart from the true value.

biologicals Medicines made from living organisms and their products, including serums, vaccines, antigens, and antitoxins.

blood component A fraction of separated whole blood, for example, red blood cell, plasma, platelets, and granulocytes.

blood derivative A pooled blood product, such as albumin, gamma globulin, or Rh immune globulin whose use is considered significantly lower in risk than that of blood or blood components.

blood usage measurement An activity that entails measuring, assessing, and improving the ordering, distributing, handling, dispensing, administering, and monitoring of blood and blood components.

Board of Commissioners The governing body of the Joint Commission. *See* Joint Commission on Accreditation of Healthcare Organizations.

business occupancy *See* occupancy.

bylaws A governance framework that establishes the roles and responsibilities of a body and its members.

capping A limit on the aggregation of an individual Joint Commission standard score that reduces the severity of its impact on the grid element score. *See also* grid element score.

care The provision of accommodations, comfort, and treatment to an individual, implying responsibility for safety, including care, treatment, services, habilitation, rehabilitation, or other programs instituted by the organization for the individual.

chemical restraint *See* restraint.

circuit testing To periodically test, in terms of their conductivity, all alarm initiating and notification appliance wiring circuits that are connected to the main fire alarm system control panel.

CLIA '88 The Clinical Laboratory Improvement Amendments of 1988.

clinical laboratory A facility that is equipped to examine material derived from the human body to provide information for use in the diagnosis, prevention, or treatment of disease; also called medical laboratory.

clinical privileges Authorization granted by the appropriate authority (for example, a governing body) to a practitioner to provide specific care services in an organization within well-defined limits, based on the following factors, as applicable: license, education, training, experience, competence, health status, and judgment.

community The individuals, families, groups, agencies, facilities, or institutions within the geographic area served by a health care organization.

competence or competency A determination of an individual's capability to perform up to defined expectations.

compliance To act in accordance with stated requirements, such as standards. Levels of compliance include noncompliance, minimal compliance, partial compliance, significant compliance, and substantial compliance.

conditional accreditation *See* accreditation decision.

confidentiality
1. Restriction of access to data and information to individuals who have a need, a reason, and permission for such access.
2. An individual's right, within the law, to personal and informational privacy, including his or her health care records.

consultation
1. Provision of professional advice or services.
2. For purposes of Joint Commission accreditation, advice that is given to staff members of surveyed organizations relating to compliance with standards that are the subject of the survey.

consultation report
1. A potential component of the medical record consisting of a written opinion

by a consultant that reflects, when appropriate, an examination of the individual and the individual's medical record(s).
2. Information given verbally by a consultant to a care provider that reflects, when appropriate, an examination of the individual. The individual's care provider usually documents those opinions in the medical record.

continuing care Care provided over an extended time, in various settings, spanning the illness-to-wellness continuum.

continuing education Education beyond initial professional preparation that is relevant to the type of care delivered in an organization, that provides current knowledge relevant to an individual's field of practice or service responsibilities, and that may be related to findings from performance-improvement activities.

continuity The degree to which the care of individuals is coordinated among practitioners, among organizations, and over time.

continuum of care Matching an individual's ongoing needs with the appropriate level and type of medical, psychological, health, or social care or service within an organization or across multiple organizations.

control chart A graphic display of data in the order they occur with statistically determined upper and lower limits of expected common-cause variation. A control chart is used to identify special causes of variation, to monitor a process for maintenance, and to determine if process changes have had the desired effect.

control limit In statistics, an expected limit of common-cause variation, sometimes referred to as either an upper or a lower limit. Variation beyond a control limit is evidence that special causes are affecting a process. Control limits are calculated from process data and are not to be confused with engineering specifications or tolerance limits. Control limits are typically plotted on a control chart.

coordination of care or services The process of coordinating care or services provided by a health care organization, including referral to appropriate community resources and liaison with others (such as the individual's physician, other health care organizations, or community services involved in care or services) to meet the ongoing identified needs of individuals, to ensure implementation of the plan of care, and to avoid unnecessary duplication of services.

creative arts therapist, qualified A person who is registered or certified as an art, dance and movement, music, poetry, drama, or psychodrama therapist by a recognized body, or has the documented equivalent in education, training, or experience, and who meets current legal requirements of licensure, registration, or certification in the state in which he or she provides services.

creative arts therapy Therapy which uses creative arts modalities and creative processes during intentional intervention in a therapeutic, rehabilitative, community, or educational setting to foster communication and expression; promote integration of physical, emotional, and cognitive states; enhance self-awareness; facilitate change; and maintain social well-being. Examples of creative arts therapies include art, dance and movement, music, poetry, drama, and psychodrama therapies.

credentialing The process of obtaining, verifying, and assessing the qualifications of a health care practitioner to provide patient care services in or for a health care organization.

credentials Documented evidence of licensure, education, training, experience, or other qualifications.

criteria
1. Expected level(s) of achievement, or specifications against which performance or quality may be compared.
2. For purposes of eligibility for a Joint Commission survey, the conditions necessary for health care organizations and networks to be surveyed for accreditation by the Joint Commission.

dance and movement therapy The use of psychotherapeutic movement, facilitated by a dance and movement therapist, to further an individual's emotional, cognitive, social, and physical integration.

data Uninterpreted material, facts, or clinical observations.

data accuracy The extent to which data are free of identifiable errors.

data capture The acquisition or recording of data and information.

data connectivity The ability to link data from different sources or systems.

data definition The identification of the data to be used in analysis.

data integrity The accuracy, consistency, and completeness of data.

data parity The degree to which data are equivalent.

data pattern An identifiable arrangement of data that suggests a systematic design or orderly formation relative to a data set.

data reliability The stability, repeatability, or precision of data.

data security The protection of data from intentional or unintentional destruction, modification, or disclosure.

data transformation The process of changing the form of data representation; for example, changing data into information using decision-analysis tools.

data transmission The sending of data or information from one location to another.

data trend One type of data pattern consisting of the general direction of data measurements.

data validity Verification of correctness; reflects the true situation.

database An organized, comprehensive collection of data elements (variables) and their values.

decentralized laboratory testing *See* point-of-care testing.

decentralized pharmaceutical services The storage, preparation, and dispensing of drugs at organization sites physically located outside the organization's central pharmacy; also called satellite pharmacies.

deemed status Status conferred by the Health Care Financing Administration (HCFA) on a health care provider when that provider is judged or determined to be in compliance with relevant Medicare Conditions of Participation because it has been accredited by a voluntary organization whose standards and survey process are determined by HCFA to be equivalent to those of the Medicare program or other federal laws, such as the Clinical Laboratory Improvement Amendments of 1988 (CLIA '88) or Conditions of Coverage.

delineation of clinical privileges The listing of the specific clinical privileges an organization's staff member is permitted to perform in the organization.

denominator The lower portion of a fraction used to calculate a rate, proportion, or ratio. The denominator statement of a clinical indicator is the population (or population experience) at risk in the calculation of a rate. For example,"Total number of deliveries" in the calculation of a cesarean section birth rate indicator. *See also* indicator; numerator; performance measure.

dental services Services, provided by a dentist or a qualified individual under the supervision of a dentist, to improve or maintain the health of an individual's teeth, oral cavity, and associated structures.

dentist An individual who has received the degree of either doctor of dental surgery or doctor of dental medicine and who is licensed to practice dentistry.

department Any structural unit of a health care organization, whether it is called a department, service, unit, or something similar.

detoxification The systematic reduction of the amount of a toxic agent in the body or the elimination of a toxic agent from the body.

diagnosis A scientifically or medically acceptable term given to a complex of symptoms (disturbances of function or sensation of which the individual is aware), signs (disturbances the physician or another individual can detect), and findings (detected by laboratory, x-ray, or other diagnostic procedures, or responses to therapy).

diagnostic testing Laboratory and other invasive, diagnostic, and imaging procedures.

dietetic services The delivery of care pertaining to the provision of optimal nutrition and quality food service for individuals.

dietitian, qualified An individual who is registered by the Commission on Dietetic Registration or the American Dietetic Association, or who has the documented equivalent in education, training, and experience, with evidence of relevant continuing education.

dimensions of performance Nine definable, measurable, and improvable attributes of organization performance related to "doing the right things right" (appropriateness, availability, and efficacy) and "doing things well" (timeliness, effectiveness, continuity, safety, efficiency, and respect and caring).

director A person who directs, controls, supervises, or manages an organization or a component thereof.

disaster A natural or man-made event that significantly disrupts the environment of care, such as damage to the organization's building(s) and grounds due to severe wind storms, tornadoes, hurricanes, or earthquakes. Also, an event that disrupts care and treatment, such as loss of utilities (power, water, telephones) due to floods, riots, accidents, or emergencies within the organization or in the surrounding community.

disaster plan *See* emergency-preparedness plan or program.

discharge The point at which an individual's active involvement with an organization or program is terminated and the organization or program no longer maintains active responsibility for the care of the individual.

documentation The process of recording information in the individual's medical record and other source documents.

drama therapy Intentional use of drama and theater processes to achieve the therapeutic goals of symptom relief, emotional and physical integration, and personal growth.

drug Any substance, other than food or devices, that may be used on or administered to persons as an aid in the diagnosis, treatment, or prevention of disease or other abnormal condition. *Synonym:* medication.

drug administration The act of giving a prescribed and prepared dose of an identified drug to an individual.

drug allergies A state of hypersensitivity induced by exposure to a particular drug antigen resulting in harmful immunologic reactions on subsequent drug exposures, such as a penicillin drug allergy.

drug dispensing   The issuance of one or more doses of a prescribed and prepared drug by a pharmacist or other authorized staff member to another person responsible for administering it.

effectiveness   The degree to which care is provided in the correct manner, given the current state of knowledge, to achieve the desired or projected outcome(s) for the individual.

efficacy   The degree to which the care of the individual has been shown to accomplish the desired or projected outcome(s).

efficiency   The relationship between the outcomes (results of care) and the resources used to deliver care.

electroconvulsive therapy   A form of somatic treatment that uses electricity to evoke a convulsive response.

emergency-preparedness plan or program   A component of an organization's environment of care program designed to manage the consequences of natural disasters or other emergencies that disrupt the organization's ability to provide care and treatment. *See also* disaster.

endemic infection   *See* infection, endemic.

enteral nutrition   *See* nutrition, enteral.

entry   The process by which an individual is screened and/or assessed by the organization or the practitioner in order to determine the capabilities of the organization or the practitioner to provide the care or services required to meet the individual's needs.

epidemic infection   *See* infection, epidemic.

epidemiologically significant infection   *See* infection, epidemiologically significant.

equipment maintenance, preventive   The planned, scheduled, visual, mechanical, engineering, and functional evaluation of equipment conducted before using new equipment and at specified intervals throughout the equipment's lifetime. The purpose is to maintain equipment performance within manufacturers' guidelines and specifications and to help ensure accurate diagnosis, treatment, or monitoring. It includes measuring performance specifications and evaluating specific safety factors.

equipment maintenance, routine   The performance of basic safety checks, that is, the visual, technical, and functional evaluations of equipment, to identify obvious deficiencies before they have a negative impact on an individual. It normally includes inspections of the case, power cord, structural frame, enclosure, wheels, controls, indicators, and so on, as appropriate. It must be performed after equipment is reprocessed and before use by another individual, and also may be performed during use.

family   The person(s) who plays a significant role in the individual's life. This may include a person(s) not legally related to the individual. This person(s) is often referred to as a surrogate decision maker if authorized to make care decisions for an individual should the individual lose decision-making capacity. *See also* guardian; surrogate decision maker.

first-generation type I recommendation   *See* recommendation, type I.

focused survey   A survey conducted during the Joint Commission accreditation cycle to assess the degree to which an organization has improved its level of compliance relating to specific recommendations. The subject matter of the survey is typically an area(s) of identified deficiency in compliance; however, other performance areas may also be assessed by a surveyor(s), even though they may not have been previously identified as deficiencies. *See also* compliance; recommendation.

function A goal-directed, interrelated series of processes, such as continuum of care or management of information.

governing body The individual(s), group, or agency that has ultimate authority and responsibility for establishing policy, maintaining care quality, and providing for organization management and planning; other names for this group include the board, board of trustees, board of governors, board of commissioners, and partners (networks).

grid element A performance area that receives a discrete score on the Joint Commission accreditation decision grid. *See also* grid element score; summary grid score.

grid element score A number representing the aggregated scores of individual standards in a grid element. *See also* summary grid score.

guardian A parent, trustee, conservator, committee, or other individual or agency empowered by law to act on behalf of or be responsible for an individual. *See also* family; surrogate decision maker.

hazardous materials and wastes Materials whose handling, use, and storage are guided or defined by local, state, or federal regulation (for example, the Occupational Safety and Health Administration's Regulations for Bloodborne Pathogens regarding the disposal of blood and blood-soaked items; the Nuclear Regulatory Commission's regulations for the handling and disposal of radioactive waste), hazardous vapors (for example, gluteraldehyde, ethylene oxide, nitrous oxide), and hazardous energy sources (for example, ionizing or nonionizing radiation, lasers, microwave, ultrasound). Though the Joint Commission considers infectious waste as falling into this category of materials, federal regulations do not define infectious or medical waste as hazardous waste.

hazardous materials and waste management process or program A management process or program that includes all materials and waste that require special handling in order to address identified occupational and environmental hazards. Infectious waste and medical waste fall into the special handling category since there are recognized occupational exposure issues that must be dealt with properly. The program is expanded, when appropriate, to residential occupancies.

health care occupancy *See* occupancy.

health care organization A generic term used to describe many types of organizations that provide health care services.

histogram A graphic display, using a bar graph, of the frequency distribution of a variable. Rectangles are drawn so that their bases lie on a linear scale representing different intervals, and their heights are proportional to the frequencies of the values within each of the intervals.

hospice An organized program that consists of services provided and coordinated by an interdisciplinary team at a frequency appropriate to meet the needs of individuals who are diagnosed with terminal illnesses and have limited life spans. The hospice specializes in palliative management of pain and other physical symptoms, meeting the psychosocial and spiritual needs of the individual and the individual's family or other primary care person(s). The program also includes a continuum of interdisciplinary team services across all settings where hospice care is provided, the availability of 24-hour access to care, utilization of volunteers, and bereavement care to the survivors, as needed, for an appropriate period of time.

housestaff Individuals, licensed as appropriate, who are graduates of medical, dental, osteopathic, or podiatric schools; who are appointed to a hospital's professional graduate training program that is approved by a nationally recognized accrediting body approved by the U.S. Department of Education; and who participate in patient care under the direction of licensed independent practitioners of the pertinent clinical disciplines who have clinical privileges in the hospital and are members of, or are affiliated with, the medical staff.

human subject research   The use of individuals in the systematic study, observation, or evaluation of factors on preventing, assessing, treating, and understanding an illness. The term applies to all behavioral and medical experimental research that involves human beings as experimental subjects.

important process   On the basis of evidence or expert consensus, a process which, when operating well, increases the probability that desired outcomes will occur.

improve   To take actions that result in the desired measurable change.

independent practitioner   *See* licensed independent practitioner.

indicator   A measure used to determine, over time, an organization's performance of functions, processes, and outcomes. *See also* denominator; numerator; performance measure.

individual   A person who receives treatment services. The term is synonymous with patient, client, resident, consumer, individual served, and recipient of treatment services.

infection   An illness produced by a microorganism or other infectious agent.

  endemic infection   The habitual presence of an infection within a geographic area; may also refer to the usual prevalence of a given disease within such an area.

  epidemic infection   An outbreak in a community or region of a group of infections of similar nature, clearly in excess of normal expectancy and derived from a common or propagated source.

epidemiologically significant infection   An outbreak in a community or region of a group of similar infections that is statistically in excess of normal expectations.

nosocomial   An infection acquired by an individual while receiving care or services in the health care organization.

  nosocomial infection rate   The ratio describing the number of individuals with nosocomial infections divided by the number of individuals at risk of developing nosocomial infections. Rates may be stratified by taking into account certain factors that may predispose a specified group of individuals to an increased risk of acquiring a nosocomial infection (also called rate stratification by infection risk).

infection control program or process   An organizationwide program or process, including policies and procedures, for the surveillance, prevention, and control of infection.

information   Interpreted set(s) of data that can assist in decision making.

infusion therapy services   Services for the provision of therapeutic agents or nutritional products to individuals by intravenous infusion for the purpose of improving or sustaining an individual's health condition. These services may be provided directly or through a written agreement with another organization or individual. *See also* nutrition.

inpatient program   A program, in a suitably equipped setting not eligible for survey as a hospital program under the *Comprehensive Accreditation Manual for Hospitals* (*CAMH*), that provides services to persons who require care that warrants 24-hour treatment or habilitation.

in-service Organized education designed to enhance the skills of staff members or teach them new skills relevant to their responsibilities and disciplines.

intent of standard A scorable, brief explanation of a standard's rationale, meaning, and significance.

interim life safety measures (ILSM) A series of 11 administrative actions required to temporarily compensate for significant hazards posed by existing National Fire Protection Association 101® 1997 *Life Safety Code®* (*LSC®*) deficiencies or construction activities. ILSM apply to appropriate staff (including construction workers), must be implemented upon project development, and must be continuously enforced through project completion. Implementation of ILSM is required in or adjacent to all construction areas and throughout buildings with existing *LSC®* deficiencies. ILSM are intended to provide a level of life safety comparable to that described in Chapters 1 through 7, 31, and the applicable occupancy chapters of the *LSC®*. Each ILSM action must be documented through written policies and procedures. Frequencies for inspection, testing, training, and monitoring and evaluation must be established by the organization. *See also Life Safety Code®;* life safety management program or process.

invasive procedure A procedure involving puncture or incision of the skin, or insertion of an instrument or foreign material into the body, including, but not limited to, percutaneous aspirations, biopsies, cardiac and vascular catheterizations, endoscopies, angioplasties, and implantations, and excluding venipuncture and intravenous therapy.

Joint Commission on Accreditation of Healthcare Organizations An independent, not-for-profit organization dedicated to improving the quality of care in organized health care settings. Founded in 1951, its members are the American College of Physicians, the American College of Surgeons, the American Dental Association, the American Hospital Association, and the American Medical Association. The major functions of the Joint Commission include developing accreditation standards, awarding accreditation decisions, and providing education and consultation to health care organizations.

knowledge-based information A collection of stored facts, models, and information found in the clinical, scientific, and management literature that can be used for designing and redesigning processes and for problem solving.

laboratory *See* pathology and clinical laboratory services.

leaders The leaders described in the leadership function include at least the leaders of the governing body; the chief executive officer and other senior managers; department leaders; the elected and the appointed leaders of the medical staff and the clinical departments and other medical staff members in organizational administrative positions; and the nurse executive and other senior nursing leaders.

licensed independent practitioner (LIP) Any individual permitted by law and by the organization to provide care and services, without direction or supervision, within the scope of the individual's license and consistent with individually granted clinical privileges.

licensed practical nurse (LPN) A nurse who has completed a practical nursing program and is licensed by a state to provide routine patient care under the direction of a registered nurse or a physician. Referred to as licensed vocational nurse (LVN) in California and Texas.

licensure A legal right that is granted by a government agency in compliance with a statute governing an occupation (such as medicine or nursing) or the operation of an activity (such as in a hospital).

***Life Safety Code*® (*LSC*®)** A set of standards for the construction and operation of buildings, intended to provide a reasonable degree of safety to life during fires; prepared, published, and periodically revised by the National Fire Protection Association and adopted by the Joint Commission to evaluate health care organizations under its life safety management program. *See also* interim life safety measures; life safety management program or process.

life safety management program or process An organization's documented management plan describing the processes for protecting patients, staff members, visitors, and property from fire and the products of combustion (smoke). *See also* interim life safety measures; *Life Safety Code*®.

loss of protective reflexes An inability to handle secretions without aspiration or to maintain a patent airway independently.

measure To collect quantifiable data about a function or process.

measurement The systematic process of data collection, repeated over time or at a single point in time.

medical equipment Fixed and portable equipment used for the diagnosis, treatment, monitoring, and direct care of individuals.

medical equipment management A component of an organization's management of the environment of care program designed to assess and control the clinical and physical risks of fixed and portable equipment used for the diagnosis, treatment, monitoring, and care of individuals.

medical history A component of the medical record consisting of an account of an individual's history, obtained whenever possible from the individual, and including at least the following information: chief complaint, details of the present illness or care needs, relevant past history, and relevant inventory by body systems.

medical laboratory *See* clinical laboratory.

medical radiation physician, qualified An individual who is certified by the American Board of Radiology in the appropriate disciplines of radiologic physics, including diagnostic, therapeutic, or medical nuclear physics, or an individual who demonstrates equivalent competency in these disciplines.

medical record The account compiled by physicians and other health care professionals of a variety of patient health information, such as assessment findings, treatment details, and progress notes.

medical record practitioner, qualified An individual who is eligible for certification as a registered record administrator or as an accredited record technician by the American Health Information Management Association (AHIMA), or who is a graduate of a school of medical record science accredited jointly by the Committee on Allied Health Education and Accreditation and the AHIMA; or an individual who has the documented equivalent education, training, or experience.

medical record review The process of measuring, assessing, and improving the quality of medical record documentation—that is, the degree to which medical record documentation is accurate, complete, and performed in a timely manner. This process is carried out with the cooperation of relevant departments or services.

medical staff A body that has the overall responsibility for the quality of the professional services provided by individuals with clinical privileges and also the responsibility of accounting, therefore, to the governing body. The medical staff includes fully licensed physicians and may include other licensed individuals permitted by law and by the organization to provide patient care services independently (that is, without clinical direction or supervision) within the organization. Members have delineated clinical privileges that allow them to provide patient care services independently within the scope of their clinical privileges. *See also* clinical privileges; licensed independent practitioner.

medical staff bylaws A document that describes the organization, roles, and responsibilities of the medical staff. The bylaws are developed, adopted, and periodically reviewed by the medical staff and approved by the governing body.

medical staff executive committee A group of medical staff members, a majority of whom are licensed physician members of the medical staff practicing in the organization, selected by the medical staff, or appointed in accordance with governing body bylaws. This group is responsible for making specific recommendations directly to the organization's governing body for approval, as well as receiving and acting on reports and recommendations from medical staff committees, clinical departments or services, and assigned activity groups.

medication Any substance, other than food or devices, that may be used on or administered to persons as an aid in the diagnosis, treatment, or prevention of disease or other abnormal condition. *Synonym:* drug.

medication-use measurement The measurement, assessment, and improvement of the prescribing or ordering, preparing and dispensing, administering, and monitoring of medications.

mental abuse *See* abuse.

minimum data set An agreed-on and accepted set of terms and definitions constituting a core of data; a collection of related data items.

mission statement A written expression that sets forth the purpose of an organization or one of its components. The generation of a mission statement usually precedes the formation of goals and objectives.

multidisciplinary team A group of clinical staff members composed of representatives of a range of professions, disciplines, or service areas.

music therapy The use of musical or rhythmic interventions specifically selected by a music therapist to restore, maintain, or improve the social or emotional functioning, mental processing, or physical health of individuals.

neglect An impaired quality of life for an individual resulting from the absence of minimal services or resources to meet basic needs. Neglect includes withholding or inadequately providing food and hydration (without physician, patient, or surrogate approval), clothing, medical care, and good hygiene. It may also include placing the individual in unsafe or unsupervised conditions. *See also* abuse.

network An entity which offers comprehensive or specialty services that provides, or provides for, integrated health care services to a defined population of individuals. Networks are characterized by a centralized structure which coordinates and integrates services provided by components and practitioners participating in the network.

nosocomial infection *See* infection, nosocomial.

nosocomial infection rate *See* infection, nosocomial.

not accredited *See* accreditation decision.

numerator The upper portion of a fraction used to calculate a rate, proportion, or ratio. The numerator statement of a clinical indicator is the population(s) of the event being measured. For example, "Total number of cesarean sections" in the calculation of a cesarean section birth rate indicator. *See also* denominator; indicator; performance measure.

nursing The health profession dealing with nursing care and services as defined in relevant state, commonwealth, or territory nurse practice acts and other applicable laws and regulations, and as permitted by a health care organization in accordance with these definitions.

nursing care Professional processes intended to assist an individual in the performance of those activities contributing to health or its recovery (or to peaceful death) that he or she would perform unaided if he or she had the necessary strength, will, or knowledge. This includes, but is not limited to, assisting individuals in carrying out therapeutic plans and understanding the health needs of individuals. The special content of nursing care varies in different countries and situations, and, as defined, it is not given solely by registered nurses, but also by other health care professionals.

nursing services Services provided to patients by an individual who is qualified by an approved postsecondary program or baccalaureate or higher degree in nursing and who is licensed or certified by the state to practice nursing. These services may be provided directly or through contract with another organization or individual.

nursing staff Registered nurses, licensed practical or vocational nurses, nursing assistants, and other nursing staff who perform nursing care in a health care organization.

nutrients Protein, carbohydrates, lipids, vitamins, electrolytes, minerals, and water.

nutrition The sum of the processes by which one takes in and uses nutrients.

enteral nutrition Nutrition provided via the gastrointestinal tract. Enteral nutrition encompasses both oral (delivered through the mouth) and tube (provided through a tube or catheter that delivers nutrients distal to the mouth) routes.

parenteral nutrition Nutrition provided intravenously to those individuals who have lost gastrointestinal function or who cannot maintain adequate nutrition care status through conventional intake of nutrients. Parenteral nutrition allows safe administration, through a variety of veins, of all daily nutrition requirements to effect protein synthesis and maintain adequate nutrition status.

parenteral product A sterile pharmaceutical preparation introduced into the body through a route other than the digestive tract, as by subcutaneous, intramuscular, or intravenous injection or infusion.

nutrition assessment A comprehensive process for defining an individual's nutrition status using medical, nutrition, and medication intake histories, physical examination, anthropomorphic measurements, and laboratory data.

nutrition care Interventions and counseling to promote appropriate nutrition intake, based on nutrition assessment and information about food, other sources of nutrients, and meal preparation consistent with the individual's cultural background and socioeconomic status. Nutrition therapy, a component of medical treatment, includes enteral and parenteral nutrition. *See also* nutrition.

nutrition criteria Characteristics known to be associated with nutrition problems. These criteria are used to pinpoint individuals who are at high nutrition risk for malnourishment or are malnourished. *See also* nutrition screening.

nutrition screening The process of using characteristics known to be associated with nutrition problems in order to determine if individuals are malnourished or at a high nutrition risk for malnourishment. *See also* nutrition criteria.

occupancy

ambulatory health care occupancy An occupancy used to provide services or treatment to four or more patients at the same time that either (1) render them incapable of taking their own means for self-preservation in an emergency or (2) provide outpatient surgical treatment requiring general anesthesia.

business occupancy An occupancy used to provide outpatient services or treatment that does not meet the criteria in the ambulatory health care occupancy definition (for example, three or fewer patients at the same time who are rendered incapable of self-preservation in an emergency or are undergoing general anesthesia).

health care occupancy An occupancy used for purposes such as medical or other treatment or care of persons suffering from physical or mental illness, disease, or infirmity; and for the care of infants, convalescents, or infirm aged persons. Health care occupancies provide sleeping facilities for four or more occupants and are occupied by persons who are mostly incapable of self-preservation because of age, physical or mental disability, or because of security measures not under the occupant's control. Health care occupancies include hospitals, nursing homes, and limited care facilities.

residential occupancy An occupancy in which sleeping accommodations are provided for normal residential purposes and include all buildings designed to provide sleeping accommodations.

occupational therapist assistant, qualified, certified An individual who is a graduate of an occupational therapy assistant program accredited by a nationally recognized accreditation body; is currently certified as an occupational therapy assistant by the American Occupational Therapy Certification Board; meets any current legal requirements of state licensure or registration; or has the documented equivalence in education, training, and experience; and is competent in the field. For purposes of Joint Commission Medicare surveys, occupational therapy assistants meet the personnel requirements as outlined in the Medicare regulations for home health agencies.

occupational therapist, qualified An individual who is a graduate of an occupational therapy program accredited by a nationally recognized accreditation body; is initially certified as an occupational therapist by a nationally recognized certification body; meets any current legal requirements of state licensure or registration; or has the documented equivalence in education, training, and experience; and is currently competent in the field. For purposes of Joint Commission Medicare surveys, occupational therapists meet the personnel requirements as outlined in the Medicare regulations for home health agencies.

occupational therapist, qualified, certified An individual who is a graduate of an occupational therapy program accredited by a nationally recognized accrediting body; is currently certified as an occupational therapist by the American Occupational Therapy Certification Board; meets any current legal requirements of licensure or registration or has the documented equivalent in education, training, and experience; and is currently competent in the field.

occupational therapy assistant, qualified An individual who is a graduate of an occupational therapy assistant program accredited by a nationally recognized accreditation body; is initially certified as an occupational therapy assistant by a nationally recognized certification body; meets any current legal requirements of state licensure or registration; or has the documented equivalence in education, training, and experience; and is competent in the field. For Medicare surveys, occupational therapy assistants meet the personnel requirements as outlined in the Medicare regulations for home health agencies.

occupational therapy services   Services that provide for goal-directed, purposeful activity to evaluate, assess, or treat persons whose function is impaired by physical illness or injury, emotional disorder, congenital or developmental disability, or the aging process. Such therapy is designed to achieve optimum functioning, to prevent disability, and to maintain health. These services are provided by a qualified occupational therapist; by a qualified occupational therapy assistant supervised by an individual who has the documented equivalent education, training, and experience and who meets any current legal requirements of licensure or registration. These services may be provided directly or through contract with another organization or individual.

Official Accreditation Decision Report   In the Joint Commission accreditation process, the report resulting from the on-site assessment of an organization or network that outlines identified deficiencies in standards compliance. It also outlines the nature of the accreditation decision including enumeration of type I recommendations, the remediation of which will be monitored by the Joint Commission through focused surveys or written progress reports. The report may also include other supplemental recommendations that are designed to assist the organization or network in improving its performance. *See also* accreditation decision; recommendation.

operative and other procedures   Includes operative, other invasive, and noninvasive procedures, such as radiotherapy, hyperbaric treatment, CAT scan, and MRI, that place the patient at risk. The focus is on procedures and is not meant to include medications that place the patient at risk.

oral and maxillofacial surgeon, qualified   An individual who has successfully completed a postgraduate program in oral and maxillofacial surgery accredited by a nationally recognized accrediting body approved by the U.S. Department of Education. As determined by the medical staff, the individual is also currently competent to perform a complete history and physical examination in order to assess the medical, surgical, and anesthetic risks of the proposed operative and other procedure(s).

organizationwide   Throughout the organization and across multiple structural and staffing components, as appropriate.

orientation   A process to provide initial training and information and to assess staff members' competence related to their job responsibilities and the organization's mission, vision, and values.

outcome   The result of the performance(or nonperformance) of a function or process(es).

outpatient program   A program that provides services to persons who generally do not need the level of care associated with the more structured environment of an inpatient or a residential program.

parenteral nutrition   *See* nutrition, parenteral.

parenteral product   *See* nutrition, parenteral product.

partial-hospitalization program   A program that provides services to persons who spend only part of a 24-hour period in a behavioral health facility. Partial-hospitalization programs do not provide overnight care.

pathology and clinical laboratory services The services that provide information on diagnosis, prevention, or treatment of disease through the examination of the structural and functional changes in tissues and organs of the body that cause or are caused by disease.

patient An individual who receives care or services, or one who may be represented by an appropriately authorized person. For hospice providers, the patient and family are considered a single unit of care. Synonyms used by various health care fields include client, resident, customer, patient and family unit, individual served, consumer, or health care consumer. *See also* individual.

performance The way in which an individual, a group, or an organization carries out or accomplishes its important functions and processes.

performance area An element of the Joint Commission accreditation decision grid that summarizes a standard or group of related standards. The performance areas identified on the accreditation decision grid are considered to be the most critical to the final accreditation decision. *See also* accreditation decision grid.

performance improvement The continuous study and adaptation of a health care organization's functions and processes to increase the probability of achieving desired outcomes and to better meet the needs of individuals and other users of services. This is the third segment of a performance measurement, assessment, and improvement system.

performance measure A quantitative tool (for example, rate, ratio, index, percentage) that provides an indication of an organization's performance in relation to a specified process or outcome. *See also* indicator; denominator; numerator.

pharmaceutical equivalence The degree to which two formulations of the same medication are identical in strength, concentration, and dosage form.

pharmacist An individual who has a degree in pharmacy and is licensed and registered to prepare, preserve, compound, and dispense drugs and chemicals.

pharmacy A licensed location where drugs are stored and compounded or dispensed.

physical abuse *See* abuse.

physical restraint *See* restraint.

physical therapist assistant, qualified An individual who is educated specifically to work under the direction and supervision of the physical therapist in the delivery of physical therapy services; who is a graduate of a physical therapist assistant associate degree program accredited by the Commission on Accreditation in Physical Therapy Education, a nationally recognized accreditation body, or has the documented equivalence in training, education, and experience; who meets any current legal requirements of licensure or registration; and who is currently competent in the field. For purposes of Joint Commission Medicare surveys, physical therapy assistants meet the personnel requirements as outlined in the Medicare regulations for home health agencies.

physical therapist, qualified An individual who is a graduate of a physical therapist education program accredited by a nationally recognized accrediting body; who meets any current legal requirements of licensure or registration or who has the documented equivalence in training, education, and experience; and is currently competent in the field. Physical therapists assess, evaluate, and treat movement dysfunction and pain resulting from injury, disease, disability, or other health-related conditions. For purposes of Joint Commission Medicare surveys, physical therapists meet the personnel requirements outlined in the Medicare regulations for home health agencies.

physical therapy aide   An individual who is trained on the job to provide support services for the physical therapy department under the direction and supervision of a physical therapist. Direct patient services may include transportation, assistance of other physical therapy staff with dependent patients, and other activities as delegated by the physical therapist. Routine duties of the physical therapy aide include equipment management, preparation and cleaning of treatment areas, and supply inventory.

physical therapy services   The health care field concerned primarily with the treatment of disorders with physical agents and methods, such as massage, manipulation, therapeutic exercises, cold, heat (including shortwave, microwave, and ultrasonic diathermy), hydrotherapy, electric stimulation, and light, to assist in rehabilitating individuals and in restoring normal function after an illness or injury.

physician licensure   The process by which a legal jurisdiction, such as a state, grants permission to a physician to practice medicine after finding that he or she has met acceptable qualification standards. Licensure also involves ongoing regulation of physicians by the legal jurisdiction, including the authority to revoke or otherwise restrict a physician's license to practice.

physician member of the medical staff   A doctor of medicine or doctor of osteopathy who, by virtue of education, training, and demonstrated competence, is granted medical staff membership and clinical privileges by the organization to perform specified diagnostic or therapeutic procedures.

physician, qualified   A doctor of medicine or doctor of osteopathy who, by virtue of education, training, and demonstrated competence, is granted clinical privileges by the organization to perform specific diagnostic or therapeutic procedure(s) and who is fully licensed to practice medicine.

plan for improvement   For purposes of Joint Commission accreditation, an organization's written statement that details the procedures to be taken to correct existing *Life Safety Code*® deficiencies and, where applicable, includes the interim life safety measures to be implemented to temporarily reduce the hazards associated with the deficiencies. *See also* interim life safety measures; *Life Safety Code*.®

plan of care   A plan, based on data gathered during patient assessment, that identifies the patient's care needs, lists the strategy for providing services to meet those needs, documents treatment goals and objectives, outlines the criteria for terminating specified interventions, and documents the individual's progress in meeting specified goals and objectives. The format of the "plan" in some organizations may be guided by patient-specific policies and procedures, protocols, practice guidelines, clinical paths, care maps, or a combination of these. The plan of care may include care, treatment, habilitation, and rehabilitation.

plan of correction, conditional accreditation   For purposes of Joint Commission accreditation, an organization's written plan, approved by Joint Commission staff, that outlines the actions the organization will take to address compliance issues that caused the Joint Commission's Accreditation Committee to make a decision of conditional accreditation. The plan is the basis for the follow-up survey at a specified time once the plan is approved. *See also* accreditation decision.

podiatrist An individual who has received the degree of doctor of podiatry medicine and who is licensed to practice podiatry.

poetry therapy The initial use of literature or writing by a qualified biblio-poetry therapist to further therapeutic goals and enhance the well-being of individuals through the integration of emotional, cognitive, and social aspects of self.

point-of-care testing Analytical testing performed at sites in the organization but physically located outside the organization's central laboratory. The testing sites are either under the jurisdiction of the organized pathology and clinical laboratory or another department or service. Examples include bedside testing and on-unit testing such as occult-blood testing, serologic screens (for example, mononucleosis, streptococcus), urine analysis, Gram stains, and glucose meter testing. For the purposes of Joint Commission standards, point-of-care testing does not include testing in "satellite laboratories" under the jurisdiction of the organized pathology and clinical laboratories that perform tests such as "stat" laboratory tests or off-site hemoglobins, hematocrits, or electrolytes (standards in the *Comprehensive Accreditation Manual for Pathology and Clinical Laboratories* apply to such satellite laboratories). Point-of-care testing also does not include "special function laboratories" such as blood gas laboratories, most sites where intraoperative testing is performed, and cytogenetic laboratories. Also called alternate site testing, decentralized laboratory testing, and distributed site testing.

policies and procedures The formal, approved description of how a governance, management, or clinical care process is defined, organized, and carried out.

practice guidelines Descriptive tools or standardized specification for care of the typical individual in the typical situation, developed through a formal process that incorporates the best scientific evidence of effectiveness with expert opinion. Synonyms include clinical criteria, parameter (or practice parameter), protocol, algorithm, review criteria, preferred practice pattern, and guideline.

preliminary nonaccreditation *See* accreditation decision.

prescribing or ordering Directing the selection, preparation, or administration of medication(s).

primary source The original source of a specific credential that can verify the accuracy of a qualification reported by an individual health care practitioner. Examples include medical school, graduate medical education program, and state medical board.

privileging The process whereby a specific scope and content of patient care services (that is, clinical privileges) are authorized for a health care practitioner by a health care organization based on evaluation of the individual's credentials and performance. *See* licensed independent practitioner.

process A goal-directed, interrelated series of actions, events, mechanisms, or steps.

program
1. An outline of work to be done or a prearranged plan or procedure.
2. A general term for an organized system of services designed to address the individual's care and treatment needs.

protective services A range of sociolegal, assistive, and remedial services that facilitate the exercise of individual rights and provide certain supportive and surrogate mechanisms. Such mechanisms are designed to help developmentally disabled individuals reach the maximum independence possible, yet protect them from exploitation, neglect, or abuse. Depending on the nature and extent of individual needs, protective services may range from counseling to full guardianship.

provisional accreditation *See* accreditation decision.

psychiatric nurse, qualified A licensed, registered nurse who has a master's degree in psychiatric nursing, who has been certified to practice psychiatric nursing by the voluntary certification process of the American Nurses' Association, or who has the documented equivalent in education, training, or experience.

psychiatrist, qualified A physician who specializes in assessing and treating persons having psychiatric disorders; is certified by the American Board of Psychiatry and Neurology or has the documented equivalent in education, training, or experience; and is fully licensed to practice medicine in the state in which he or she practices.

psychodrama therapy The use of action methods of enactment, sociometry, group dynamics, role theory, and social systems analysis to facilitate constructive change in individuals and groups by developing new perceptions or reorganizing old cognitive patterns and concomitant changes in behavior.

psychologist, qualified An individual who specializes in psychological research, testing, or therapy.

psychotropic medication Any drug that alters perception or behavior. These include, but are not limited to, those drugs that produce drug dependence. *See also* medication.

public information policy A Joint Commission policy governing the release of information about the performance of a health care organization or network. This policy describes information that will be released in performance reports as well as other information that will be publically disclosed on request. The policy also addresses the release of complaint information, aggregate performance data, and information that will be provided to government agencies.

qualified individual An individual or staff member who is qualified to participate in one or all of the mechanisms outlined in Joint Commission standards by virtue of the following: education; training; experience; competence; registration; certification; or applicable licensure, law or regulation.

qualified individual, infection control An individual who is qualified to participate in one or all of the mechanisms outlined in the standards by virtue of one or more of the following: education, training, certification or licensure, or experience. Certification by the Certification Board for Infection Control is often a requirement for infection control practitioners.

quality improvement An approach to the continuous study and improvement of the processes of providing health care services to meet the needs of individuals and others. Synonyms include continuous quality improvement, continuous improvement, organizationwide performance improvement, and total quality management.

quality of care The degree to which health services for individuals and populations increase the likelihood of desired health outcomes and are consistent with current professional knowledge. Dimensions of performance include the following: resident perspective issues; safety of the care environment; and accessibility, appropriateness, continuity, effectiveness, efficacy, efficiency, and timeliness of care.

radiologic technologist, qualified An individual who is a graduate of a radiologic technology program accredited by an accreditation body recognized by the U.S. Department of Education; is currently certified as a radiologic technologist by the American Registry of Radiologic Technologists; meets any current legal requirements of licensure or registration or has the documented equivalent in education, training, and experience; and is currently competent in the field.

reassessment Ongoing data collection that begins on initial assessment, comparing the most recent data with the data collected on the previous assessment.

recommendation A citation requiring corrective action based on the nature, severity, or number of compliance problems which is accompanied by appropriate follow-up monitoring.

> **type I recommendation** A recommendation or group of recommendations that addresses insufficient or unsatisfactory standards compliance in a specific performance area. Resolution of type I recommendations must be achieved within stipulated time frames for an organization to maintain its accreditation.
>
> **first-generation type I recommendation** The first opportunity an organization surveyed by the Joint Commission has to correct a type I recommendation either through a written progress report or through a focused survey, that is, the first follow-up to a triennial or unannounced/unscheduled survey.
>
> **second-generation type I recommendation** An organization's second opportunity to correct a deficiency either through a written progress report or through a focused survey, that is, the second follow-up to a triennial or unannounced/unscheduled survey.
>
> **third-generation type I recommendation** The third opportunity an organization has to correct a deficiency either through a written progress report or through a focused survey, that is, the third follow-up to a triennial or unannounced/unscheduled survey.

supplemental recommendation A recommendation or group of recommendations that encompasses a standard(s) that was scored in less than substantial compliance (that is, less than a score 1) but did not result in a type I recommendation. If not resolved, a supplemental recommendation may affect a future accreditation decision.

recreational therapist assistant or technician, qualified An individual who, at a minimum, is a graduate of an associate degree program in recreational therapy; meets any current legal requirements of licensure, registration, or certification or has the documented equivalence in education, training, and experience; and is competent in the field. Recreational therapy assistants or technicians assist recreational therapists to assess and treat patients individually using interventions to restore, remediate, or rehabilitate to improve functioning and independence in life activities as well as to reduce or eliminate the effects of illness or disability. A qualified recreational therapist clinically supervises the work of recreational therapy assistants or technicians.

recreational therapist, qualified An individual who, at a minimum, is a graduate of a baccalaureate degree program in recreational therapy accredited by a nationally recognized accreditation body; is currently a Certified Therapeutic Recreation Specialist by the National Council for Therapeutic Recreation Certification; meets any current legal requirements of licensure, registration, or certification or has the documented equivalent in education, training, and experience; and is currently competent in the field. Recreational therapists assess and treat patients individually using interventions to restore, remediate, or rehabilitate to improve functioning and independence in life activities as well as to reduce or eliminate the effects of illness or disability.

reference database An organized collection of similar data from many organizations that can be used to compare an organization's performance to that of others.

referral The sending of an individual (1) from one clinician to another clinician or specialist, (2) from one setting or service to another, or (3) by one physician (the referring physician) to another physician(s) or other resource, either for consultation or care.

registered dietitian As defined by the Commission on Dietetic Registration, the credentialing agent of the American Dietetic Association, an individual who completed the minimum of a baccalaureate degree granted by a U.S. regionally accredited college or university; meets current academic requirements (Didactic Program in Dietetics) as approved by the American Dietetic Association; completed preprofessional experience accredited or approved by the American Dietetic Association; successfully completed the Registration Examination for Dietitians; and accrues 78 hours of approved continuing education every five years.

registered nurse An individual who is qualified by an approved postsecondary program or baccalaureate or higher degree in nursing and licensed by the state, commonwealth, or territory to practice professional nursing.

residential occupancy *See* occupancy.

residential program A program that provides services to individuals who need a less structured environment than that of an inpatient program and who are capable of self-preservation in the event of an internal disaster. *See also* inpatient program; outpatient program.

respect and caring The degree to which those providing services do so with sensitivity for the individual's needs, expectations, and individual differences, and the degree to which the individual or a designee is involved in his or her own care decisions.

respiratory care services Delivery of care to provide ventilatory support and associated services for individuals.

respiratory care technician, certified An individual who is certified by the National Board for Respiratory Care after successfully completing all education, experience, and examination requirements.

respiratory therapist An individual who has successfully completed a training program accredited by the American Medical Association Committee on Allied Health Education and Accreditation in collaboration with the Joint Review Committee for Respiratory Therapy Education and is eligible to take the registry examination administered by the National Board for Respiratory Care or has the documented equivalent in training or experience.

respiratory therapy technician An individual who has successfully completed a training program accredited by the American Medical Association Committee on Allied Health Education and Accreditation in collaboration with the Joint Review Committee for Respiratory Therapy Education and is eligible to take the certification examination administered by the National Board for Respiratory Care or has the documented equivalent in training or experience.

restraint Any method (chemical or physical) of restricting an individual's freedom of movement, physical activity, or normal access to the body.

chemical restraint The inappropriate use of a sedating psychotropic drug to manage or control behavior.

physical restraint Any method of physically restricting a person's freedom of movement, physical activity, or normal access to his or her body.

risk management activities Clinical and administrative activities that organizations undertake to identify, evaluate, and reduce the risk of injury to patients, staff, and visitors and the risk of loss to the organization itself.

run chart A display of data in which data points are plotted as they occur over time (for example, observed weights over time) to detect trends or other patterns and variation occurring over time. Run charts, as opposed to tabular frequency displays, are capable of time-order analytic studies.

safety The degree to which the risk of an intervention (for example, use of a drug or a procedure) and risk in the care environment are reduced for a patient and other persons, including health care practitioners.

safety management A component of an organization's management of the environment of care program that maintains and improves the general safety of the care environment.

scope of care or services The activities performed by governance, managerial, clinical, or support staff.

second-generation type I recommendation *See* recommendation, second-generation type I.

sentinel event Sentinel event is an event that has resulted in an unanticipated death or major permanent loss of function, not related to the natural course of the patient's illness or underlying condition (refer to 1 and 2, below). The following events are also considered sentinel events even if the outcome was not death or major permanent loss of function: suicide of a patient in a setting where the patient receives around-the-clock care (for example, hospital, residential treatment center, crisis stabilization center); infant abduction or discharge to the wrong family; rape; hemolytic transfusion reaction involving administration of blood or blood products having major blood group incompatibilities; and surgery on the wrong patient or wrong body part (refer to 3 and 4, below).

Use the above definition as well as the four additional explanations below.

1. A distinction is made between an adverse outcome that is related to the natural course of the patient's illness or underlying condition (not reportable) and a death or major permanent loss of function that is associated with the treatment, *or lack of treatment*, of that condition (voluntarily reportable).

2. "Major permanent loss of function" means sensory, motor, physiologic, or intellectual impairment not present on admission requiring continued treatment or life-style change. When "major permanent loss of function" cannot be immediately determined, reporting is not expected until either the patient is discharged with continued major loss of function, or two weeks have elapsed with persistent major loss of function, whichever occurs first.

3. The determination of "rape" is to be based on the health care organization's definition, consistent with applicable law and regulation. Reporting of an allegation of rape is not expected. The five-day time frame for voluntarily reporting begins when a determination is made that a rape has occurred. Reporting of a rape is not expected where such reporting is prohibited by law.

4. All events of surgery on the wrong patient or wrong body part are voluntarily

reportable, regardless of the magnitude of the procedure.

services Structural divisions of an organization, its medical staff, or its licensed independent practitioner staff; also, the delivery of care.

sexual abuse *See* abuse.

significant medication errors and significant adverse drug reactions Unintended, undesirable, and unexpected effects of prescribed medications or of medication errors that require discontinuing a medication or modifying the dose; require initial or prolonged hospitalization; result in disability; require treatment with a prescription medication; result in cognitive deterioration or impairment; are life threatening; result in death; or result in congenital anomalies. *See also* drug; medication.

social work assistant An individual with a bachelor's degree, preferably with a social work sequence, who is given training on the job for specific assignments and responsibilities in the provision of social work services or who has the documented equivalent in education, training, or experience. For purposes of Joint Commission Medicare surveys, social work assistants meet the personnel requirements outlined in the Medicare regulations for home health agencies.

social work services Services to assist individuals and their families in addressing social, emotional, and economic stresses associated with illness or injury. Such services are provided by a qualified social worker or a social work assistant under the supervision of a qualified social worker. These services may be provided directly or through contract with another organization or individual.

social worker, qualified An individual who either has met the requirements of a graduate curriculum (leading to a master's degree) in a school of social work that is accredited by the Council on Social Work Education or has the documented equivalent in education, training, or experience. For purposes of Joint Commission Medicare surveys, social workers meet the personnel requirements outlined in the Medicare regulations for home health agencies.

speech-language pathologist, qualified An individual who holds either a master's or doctoral degree; the Certificate of Clinical Competence (CCC) of the American Speech-Language-Hearing Association (ASHA); or has the documented equivalent education, training, or experience, and, where applicable, state licensure.

speech-language pathology services Services provided to assist individuals in speech, language, oral and pharyngeal sensorimotor function, cognitive or communicative function, and their underlying processes. Such services are provided by a qualified speech-language pathologist and may be provided directly or through contract with another organization or individual.

staff Individuals, including employees, volunteers, contractors, or temporary agency personnel, who successfully complete a credentialing process and are granted clinical privileges by the organization.

standard A statement that defines the performance expectations, structures, or processes that must be substantially in place in an organization to enhance the quality of care.

Statement of Conditions™ (SOC™) A proactive document that helps an organization to do a critical self-assessment of its current level of compliance and describe how to resolve any *Life Safety Code*® (*LSC*®) deficiencies. The SOC™ was created to be a "living, ongoing" management tool that should be used in a management process that continually identifies, assesses, and resolves *LSC*® deficiencies.

subacute care Care that is rendered immediately after, or instead of, acute hospitalization to treat one or more specific, active, complex medical conditions or to administer one or more technically complex treatments in the context of an individual's underlying long-term conditions and overall situation. Subacute care requires the coordinated services of an interdisciplinary team. It is given as part of a specifically defined program, regardless of the site.

Subacute care is generally more intensive than traditional nursing facility care and less intensive than acute inpatient care. It requires frequent (daily to weekly) patient assessment and review of the clinical course and treatment plan for a limited time period (several days to several months), until a condition is stabilized or a predetermined treatment course is completed.

summary grid score A number that indicates an organization's overall accreditation performance. The grid score is calculated from the grid element scores. Also referred to as the grid score. *See also* accreditation decision grid; grid element score.

supplemental recommendation *See* recommendation, supplemental.

surrogate decision maker Someone appointed to act on behalf of another. Surrogates make decisions only when an individual is without capacity or has given permission to involve others. *See also* advocate; family.

survey team The group of health care professionals who work together to perform a Joint Commission accreditation survey.

surveyor For purposes of Joint Commission accreditation, a physician, nurse, administrator, laboratorian, or any other health care professional who meets the Joint Commission's surveyor selection criteria, evaluates standards compliance, and provides education and consultation regarding standards compliance to surveyed organizations or networks.

tailored survey A Joint Commission survey in which standards from more than one accreditation manual are used in assessing compliance. This type of survey may include using specialist surveyors appropriate to the standards selected for survey.

therapeutic equivalence The degree to which two formulations of different active ingredients are judged by the clinical staff to have acceptably similar therapeutic effects.

third-generation type I recommendation *See* recommendation, type I.

timeliness The degree to which care is provided to the individual at the most beneficial or necessary time.

transfer The formal shifting of responsibility for the care of an individual (1) from one care unit to another, (2) from one clinical service to another, (3) from one licensed independent practitioner to another, or (4) from one organization to another organization.

type I recommendation *See* recommendation, type I.

type II recommendation *See* recommendation, supplemental.

utilities management A component of an organization's management of the environment of care program designed to ensure the operational reliability, assess the special risks, and respond to failures of utility systems that support the patient care environment.

utility systems Organization systems for life support; surveillance, prevention, and control of infection; environment support; and equipment support. May include electrical distribution; emergency power; vertical and horizontal transport; heating, ventilating, and air conditioning; plumbing, boiler, and steam; piped gases; vacuum systems; or communication systems including data exchange systems.

utilization management The examination and evaluation of the appropriateness of the utilization of an organization's resources. Also referred to as a utilization review.

variance
1. A measure of the differences in a set of observations.
2. In statistics, equal to the square of the standard deviation.

variation The differences in results obtained in measuring the same phenomenon more than once. The sources of variation in a process over time can be grouped into two major classes: common causes and special causes.

waived testing Tests that meet the Clinical Laboratory Improvement Amendments of 1988 (CLIA '88) requirements for waived tests; are cleared by the Food and Drug Administration for home use; employ methodologies that are so simple and accurate as to render the likelihood of erroneous results negligible; or pose no risk of harm to the individual if the test is performed incorrectly. *See also* CLIA '88.

written progress report (WPR) For purposes of Joint Commission accreditation, a postsurvey activity that involves preparing a report documenting evidence that correction of a compliance problem(s) is complete. Preparing a WPR involves summarizing, documenting, and collecting facts and other evidence that prove an organization's current compliance with the standards that caused a type I recommendation. *See also* recommendation.

Index

This index is designed to help the user find items quickly and efficiently. The majority of entries are referenced to specific standards. The standards numbers are listed in parentheses after the page number references. For example, if you are looking for information on dispensing medications, you would look up "medication" in this index. Under this heading you would find the subheading "dispensing of" and be directed to standards TX.3.4 and TX.3.5 on pages 88 and 89, respectively.

A

Abuse
  defined, 281
  patient assessment of, 68 (PE.1.8); 76 (PE.8)
Accreditation
  annual update process, 40
  award display and use, 34, 37
  with commendation, 35, 281
  conditional, 36, 281–282
  continuing, 38–39
  continuous, 5–6
  cycle, 7–40, 281
  decision, 281
  defined, 281
  duration, 38, 282
  eligibility requirements, 8
  extension, 39
  history, 282
  manuals, 282
  notification of changes made between surveys, 39
  official policies and procedures, 7–40
  participation requirements, 41–46
  provisional, 11–12, 36, 281
  renewal process, 38–39
  with type I recommendation, 35, 281
  unscheduled and unannounced surveys, 40
Accreditation appeal, defined, 281
Accreditation Committee, defined, 281
Accreditation cycle, 7–40; defined, 281
Accreditation decision, 34; defined, 281
  appealing, 34
  grid, defined, 282
  rules, defined, 282
  types of, 35–37
Accreditation Manual for Preferred Provider Organizations, 9; defined, 282
Accreditation service specialist, 26
Accreditation survey, 8–10; defined, 282
  acceptance of, 42
  agenda, 27
  application for, 25–26, 42
  document review, 31
  eligibility requirements, 8
  feedback sessions, 32
  fees, 24
  function interviews, 31
  interviews with organization leaders, 31
  leadership exit conference, 33
  misrepresentation of information, 45–46
  notifying the public, 27–29
  opening conference, 31
  patient care or safety concerns, 32
  performance improvement overview, 31
  performance measurement, 43–44
  preliminary reports, 33
  process, 30–32
  public information interview, 28–30, 44–45
  purpose of, 8
  scheduling and postponements, 26–27
  scope of, 8–9
  scoring, 32
  team, 31
  unscheduled and unannounced, 40
  visits to patient care settings, 31
Accreditation Watch, 14, 17; defined, 283
Acquisitions, 39
Action plan, 18–19
Activities coordinator, qualified, defined, 283
Activity services, defined, 283
Administration, defined, 283
Admissions
  code of ethics, 57–58 (RI.4.1)
  information exchange, 126 (CC.7)
  medical record access, 209 (IM.7.9)
Admitting privileges, 267–268, 273 (MS.6–MS.6.1); defined, 283
Adolescent, patient assessment, 74 (PE.5)
Advance directive, 53 (RI.1.2.4)
  defined, 283
Advocate, defined, 283
Aggregate, defined, 283
Aggregate survey data, defined, 283
Aggregation, defined, 283
  data for performance improvement, 139–141 (PI.4–PI.4.4)
Aggregation rules, defined, 283
Alcoholism, patient assessment, 75–76 (PE.7)
Algorithm, defined, 283–284
Ambulatory care, medical record for, 207 (IM.7.4–IM.7.4.1); 209 (IM.7.9)

309

American Board of Medical Specialties (ABMS), 255, 257
American College of Physicians, 212; defined, 292
American College of Surgeons, defined, 292
American Dental Association, defined, 292
American Dietetic Association, defined, 303
American Health Information Management Association (AHIMA), defined, 293
American Hospital Association, defined, 292
American Institute of Architects, 167
American Medical Association, defined, 292
  Physician Masterfile, 255, 256, 257
American Speech-Language-Hearing Association (ASHA), defined, 305
Americans with Disabilities Act (ADA), 254
Analysis
  data, 140 (PI.4.1)
  environment of care management issues, 182–183 (EC.3.2)
  intense, 140–141 (PI.4.3)
  root cause, 18, 141 (PI.4.3)
Anesthesia, defined, 284
  discussion of options and risks, 86 (TX.2.2)
  patient assessment for, 67–68 (PE.1.7.1–PE.1.7.3); 85 (TX.2)
  physiological monitoring, 86 (TX.2.3)
  planning, 85 (TX.2.1)
  postprocedure assessment, 86 (TX.2.4)
Anesthetizing location, defined, 284
Annals of Internal Medicine, 212
Appeals
  credentialing, 235 (MS.5.2–MS.5.2.1)
  requests for accreditation, 34
Appropriateness, 130, 284
Art therapy, defined, 284
Assessment, defined, 284
  abuse or neglect, 68 (PE.1.8); 76 (PE.8)
  adolescent patients, 74 (PE.5)
  alcohol/substance-abusing patients, 75–76 (PE.7)
  anesthesia, 67–68 (PE.1.7–PE.1.7.4)
  audiological, defined, 284
  care setting in, 65 (PE.1.1)
  children, 74 (PE.5)
  comparisons, 73 (PE.4.2–PE.4.3)
  continuum of care, 124 (CC.2)
  education needs of patient and family, 116 (PF.1–PF.1.2)
  entry, 124 (CC.2)
  functional, 65–66 (PE.1.3)
  nursing, 66–67 (PE.1.6.1)
  nutrition, 65–66 (PE.1.2); defined, 295
  operative and other procedures, 67–68 (PE.1.7); 94 (TX.5.1–TX.5.1.4)
  patient, 61–76
  preanesthesia, 85 (TX.2)
  safety, 182–183 (EC.3.2)
  statistical quality control for, 140 (PI.4.1)
Audiological assessment, defined, 284

Audiologist, qualified, defined, 284
Audiology services, defined, 284
Audiometric screening, defined, 284
Audit, 152 (LD.1.5.3)
Authentication, defined, 284
Autopsies, role of medical staff in, 272 (MS.8.5–MS.8.5.3)
Availability, 130; defined, 284
Average daily census (ADC)
  less than 10, 41
  30 or fewer, 44

B

Bathing, 84 (TX.1.2.1)
Behavior management, defined, 284
  procedures, 106 (TX.7.4–TX.7.4.1)
Behavioral disorders, patient assessment for, 74–75 (PE.6)
Behavioral health, defined, 284
Behavioral health patients, restraint and seclusion, 99–100
Behavioral health services, defined, 101
Bias, defined, 284
Billing, code of ethics, 57–58 (RI.1.4.1)
Biologicals, 284
Blood component, defined, 285
Blood derivative, defined, 285
Blood usage measurement, defined, 285
Board of Commissioners, defined, 285
Brandon-Hill list, 212
Budget, annual operating, 152 (LD.1.5–LD.1.5.2)
Buildings, design of, 166–167 (EC.1.1–EC.1.2)
Bulletin of the MLA, 212
Business, code of ethics, 57–59 (RI.4–RI.4.4)
Bylaws, defined, 285
  hospital governing body, 221 (GO.2.1)
  medical staff, 244–246 (MS.2–MS2.4.2); defined, 294

C

Capping, defined, 285
Care, defined, 285
Care of patients. *See* Patient care
Certificate of accreditation, 34
Certification Board of Infection Control (CBIC), 217 (IC.1.1)
Chemical restraint, defined, 304
Chief executive officer, 225–228 (MA.1–MA.4)
  authority to grant temporary clinical privileges, 265 (MS.5.14.4)
  relations with governing body, 227 (MA.1, MA.2.1); 228 (MA.4)
  selection process, 222 (GO.2.3)
Child, patient assessment, 74 (PE.5)
Circuit testing, defined, 285
Clinical decisions, integrity of, 58–59 (RI.4.4)
Clinical information, 66 (PE.1.4.1). *See also* Medical record
Clinical laboratory, defined, 285. *See also* Pathology and clinical laboratory services

Index

Clinical Laboratory Improvement Amendments of 1988 (CLIA '88), defined, 285
Clinical privileges
   appeal of adverse decisions, 253 (MS.5.2–MS.5.2.1)
   applicant promises, 260–261 (MS.5.10–MS.5.10.3)
   application for, 251–253 (MS.5.1.1–MS.5.1.2); 256–258 (MS.5.4.3.1–MS.5.4.3.2); 260 (MS.5.8–MS.5.8.2)
   categories of, 266 (MS.5.15.4)
   criteria, 253–260 (MS.5.4–MS.5.9)
   defined, 285
   delineated, 243 (MS.1.1.2); 263–265, 273 (MS.5.14–MS.5.14.3)
   department structure, 266–267, 273 (MS.5.15.5–MS.5.15.7)
   duration, 261–262 (MS.5.11)
   granting and renewal mechanisms, 253–256 (MS.5.3–MS.5.3.3)
   limitations, 264 (MS.5.14.1); 265–266 (MS.5.15–MS.5.15.3)
   renewal, 262 (MS.5.12–MS.5.13)
   suspension, 245 (MS.2.3.3)
   temporary, 265 (MS.5.14.4)
Clinical trials, patient rights in, 57 (RI.3–RI.3.1)
Clothing, suitable to patient clinical condition, 184 (EC.4.2)
Coaching, 158 (LD.3.2)
Code of ethical behavior, 57–59 (RI.4–RI.4.4)
Committee on Allied Health Education and Accreditation, 293
"Committee of the whole," 248
Communication
   effective, 54
   individuals and departments, 157–158 (LD.3.2–LD.3.4)
   patient right to, 54–55 (RI.1.3.6–RI.1.3.6.1.1)
Community, defined, 285
Community resources education, patient and family, 116–117 (PF.1.7)
Comparative data, 213 (IM.10–IM.10.3)
Competence, 255, defined, 285
   staff, 189–190 (HR.3); 191 (HR.4.3); 192 (HR.5)
Competency, defined, 285
Complaint
   patient right to resolution of, 54–55 (RI.1.3.4)
   public release of, 22
Compliance, defined, 285
   continuous, 38
Comprehensive Accreditation Manual for Ambulatory Care, 8; defined, 282
Comprehensive Accreditation Manual for Behavioral Health Care, 8; defined, 282
Comprehensive Accreditation Manual for Health Care Networks, 8; defined, 282
Comprehensive Accreditation Manual for Home Care, 8; defined, 282
Comprehensive Accreditation Manual for Hospitals: The Official Handbook, 8; defined, 282
Comprehensive Accreditation Manual for Long Term Care, 9; defined, 282
Comprehensive Accreditation Manual for Long Term Care Pharmacies, 9; defined, 282
Comprehensive Accreditation Manual for Managed Behavioral Health Care, 9; defined, 282
Comprehensive Accreditation Manual for Pathology and Clinical Laboratory Services (CAMPCLS), 9, 157 (LD.2.11.3); defined, 282
Computers, laptops. *See* Surveyor laptop technology project
Conditional accreditation, 36; defined, 281–282
Confidentiality
   data and information, 200–201 (IM.2–IM.2.3)
   defined, 285
   patient right to, 54–55 (RI.1.3.1)
Consent forms, 57 (RI.3.1)
Consolidations, 39
Consultation, defined, 285
   criteria, 268–269 (MS.6.5.2)
   procedures, 125–126 (CC.6)
Consultation report, defined, 285–286
Continuing care, defined, 286
Continuing education, defined, 286
Continuity, 125 (CC.4); 131, 286
Continuous accreditation, 5–6
Continuous compliance, 38
Continuous Survey Readiness (CSR) Project, 6
Continuum of care
   assessment, 124 (CC.2–CC.2.1)
   continuity, 125 (CC.4)
   coordination, 125 (CC.5)
   defined, 286
   denial-of-care conflicts, 126–127 (CC.8)
   goal of, 121
   information exchange, 126 (CC.7)
   patient access, 124 (CC.1)
   patient education, 125 (CC.3)
   referral, transfer, discharge, 125–126 (CC.6–CC.6.1)
Contract laboratory services, 69–70 (PE.1.9.2.1–PE.1.9.2.2)
Contracted services, 10
Control chart, defined, 286
Control limit, defined, 286
Coordination, of care or services, 125 (CC.5); defined, 286
Core criteria, for medical staff membership or clinical privileges, 254–256 (MS.5.4.3)
   ability to perform privileges requested, 255–256
   current competence, 255
   current licensure, 255
   relevant training or experience, 255
Creative arts therapist, qualified, defined, 286
Creative arts therapy, defined, 286
Credentialing, 251–267 (MS.5–MS.5.15.7)
   defined, 286
Credentials, defined, 286
Credentials verification organization (CVO), 255, 257
Criteria, defined, 287

D

Dance and movement therapy, defined, 287
Data, defined, 287
  accuracy, defined, 287
  aggregation, 139–141 (PI.4–PI.4.4)
  analysis, 140–141 (PI.4.1, PI.4.3)
  capture, 201 (IM.3); defined, 287
  collection, 135–138 (PI.3–PI.3.1.3)
  connectivity, defined, 287
  definition, 201 (IM.3); defined, 287
  integrity, 200–201 (IM.2.2–IM.2.3); defined, 287
  parity, defined, 287
  pattern, defined, 287
  release to government agencies, defined, 23
  reliability, defined, 287
  security, 200–201 (IM.2–IM.2.3); defined, 287
  transformation, defined, 287
  transmission, defined, 287
  trend, defined, 287
  validity, defined, 287
Data collection
  areas for further study, 138 (PI.3.1.2)
  autopsies, 242 (MS.8.5)
  improvement priorities and continuing measurement, 136 (PI.3)
  outcomes and performance, 136 (PI.3–PI.3.1)
  problem-prone areas, 137 (PI.3.1.1)
  timely, economic and efficient, 201 (IM.3.2)
Database, defined, 287
Decentralized laboratory testing. *See* Point-of-care testing
Decentralized pharmaceutical services, defined, 287
Decision making, clinical, 58–59 (RI.4.4)
Deemed status, defined, 287
Delineation of clinical privileges, defined, 287
Denial of care, 126–127 (CC.8)
Denominator, defined, 287
Dental services, defined, 287–288
Dentist, 268, 269, 274 (MS.6.2.2.2); defined, 288
Department
  clinical privileges within, 266–267 (MS.5.15.5–MS.5.15.7)
  collaborative development of policies and procedures, 158 (LD.3.4)
  defined, 288
  directors, 155–157 (LD.2–LD.2.11.3); 248–251 (MS.4–MS.4.2.1.15)
  input to medical staff reappointment and clinical privilege renewal, 262–263 (MS.5.13)
  relationships among, 157 (LD.3.1)
  scope of services, 153–154 (LD.1.7–LD.1.7.1)
Designated requestor, 56
Detoxification, defined, 288
Diagnosis, defined, 288
  preoperative, 67–68 (PE.1.7)
Diagnosis-related groups (DRGs), 136
Diagnostic testing, defined, 288
  in patient assessment, 66 (PE.1.4–PE.1.4.1)

Diet. *See* Nutrition
Dietetic services, defined, 288
Dietitian, qualified, defined, 288
Dimensions of performance, 130–131; defined, 288
Director
  defined, 288
  department, 155–157 (LD.2–LD.2.11.3)
  medical staff, 248–251 (MS.4–MS.4.2.1.15)
  nursing, 277–278 (NR.1)
  safety management, 183 (EC.3.3)
Disaster, defined, 288
Discharge, defined, 288
  code of ethics, 57–58 (RI.4.1)
  information exchange, 126 (CC.7)
  planning, 118 (PF.3)
  process, 126 (CC.6.1)
Discharge planning assessment, 66 (PE.1.5)
Document review, 31
Documentation, defined, 288
Domestic abuse. *See* Abused patients
Drama therapy, defined, 288
Drug administration, defined, 288
Drug allergies, defined, 288
Drug dependencies
  patient assessment, 75–76 (PE.7)
  treatment plans, 269 (MS.6.6)
Drug dispensing, defined, 289
Drug-food interactions, 116 (PF.1.5)
Drugs. *See also* Medication
  defined, 288
  significant adverse reaction, 140 (PI.4.3); defined, 305

E

Early Survey Policy Options, 13
  Option 1 (provisional accreditation), 11–12
  Option 2, 12–13
Education
  information management, 202 (IM.4)
  leadership, 159 (LD.4.1)
  medical staff, 270 (MS.7–MS.7.2.1)
  patient and family, 113–118 (PF.1–PF.1.10); 125 (CC.3)
    activities and resources, 118–119 (PF.4–PF.4.1)
    assessment of needs, 116 (PF.1–PF.1.2)
    care responsibilities, 117 (PF.9)
    collaborative, 119–120 (PF.4.2)
    community resources, 116–117 (PF.1.7)
    continuing care, 118 (PF.3)
    discharge, 118 (PF.3)
    interactive, 118 (PF.2)
    medical equipment, 116 (PF.1.4)
    medication, 116, (PF.1.3)
    personal hygiene, 117 (PF.1.10)
    rehabilitation, 116 (PF.1.6)
  staff, 174–175 (EC.2.1); 190–191 (HR.4–HR.4.3)
Education Commission for Foreign Medical Graduates (ECFMG), 257

Index

Effective communication, 54
Effectiveness, 130; defined, 289
Efficacy, 130; defined, 289
Efficiency, 130, 271
Electroconvulsive therapy, 105–106 (TX.7.2); defined, 289
Emergency drills, 178 (EC.2.9–EC.2.10)
Emergency-preparedness plan, 169–170 (EC.1.6); defined, 289
Emergency services
   house staff, 265 (MS.5.14.4)
   medical record, 207–208 (IM.7.5–IM.7.5.3)
Emotional disorder, patient assessment, 74–75 (PE.6)
End of life, care at, 54 (RI.1.2.7)
Enteral nutrition, defined, 295
Entry, defined, 289
Environment of care
   analysis of management issues, 182–183 (EC.3.2)
   buildings, 166–167 (EC.1.1–EC.1.2)
   design, 166–173 (EC.1–EC.1.9)
   emergency drills, 178 (EC.2.9–EC.2.10)
   goal, 163
   implementation, 173–181 (EC.2–EC.2.14)
   maintenance, testing, inspection, 179–181 (EC.2.11–EC.2.14)
   management plans, 167–173 (EC.1.3–EC.1.9)
   measuring outcomes of implementation, 182–183 (EC.3–EC.3.3)
   nonsmoking policy, 185–186 (EC.5–EC.5.1)
   other environmental considerations, 183–186 (EC.4–EC.5.1)
   patient self-image and dignity, 184–185 (EC.4.2)
   space for patient services, 184 (EC.4.1)
   staff orientation and education, 174–175 (EC.2.1)
Equipment. *See* Medical equipment
Equipment maintenance
   preventive, defined, 289
   routine, defined, 289
Extension of accreditation survey, 39

F
Falsification of information, 15–16, 45
Family, defined, 289
   education, 113–120 (PF.1–PF.4.2)
   participation in care decisions, 52 (RI.1.2.2)
Federation of State Medical Boards
   Action Data Bank, 255
   Physician Disciplinary Data Bank, 258
Fees, 24
Fire drills, 178 (EC.2.10)
Fire safety
   maintenance, testing, inspection, 179–180 (EC.2.12)
   management plan, 170–171 (EC.1.7); 176–177 (EC.2.6)
Focused survey, defined, 289
Food and nutrition. *See* Nutrition care
Forensic services, 191 (HR.4.1)
Function, defined, 290
Functional assessment, 65–66 (PE.1.3–PE.1.3.1)

G
Governance, 219–223 (GO.1–GO.2.6)
   identification of, 221 (GO.1)
   medical staff participation in, 222 (GO.2.2–GO.2.2.2)
Governing body, 221–223 (GO.2–GO.2.6); defined, 290
   and chief executive officer, 222 (GO.2.3); 227 (MA.1, MA.2.1); 228 (MA.4)
   and conflict resolution, 223 (GO.2.6)
   credentialing authority, 251–253 (MS.5.1–MS.5.1.2)
   law and regulations compliance, 222 (GO.2.4); 227 (MA.2–MA.2.1)
   policies and procedures, 223 (GO.2.5)
   responsibilities of, 221 (GO.2–GO.2.1)
Grid element, defined, 290
Grid element score, defined, 290
Guardian, defined, 290
Guidelines for Design and Construction of Hospitals and Health Care Facilities, 167

H
Hazardous materials and wastes, defined, 290
   management, defined, 290
   management plan, 168–169 (EC.1.5); 175 (EC.2.4)
Health Care Financing Administration (HCFA), defined, 287
Health care organization, defined, 290
Health Care Quality Improvement Act of 1986, 256
Histogram, defined, 290
Hospice, defined, 290
House staff, defined, 290–291
   emergency care, 265 (MS.5.14.4)
   supervision by medical staff, 246 (MS.2.5)
Human resources, goal, 187. *See also* Staff
Human subject research, defined, 291

I
Important process, defined, 291
Improvement, defined, 291
In-service education, 191 (HR.4.2); defined, 292
Individual, defined, 291
Infant, patient assessment, 74 (PE.5)
Infection, defined, 291
   endemic, defined, 291
   epidemic, defined, 291
   epidemiologically significant, defined, 291
   nosocomial, defined, 291
   report of, 217–218 (IC.3)
   surveillance, prevention, and control of, 215–218 (IC.1–IC.6.2)
      case findings, 217–218 (IC.2)
      management of, 217 (IC.1.1)
Infection control
   program or process, defined, 291
   qualified individual, defined, 301
Information, defined, 291
   accuracy and truthfulness, 15–16, 20
   misrepresentation of, 45–46

313

patient, 124 (CC.2.1)
publicly disclosed on request, 22
Information Accuracy and Truthfulness Policy, 15–16, 20
Information Collection and Evaluation System (ICES), 163, 182 (EC.3)
Information management
 aggregate data and information, 209–210 (IM.8)
 comparative data and information, 213 (IM.10–IM.10.3)
 decision maker training in, 202–203 (IM.4)
 goal, 193
 integration and interpretation, 203 (IM.6–IM.6.1)
 knowledge-based information, 211–212 (IM.9–IM.9.2)
 patient-specific data and information, 204–209 (IM.7–IM.7.9)
 planning, 199–203 (IM.1–IM.6.1)
 transmission of data and information, 203 (IM.5–IM.5.1)
Informed consent, 51 (RI.1.2.1); 57 (RI.3.1)
 operative and other procedures, 94–95 (TX.5.2–TX.5.2.2)
Infusion therapy services, defined, 291
Initial assessment of patient, time frame, 66–67 (PE.1.6–PE.1.6.1.1)
Initial survey, 13–14
Inpatient program, defined, 291–292
Integrated Survey Process (ISP), 9
Intense analysis, 140–141 (PI.4.3)
Intent of standard, defined, 292
Interim life safety measures (ILSM), 176–177 (EC.2.6); defined, 292
Invasive procedure, defined, 292

J

Joint Commission on Accreditation of Healthcare Organizations, defined, 292
 information resources at, 2–3
 Web site, 3

K

Knowledge-based information, defined, 292
 information management, 211–212 (IM.9–IM.9.2)

L

Laptop technology, 1, 33
Leaders
 defined, 292
 interviews with, 31
Leadership
 audit, 152–153 (LD.1.5.3)
 budget, 152 (LD.1.5–LD.1.5.2)
 collaboration, 149–150 (LD.1.3.1); 154 (LD.1.8)
 communicating hospital mission, vision, and plan, 149 (LD.1.2)
 decision making, 154 (LD.1.8)
 departments, 153–154 (LD.1.7–LD.1.7.1); 155–157 (LD.2–LD.2.11.3)
 goal of, 143
 hospital planning, 148 (LD.1–LD.1.1.1)

 integrating and coordinating patient care services, 157–158 (LD.3–LD.3.4)
 medical staff, 233–234 (MS.4–MS.4.2.1.1.5)
 mission, 149 (LD.1.2–LD.1.3)
 multihospital system, 148–149 (LD.1.1.2)
 performance improvement, 133 (PI.1–PI.1.1); 151 (LD.1.4), 158–162 (LD.4–LD.4.5)
 planning patient care, 149, 150 (LD.1.1.3, LD.1.3, LD.1.3.2–LD.1.3.3.1)
 providing services, 150–151 (LD.1.3.4–LD.1.3.4.2)
 response to patient and family needs, 150 (LD.1.3.3.1)
 scope of services, 153 (LD.1.7–LD.1.7.1)
 staff development, 154 (LD.1.9–LD.1.9.1)
 systemwide policy decisions, 148–149 (LD.1.1.2)
 uniform performance of patient care, 153 (LD.1.6)
Leadership exit conference, 33
Library for Internists, 212
Licensed independent practitioner (LIP)
 defined, 243 (MS.1.1.1); defined, 292
 delineated clinical privlieges, 238 (MS.5.14–MS.5.14.1)
 documentation of operative procedures, 206–207 (IM.7.3.1–IM.7.3.5)
 medical staff department assignments, 239 (MS.5.15.5)
 required to order restraint or seclusion, 104 (TX.7.1.3.1.7)
 treatment management, 240 (MS.6.5–MS.6.5.2)
Licensed practical nurse (LPN), defined, 292
Licensed vocational nurse (LVN), defined, 292
Licensure, 255; defined, 293
Life safety
 maintenance, testing, inspection, 179–180 (EC.2.12)
 management program or process, 170,–171 (EC.1.7); 176–177 (EC.2.6); defined, 293
Life Safety Code® (*LSC*®), 166 (EC.1.1); 176 (EC.2.6); 184 (EC.4.2); defined, 293
Life-sustaining treatment, forgoing or withdrawing, 53 (RI.1.2.6)
Literature. *See* Knowledge-based information
Loss of protective reflexes, defined, 293

M

Maintenance, testing, and inspection
 life safety components, 179–180 (EC.2.12)
 medical equipment, 180 (EC.2.13)
 safety components, 179 (EC.2.11)
 utility systems, 181 (EC.2.14)
Management plans
 emergency preparedness, 169–170 (EC.1.6); 176 (EC.2.5)
 fire safety, 170–171 (EC.1.7); 176–177 (EC.2.6)
 hazardous materials and waste, 168–169 (EC.1.5); 175 (EC.2.4)
 life safety, 170–171 (EC.1.7); 176–177 (EC.2.6)
 medical equipment, 171–172 (EC.1.8); 177 (EC.2.7)
 safety, 167 (EC.1.3)
 security, 168 (EC.1.4)
 utility systems, 172–173 (EC.1.9); 177 (EC.2.8)
Marketing, code of ethics, 57–58 (RI.4.1)

Index

Meals, 92 (TX.4.1.1)
Measure, defined, 293
  designing into processes, 133–135 (PI.2–PI.2.2)
Measurement, defined, 293
  systematic data collection, 136 (PI.3)
Medical equipment, defined, 293
  maintenance, testing, inspection, 180 (EC.2.13)
  management, defined, 293
  management plan, 171–172 (EC.1.8); 177 (EC.2.7)
  patient and family education, 116–117 (PF.1.5)
Medical history, 66–67 (PE.1.6.1–PE.1.6.1.1); 67–68 (PE.1.7)
  defined, 293
  persons authorized to take, 267–268, 269, 273–274 (MS.6.2–MS.6.2.2.3)
Medical Library Association (MLA), 212
Medical radiation physician, qualified, defined, 293
Medical record, 204–205 (IM.7.1–IM.7.2)
  accessibility of, 209 (IM.7.9)
  ambulatory care, 207 (IM.7.4–IM.7.4.1)
  before surgery, 67–68 (PE.1.7)
  completeness, 201 (IM.3.2.1)
  defined, 293
  documentation
    emergency care, 207 (IM.7.5–IM.7.5.3)
    operative or other procedures, 205–206 (IM.7.3)
    plans of care, 95 (TX.5.3)
    psychosurgery, 106 (TX.7.3)
  emergency services, 207–208 (IM.7.5–IM.7.5.3)
  entry authentication, 208–209 (IM.7.8)
  entry, authorized, 204–205 (IM.7.1.1)
  management, 208 (IM.7.6); 209 (IM.7.9)
  operative or other procedures, 205–207 (IM.7.3–IM.7.3.5)
  restraint or seclusion recorded in, 105 (TX.7.1.3.2); 111 (TX.7.5.5)
  review, 201–202 (IM.3.2.1–IM.3.2.1.1); defined, 293
  verbal orders, 208 (IM.7.7)
Medical record practitioner, qualified, defined, 293
Medical staff, defined, 293–294
  appointment and reappointment mechanisms, 253–256 (MS.5.3–MS.5.3.3)
  autopsy, 272 (MS.8.5–MS.8.5.3)
  bylaws, 244–246 (MS.2–MS.2.4.2); defined, 294
  clinical privileges, 230 (MS.1.1.2–MS.1.1.3)
    ability to perform, 237 (MS.5.10.11)
    assignment of, 239 (MS.5.15.5)
    based on competence, 238 (MS.5.15–MS.5.15.3)
    classification of, 239 (MS.5.15.4)
    exercise of, 239 (MS.5.15.6)
    scope of, 238 (MS.5.14.2)
  competence, 237 (MS.5.6)
  continuing medical education, 270 (MS.7–MS.7.2.1)
  credentialing, 251–267 (MS.5–MS.5.15.7)
  department directors, 248–251 (MS.4–MS.4.2.1.15)
  executive committee, 245 (MS.2.3.1); 246–248 (MS.3–MS.3.1.7); defined, 294
  hospital governance, 222 (GO.2.2–GO.2.2.2)

membership
  appeal of adverse decisions, 253 (MS.5.2–MS.5.2.1)
  applicant promises, 260–261 (MS.5.10–MS.5.10.3)
  application, 251–253 (MS.5.1.1–MS.5.1.2); 256–258 (MS.5.4.3.1–MS.5.4.3.2); 260 (MS.5.8–MS.5.8.2)
  criteria, 253–260 (MS.5.4–MS.5.9)
  duration, 261–262 (MS.5.11)
  reappointment, 262–263 (MS.5.12–MS.5.13)
  suspension, 245 (MS.2.3.3)
  multiple, within organization, 243–244 (MS.1)
  organized, 243–244 (MS.1–MS.1.1.3)
  patient care, 267–270 (MS.6–MS.6.8)
  performance improvement, 270–272 (MS.8–MS.8.4)
  physician member of, 298–299
  supervision of house staff, 246 (MS.2.5)
Medication, defined, 294
  alternative, 90 (TX.3.7)
  dispensing of, 88–89 (TX.3.4–TX.3.5)
  dose system, 88–89 (TX.3.5.1)
  emergency, 89 (TX.3.5.5)
  investigative, 90 (TX.3.8)
  law, regulation, professional standards in, 88 (TX.3.4)
  monitoring of effects on patients, 90 (TX.3.9)
  patient and family education, 116–117 (PF.1.3)
  patient information, 89 (TX.3.5.3)
  pharmacy services after hours, 89 (TX.3.5.4)
  preparation and dispensing, 88–89 (TX.3.5–TX.3.5.2)
  prescription and ordering, 88 (TX.3.3)
  recall system, 89 (TX.3.5.6)
  significant error, 140 (PI.4.3), 305
  use processes, 87 (TX.3–TX.3.1)
  verification and identification, 90 (TX.3.6)
Medication-use measurement, defined, 294
Mental abuse, defined, 281
Mergers, 39
Minimum data set, 201 (IM.3.1); defined, 294
Misrepresentation of information, 45–46
Mission statement, defined, 294
Multidisciplinary team, defined, 294
Multidisciplinary treatment plan, 269 (MS.6.6–MS.6.6.1)
Multihospital systems, 10–11
Music therapy, defined, 294

N

National Practitioner Data Bank (NPDB), 256
Neglect. *See also* Abuse
  assessment of possible victims of, 76 (PE.8)
  defined, 294
Network, defined, 294
Nonaccreditation, preliminary, 36; defined, 282
Nosocomial infection, defined, 291
Not accredited, 37; defined, 282
  appeal, 34
Numerator, defined, 294–295
Nurse executive, 277–279 (NR.2–NR.4)
Nursing, 275–279 (NR.1–NR.4); defined, 295

Nursing assessment, 66–67 (PE.1.6.1); 73 (PE.4.3)
Nursing care, defined, 295
Nursing services, defined, 295
Nursing staff, defined, 295
Nutrients, defined, 295
Nutrition, defined, 295
  distribution and administering, 92–93 (TX.4.4)
  enteral, defined, 295
  meals and snacks, 92 (TX.4.1.1)
  monitoring patient response, 93 (TX.4.5)
  parenteral, defined, 295
  patient and family education, 116–117 (PF.1.5)
  planning, 91–92 (TX.4–TX.4.1)
  responsibilities for provision, 92 (TX.4.3)
  special diets and schedules, 93 (TX.4.6)
  standardized practices, 93 (TX.4.7)
  timely prescription and ordering, 92 (TX.4.2)
Nutrition assessment, 65–66 (PE.1.2); 91, 295
Nutrition care, defined, 295
Nutrition screening, 91; defined, 295–296

O

Occupancy, defined, 296
  ambulatory health care, defined, 296
  business, defined, 296
  health care, defined, 296
  residential, defined, 296
Occupational therapist
  assistant, defined, 296
  qualified, certified, defined, 296
  qualified, defined, 296
Occupational therapy assistant, qualified, defined, 296–297
Occupational therapy services, defined, 297
Official ABMS Directory of Board Certified Medical Specialists, 255
Official Accreditation Decision Report, 23, 34; defined, 297
  appeal, 34
  requests for revision, 34
Operative and other procedures
  assessment for, 94 (TX.5–TX.5.1.5)
  documentation of, 95 (TX.5.3); 205–207 (IM.7.3–IM.7.3.5)
  defined, 297
  informed consent, 94–95 (TX.5.2–TX.5.2.2)
  medical record, 205–207 (IM.7.3–IM.7.3.5)
  monitoring of patient, 95 (TX.5.4)
  patient assessment for, 67–68 (PE.1.7); 94 (TX.5–TX.5.1.5)
  plan of care, 95 (TX.5.3)
  postoperative documentation, 206–207 (IM.7.3.3–IM.7.3.5)
  postprocedure monitoring, 95 (TX.5.4)
Oral and maxillofacial surgeon, qualified, 268, 269, 273 (MS.6.2.1); defined, 297
Ordering, defined, 300
Organ and tissue donation, policies and procedures, 56–57 (RI.2)

Organ Procurement and Transplantation Network (OPTN), 56
Organ procurement organization (OPO), 56
Organization ethics, 47–60
  code of ethical behavior, 57–59 (RI.4–RI.4.4)
  integrity of clinical decision making, 58–59 (RI.4.4)
  organ and tissue donation policies, 56–57 (RI.2)
  respect for patient needs, 54–55 (RI.1.3–RI.1.3.6.1.1)
Organizationwide, defined, 297
Orientation, defined, 297
  staff, 174–175 (EC.2.1); 190–191 (HR.4)
Outcome, defined, 297
Outpatient program, defined, 297
Outpatient services, 210

P

Parenteral nutrition, defined, 295
Parenteral product, defined, 295
Partial-hospitalization program, defined, 297–298
Pastoral care, 54–55 (RI.1.3.5)
Pathology and clinical laboratory services, defined, 298
  availability, 69 (PE.1.9–PE.1.9.1)
  contract laboratories, 69–70 (PE.1.9.2.1–PE.1.9.2.2)
  hospital laboratories, 69–70 (PE.1.9.2)
  patient assessment, 69–70 (PE.1.9–PE.1.9.2.2)
Patient
  defined, 298
  human dignity of, 184–185 (EC.4.2)
  interests, skills, opportunities, 185 (EC.4.4)
  self-image of, 184–185 (EC.4.2)
Patient assessment
  alcoholism or drug dependency, 75–76 (PE.7)
  before anesthesia, 67–68 (PE.1.7.1–PE.1.7.3); 85 (TX.2)
  defined in writing, 73 (PE.4)
  diagnostic testing, 66 (PE.1.4–PE.1.4.1)
  discharge planning, 66 (PE.1.5)
  emotional or behavioral disorders, 74–75 (PE.6)
  functional status, 65–66 (PE.1.3–PE.1.3.1)
  goal of, 61
  infant, child, or adolescent, 74 (PE.5)
  initial, 66–67 (PE.1.6–PE.1.6.1.1)
  nursing, 66–67 (PE.1.6.1); 73 (PE.4.3)
  nutritional status, 65–66 (PE.1.2)
  operative and other procedures, 67–68 (PE.1.7); 94 (TX.5.1–TX.5.1.4)
  patient and family education, 116–117 (PF.1–PF.1.8)
  physical, psychological, and social status, 65 (PE.1)
  postoperative, 67–68 (PE.1.7.4); 86 (TX.2.4–TX.2.4.1)
  reassessment, 72 (PE.2–PE.2.4)
  scope and intensity of, 65 (PE.1.1); 73 (PE.4.1–PE.4.3)
  victims of abuse or neglect, 76 (PE.8)
  waived testing, 70–72 (PE.1.10–PE.1.14.2)
Patient care
  anesthesia, 85–86 (TX.2–TX.2.4.1)
  appropriate for patient needs, 83–84 (TX.1–TX.1.1.1)

Index

collaborative planning, 84 (TX.1.2)
ethical issues in, 50 (RI.1)
evaluation of plans and goals, 84 (TX.1.3)
family participation in decisions, 52 (RI.1.2.2)
goal of, 77
information from patient assessment, 72 (PE.3–PE.3.1)
integrating and coordinating, 157–158 (LD.3–LD.3.4)
hospitalwide plan, 149 (LD.1.3)
medical staff role in, 267–270, 274 (MS.6.5–MS.6.8)
medication, 86–90 (TX.3–TX.3.9)
nutrition, 90–93 (TX.4–TX.4.7)
operative and other procedures, 93–95 (TX.5–TX.5.4)
patient involvement in, 51 (RI.1.2)
patients under legal or correctional restrictions, 149 (LD.1.1.3)
practitioner authorized to manage, 268–269 (MS.6.5–MS.6.5.2)
privacy, 84 (TX.1.2.1)
rehabilitation care and services, 96–98 (TX.6–TX.6.4)
resolving dilemmas, 52–53 (RI.1.2.3)
self-administration of medications, 90 (TX.3.7)
settings and services, 83 (TX.1.1)
sources outside hospital, 150–151 (LD.1.3.4.2)
special interventions, 98–111 (TX.7–TX.7.5.5)
uniform quality of, 153 (LD.1.6); 269–270 (MS.6.8)
Patient needs
care, treatment, rehabilitation appropriate to, 83 (TX.1–TX.1.1)
decisions not to address, 84 (TX.1.1.1)
restraint or seclusion, 104 (TX.7.1.3.1.6)
Patient responsibilities, 116 (PF.1.9)
Patient rights, 47–60
advance directives, 53 (RI.1.2.4)
care at the end of life, 54 (RI.1.2.7)
in clinical trials, 57 (RI.3–RI.3.1)
communication, 54–55 (RI.1.3.6–RI.1.3.6.1.1)
confidentiality, 54–55 (RI.1.3.1)
ethical issues, 50 (RI.1)
family participation, 52 (RI.1.2.2)
life-sustaining treatment, 53 (RI.1.2.6)
pastoral care and spiritual services, 54–55 (RI.1.3.5)
to perform or refuse to perform tasks, 57–58 (RI.4.3)
privacy, 54–55 (RI.1.3.2)
protective services, 55 (RI.1.5)
research project, 51–52 (RI.1.2.1.1–RI.1.2.1.5); 57 (RI.3–RI.3.1)
resolution of complaints, 54–55 (RI.1.3.4)
restraint and seclusion, 102–103 (TX.7.1.3.1.1)
security, 54–55 (RI.1.3.3)
treatment or service, 50 (RI.1.1)
withholding resuscitative services, 53 (RI.1.2.5)
written statement of, 55 (RI.1.4)
Peer input to credentialing, 259–260 (MS.5.7)
Perception of care and service, 137
Performance
defined, 298
dimensions of, 130–131
Performance area, 298

Performance improvement
achievement and sustenance, 142 (PI.5)
changes identified, 141 (PI.4.4)
data aggregation, 139–140 (PI.4–PI.4.2)
data collection, 135–138 (PI.3–PI.3.1.3)
defined, 298
designing measures into processes, 133–135 (PI.2.1–PI.2.2)
dimensions of performance, 130–131
goal of, 129
intense analysis, 140–141 (PI.4.3)
leadership role in, 133 (PI.1–PI.1.1); 151 (LD.1.4); 158–162 (LD.4–LD.4.5)
medical staff role in, 270–272 (MS.8–MS.8.4)
planning priorities, 151 (LD.1.4)
Performance measure, 298
Performance Report, 21, 23–24
Personal hygiene
hospital support, 184–185 (EC.4.2)
patient education, 117–118 (PF.1.10)
Pharmaceutical equivalence, defined, 298
Pharmacist, defined, 298
Pharmacy, defined, 298
Physical abuse, defined, 281
Physical examination, 66–67 (PE.1.6.1–PE.1.6.1.1); 67–68 (PE.1.7)
persons authorized to perform, 267–268, 269, 273–274 (MS.6.2–MS.6.2.2.3)
Physical restraint, defined, 304
Physical therapist
assistant, qualified, defined, 298
qualified, defined, 298–299
Physical therapy aide, defined, 299
Physical therapy services, 29
Physician, qualified, defined, 299
Physician licensure, 29
Physiological monitoring
during anesthesia, 86 (TX.2.3)
Plan for improvement, defined, 299
Plan of care
defined, 299
operative and other procedures, 95 (TX.5.3)
Plan of correction, defined, 299
in conditional accreditation, defined, 299
Planning
design process, 134 (PI.2)
hospitalwide, 133 (PI.1–PI.1.1)
leadership, 148 (LD.1–LD.1.1.1)
legal or correctional restrictions, 149 (LD.1.1.3)
patient care services, 149 (LD.1.3)
Podiatrist, 268, 269 (MS.6.2.2.3); defined, 300
Poetry therapy, defined, 300
Point-of-care testing, defined, 300
Policies and procedures, defined, 300
collaborative, 158 (LD.3.4)
governance responsibilities and, 223 (GO.2.5)
nursing, 278–279 (NR.2–NR.4)

317

Practice guidelines, defined, 300
Preliminary nonaccreditation, 36; defined, 282
    appeal, 34
Preliminary reports, 1–3, 33
Prescribing, defined, 300
Primary source, defined, 300
Prisoners, care of, 149 (LD.1.1.3)
Privacy
    environment of care, 185 (EC.4.3)
    patient care procedures, 84 (TX.1.2.1)
    patient right to, 54–55 (RI.1.3.2)
Privileging, defined, 300
Process
    defined, 300
    design of, 133–135 (PI.2–PI.2.2)
Program, defined, 300
Protective services
    defined, 300–301
    patient right to access, 55 (RI.1.5)
Provisional accreditation, 11–12, 36; defined, 281
Psychiatric nurse, qualified, defined, 301
Psychiatric services, 269 (MS.6.6–MS.6.7)
Psychiatrist, qualified, defined, 301
Psychodrama therapy, defined, 301
Psychologist, qualified, defined, 301
Psychosurgery, 106 (TX.7.3)
Psychotropic medication, defined, 301
Public information interview, 28–29, 44–45
    conduct of, 29–30
    eligibility, 30
    scheduling, 30
Public Information Policy, 20–23, 301
    performance reports, 21

Q
Qualified individual, defined, 301
    infection control, defined, 301
Quality improvement, defined, 301
Quality of care, defined, 301

R
Radiologic technologist, qualified, defined, 301–302
Reassessment, 72 (PE.2–PE.2.4); defined, 302
Recommendation, defined, 302
    supplemental, defined, 302
    type I, defined, 302
Recreational therapist
    assistant or technician, qualified, defined, 302
    qualified, defined, 302–303
Reference database, defined, 303
Reference laboratories, 69–70 (PE.1.9.2–PE.1.9.2.2)
Referral, defined, 303
    information exchange, 126 (CC.7)
    procedures, 125–126 (CC.6)
Registered dietitian, defined, 303

Registered nurse, defined, 303
Rehabilitation care and services
    discharge planning, 98 (TX.6.4)
    education of patient and family, 116 (PF.1.6)
    plan, 97–98 (TX.6.1–6.2)
    provided by qualified professionals, 96 (TX.6)
    purpose, 98 (TX.6.3)
Rehabilitation techniques, patient and family education, 116–117 (PF.1.6)
Research project, patient rights in, 51–52 (RI.1.2.1.1–RI.1.2.1.5); 57 (RI.3)
Residential program, defined, 303
Respect and caring, 131; defined, 303
Respiratory care services, defined, 303
Respiratory care technician, certified, defined, 303
Respiratory therapist, defined, 303
Respiratory therapy technician, defined, 303
Restraint. *See also* Restraint and seclusion
    appropriate and safe use, 109 (TX.7.5.2)
    chemical, defined, 304
    criteria for clinically justified use, 110 (TX.7.5.3.2)
    defined, 99, 303–304
    documentation, 111 (TX.7.5.5)
    individual order, 109–110 (TX.7.5.3–TX.7.5.3.1)
    nonpsychiatric care, 107–111 (TX.7.5–TX.7.5.5)
    opportunities to reduce risk, 108–109 (TX.7.5.1)
    organizational oversight of, 108 (TX.7.5)
    patient monitoring, 111 (TX.7.5.4)
    physical, defined, 304
Restraint and seclusion. *See also* Restraint; Seclusion
    based on assessed needs of patient, 103 (TX.7.1.3.1.2)
    correct use, 103–104 (TX.7.1.3.1.4)
    documentation in medical records, 105 (TX.7.1.3.2)
    individual orders for, 102 (TX.7.1.3.1)
    least-restrictive, 103 (TX.7.1.3.1.3)
    limiting to clinically justified situations, 100–101 (TX.7.1–TX.7.1.1.7)
    opportunities to reduce reliance on, 101 (TX.7.1.2)
    ordered by LIP, 104–105 (TX.7.1.3.1.7)
    organization policies and procedures, 102 (TX.7.1.3)
    patient monitoring, 104 (TX.7.1.3.1.5)
    patient needs, 104 (TX.7.1.3.1.6)
    patient rights, 102–103 (TX.7.1.3.1.1)
    time limits, 105 (TX.7.1.3.1.8)
Resuscitative services, withholding, 53 (RI.1.2.5)
Risk management activities, defined, 304
Root cause analysis, 18, 141 (PI.4.3)
Run chart, defined, 304

S
Safety, 131, defined, 304. *See also* Life safety
    assessment, 182–183 (EC.3.2)
    maintenance, testing, inspection, 179 (EC.2.11)
    management plan, 167 (EC.1.3); 175 (EC.2.2)
Safety committee, 183 (EC.3.2–EC.3.3)
Safety director. *See* Safety officer

Index

Safety management, defined, 304
Safety officer, 182 (EC.3.1)
Satisfaction, 137
Scope of care or services, defined, 304
Seclusion
    defined, 99
    See also Restraint and seclusion
Security
    data and information, 200–201 (IM.2–IM.2.3)
    management plan, 168 (EC.1.4); 175 (EC.2.3)
Selected List of Books and Journals for the Small Medical Library, 212
Sentinel event, 14; defined, 304–305
    data collection, 137–138 (PI.3.1.1)
    identifying and managing, 161 (LD.4.3.4)
    procedures, 17–20
    process flow, 16
    reporting of, to Joint Commission, 14–15
Setting patient care goals, 83 (TX.1.1)
Sexual abuse, defined, 281
Significant adverse drug reaction, 140 (PI.4.3); defined, 305
Significant medication error, 140 (PI.4.3); defined, 305
Single accreditation awards, 9–10
Smoking, 185–186 (EC.5–EC.5.1)
Snacks, 92 (TX.4.1.1)
Social work assistant, defined, 305
Social work services, defined, 305
Social worker, qualified, defined, 305
Special procedures, safe and appropriate use, 98 (TX.7).
    See also Behavior management; Electroconvulsive therapy; Psychosurgery; Restraint; Restraint and Seclusion
Specialty board, 249
Speech-language pathologist, qualified, defined, 305
Speech-language pathology services, defined, 305
Spiritual services, patient right to, 54–55 (RI.1.3.5)
Staff. *See also* Medical staff; Nursing staff
    competence, 189–190 (HR.3); 191 (HR.4.3); 192 (HR.5)
    defined, 305
    forensic, 191 (HR.4.1)
    leadership role in development, 154 (LD.1.9–LD.1.9.1)
    number of, 189 (HR.2)
    orientation and education, 174–175 (EC.2.1); 190–191 (HR.4–HR.4.3)
    performance expectations, 189 (HR.1)
    qualifications, 189 (HR.1)
    requests not to participate in procedure, 192 (HR.6–HR.6.2)
    self-development, 190 (HR.3.1)
Standard, defined, 305
Statement of Conditions™ (SOC™), defined, 305
    compliance document, 166 (EC.1.1)

Subacute care, defined, 306
Substance-abuse services, 269 (MS.6.6–MS.6.7)
Summary grid score, defined, 306
Surgery, patient assessment for, 67–68 (PE.1.7–PE.1.7.4). *See also* Operative and other procedures
Surrogate decision maker, defined, 306
Survey fees, 24
Survey team, defined, 306
Surveyor, defined, 306
Surveyor Laptop Technology Project, 1

T

Tailored survey, 9; defined, 306
Therapeutic equivalence, defined, 306
Timeliness, 130; defined, 306
Transfer, defined, 306
    code of ethics, 57–58 (RI.4.1)
    information exchange, 126 (CC.7)
    procedures, 125 (CC.6)
Transfusion, 94–95 (TX.5.2–TX.5.2.2)
    reaction, 140 (PI.4.3)
Transplantation services, 57 (RI.2)
Type I recommendation, defined, 302
    accreditation with and without, 35
    first-generation, defined, 302
    resolving, 38
    second-generation, defined, 302
    special, 11
    third-generation, defined, 302

U

Utilities management, defined, 306
Utility systems, defined, 306–307
    maintenance, testing, inspection, 181 (EC.2.14)
    management plan, 172–173 (EC.1.9); 177 (EC.2.8)
Utilization management, defined, 307

V

Variance, defined, 307
Variation, defined, 307
Verbal orders, 208 (IM.7.7)

W

Waived testing
    defined, 307
    patient assessment, 70–72 (PE.1.10–PE.1.14.2)
Ward, of legal system, 149 (LD.1.1.3)
World Wide Web, Joint Commission site, 3
Written progress report (WPR), defined, 307

Educational Products from the Joint Commission

The Joint Commission offers a wide variety of educational products to support your compliance, performance improvement, and survey preparation efforts. Some of these products are described below and on the following pages. To place an order or to request a free publications or hospital education programs catalog, call our Customer Service Center at 630/792-5800.

Accreditation Resources

Comprehensive Accreditation Manual for Hospitals: The Official Handbook (CAMH)

Updates for 1999!
These quarterly updates to the *CAMH* provide you more than an occasional change in standards—they give you new information on the accreditation process as it evolves, additional examples for all types of hospitals, the latest on performance measurement initiatives, and much more. They make the *CAMH* more than just a standards manual—it's your guidebook for ongoing accreditation compliance and performance improvement. Available in print or electronic formats (site licenses available).

Print
Refreshed *CAMH* Core (includes 1998 updates) (CAH-99) $325
1999 Subscription Update Service (CAH-99S) $225
Refreshed Core Manual and 1999 Subscription Update Service (CAH-991) $538

Electronic
Automated Refreshed *CAMH* Core (includes 1998 updates) (Disk: A-99; CD: A-99CD) $595
1999 Automated Subscription Update Service (Disk: A-99S; CD: A-99CDS) $395
Refreshed Automated Manual and 1999 Subscription Update Service (Disk: A-991;
CD: A-99CD1) $970

The Complete Guide to the 1999 Hospital Survey Process
Based on actual survey protocols, *The Complete Guide* explains exactly what happens, and when, on a hospital survey. This book guides you step-by-step through the entire survey process, with practical, relevant information to help all levels of staff prepare for survey.
SP-99 $55

The 1999 Hospital Survey Self-Assessment Checklist
Find out how ready you are for survey using this comprehensive self-assessment tool covering the standards in the *CAMH*. The easy-to-use design provides a tool for hospital staff to gauge their compliance with all hospital standards. The questions engage the reader to identify poor or noncompliance areas, note actions needed, identify who is responsible for implementing improvements, and track progress toward compliance. The yes/no format of the checklist provides clear, definitive answers regarding compliance.
SAC-100 $55

SCORE 100 for Hospitals, 1999 (software)
Released annually, *SCORE 100 for Hospitals* is an easy-to-use tool that provides everything an organization needs for effective assessment during survey preparation. Incorporating the information from the *CAMH*, *SCORE 100* uses the input you provide from your organizational self-assessment to project an accreditation decision and identify problem areas using the Joint Commission's aggregation and decision rules.
1999 Edition (S-99) $1,295
1999 Update to 1998 Edition (S-99U) $ 495

The Power Statement of Conditions™ (software)
The first electronic Statement of Conditions was developed to assist your efforts in creating and maintaining a fire-safe environment of care and in demonstrating compliance with Environment of Care standards. The Power SOC will help you survey your own facility, enter scores for the Statement of Conditions, and enter/track plans for improvements—freeing you from the need to hire expensive outside consulting services.
PC version (SOC-99) $495
Network version (SOCS-99) $995

General Resources
Medication Use: A Systems Approach to Reducing Errors
Appropriate medication prescribing, accurate dispensing and administration, and optimal medical use outcomes are becoming increasingly difficult to achieve in an environment of cost cutting and downsizing. Written by nationally recognized experts, this book provides a road map for developing or improving an effective medication use system that will help your organization provide high quality, cost-effective care.
MU-100 $60

Ethical Issues and Patient Rights Across the Continuum of Care
Health care professionals encounter ethical issues almost daily, yet many are uncertain about how to recognize and address them. This book provides a comprehensive guide to understanding ethical tenets and decision making, as well as meeting Joint Commission standards requirements.
EI-100 $45

Sentinel Events: Evaluating Cause and Planning Improvement
Serious and undesirable events in health care organizations should trigger analysis and response to minimize the risk of recurrence. *Sentinel Events* describes the types of errors and sentinel events that have been reported in health care organizations, how organizations can respond to these events, how sentinel events are investigated through root cause analysis, and the Joint Commission's policy on sentinel events.
SE-101 $50

Care of Patients: Examples of Compliance
This new publication will help you understand and meet standards by presenting actual examples of compliance in areas including preparation and dispensing of medications, emergency medications, and restraint and seclusion. Organized by Care of Patients grid elements, you can use the examples as models for adaptation to your own organization and patient population. This book also provides an overview

of appropriate Joint Commission standards and the survey process, and it identifies ways to demonstrate competence related to care of patients during a survey.
TX-100 $45

Information Management: Questions & Answers for Hospitals

Find answers to your questions about meeting Information Management standards for all types of hospitals. This practical, easy-to-understand Q & A guide covers the important issues your hospital faces every day in managing information. This book is directed to all hospital staff who use data and information to plan, provide, and improve patient care and organization processes.
IM-100 $55

The Medical Staff Handbook: A Guide to Joint Commission Standards

This new book gives your medical staff leaders and medical staff service professionals a comprehensive and practical resource to meet Joint Commission standards and to apply the standards to day-to-day activities. *The Medical Staff Handbook* discusses bylaws, rules and regulations, policy and procedure manuals, initial appointment and credentials review, competency assessment and clinical privileging, reappointment, and allied health professionals. Includes a complimentary copy of *The LIP's Guide to Credentials Review and Privileging*.
MS-500 $50

The LIP's Guide to Credentials Review and Privileging

Licensed independent practitioners will love this compact, easy-to-use pocket book. This companion to *The Medical Staff Handbook* outlines Joint Commission expectations, walks through the credentials review and privileging process from the LIP's perspective, and provides a checklist from common LIP activities and responsibilities. Available in a convenient 10-pack, which allows for distribution to all practicing LIPs.
MS-600 $49.50 per 10 pack

Addressing Staffing Needs for Patient Care

This new books provides a complete overview of Joint Commission staffing standards and how they are surveyed. *Addressing Staffing Needs* answers frequently asked questions about staffing requirements. It also describes the basic components of the survey process that pertain to staffing and includes example questions from surveyors. Case studies show cutting edge staffing methodologies for a variety of settings and populations served.
PC-100 $40

Maintaining Your Quality Edge

This three-ring binder addresses the how to's of standards compliance. It provides an assessment tool to help evaluate the strengths and weaknesses of your hospital's performance improvement system. *Maintaining Your Quality Edge (MQE)* is truly an indispensable companion to the *Comprehensive Accreditation Manual for Hospitals: The Official Handbook (CAMH)*. This three-in-one resource for ongoing survey preparation includes a self-assessment component, examples of compliance, and a networking directory. Like the *CAMH*, *MQE* offers updates. You'll receive updates and enhancements to the self-assessment tools, new examples of compliance from across the country, and updated names and numbers for the networking directory.

Base book (M-97)	$220
Base book and 4 updates (M-971)	$338
Updates only (M-97S)	$125

Clinical Improvement Action Guide
Edited by Eugene C. Nelson, DSc, MPH, Paul B. Batalden, MD, and Jeanne Ryer, MS
The *Clinical Improvement Action Guide* offers clinicians a practical workbook that can be used by front-line clinical teams for rapidly improving quality, reducing costs, and getting better results. This book includes contributions by nationally recognized experts on health care quality: Eugene C. Nelson, DSc, MPH; Paul B. Batalden, MD; Jeanne Ryer, MS; Brent James, MD, MStat; Christina C. Mahoney, RN, MSN; Julie J. Mohr, MSPH: and Stephen K. Plume, MD; with a foreword by Donald Berwick, MD, MPH.
AG-100 $45

Topics in Clinical Care Improvement
This new series of monographs explores the latest thinking on how to improve performance in challenging compliance areas related to Joint Commission standards. Each new monograph presents an overview of the topic and major issues, discusses standards requirements and common problem areas, relates the topic to performance improvement, and provides strategies to address problems and improve performance.

Advance Directives (CC-900)	$19.95
Age-Specific Competence (CC-300)	$19.95
Discharge Planning (CC-800)	$19.95
Geriatric Assessment in Hospitals (CC-700)	$19.95
Infection Control: Meeting Joint Commission Standards (CC-400)	$19.95
Medical Record Review (CC-600)	$19.95
Reducing Restraint Use in the Acute Care Environment (CC-100)	$19.95
Storing and Securing Medications (CC-200)	$19.95
Purchase all eight monographs for a special price (CC-1000)	$130.00

Lexikon: Dictionary of Health Care Terms, Organizations, and Acronyms, Second Edition
The *Lexikon* is a user-friendly reference to the health care language that will be used through the end of the millennium. It gathers thousands of health care words and phrases you will encounter in your day-to-day work. Terms from a broad variety of disciplines involved in health care are included. Main categories include health care quality terms, clinical terms, and business and organizational terms, including statistics, managed care, risk management, administration, legal cases and legislation, human resources, and more.
JC-600 $55

Periodicals
To order Joint Commission periodicals, please call 800/346-0085, ext. 558.

Environment of Care News
A new, information-filled newsletter publishes six times per year. It
- provides the latest information on environment of care standards and survey process;
- answers tough EC compliance questions;
- provides success stories, tips, and examples to help hospitals succeed on their next survey; and

- offers special tips for EC in multiple settings, including hospitals, ambulatory care, laboratories, long term care, and behavioral health care.

EC-98 $120.00
Canadian Rate: $142.40
International Rate: $132.00

Joint Commission Perspectives

The official newsletter of the Joint Commission brings you readable and useful information about accreditation, performance measurement, and quality improvement. Its mission is to support your efforts to improve the quality of care you provide. Six issues per year contain a variety of clear, accurate, and helpful articles about

- accreditation standards, revisions, and updates;
- interpretation of standards and scoring guidelines by authoritative Joint Commission experts;
- success stories from accredited organizations showing how they achieved high compliance scores;
- accreditation policy and procedure updates;
- theory and practical application of continuous quality improvement; and
- Joint Commission updates.

Price: $100.00
Canadian Rate: $119.84
International Rate: $112.00

The Joint Commission Journal on Quality Improvement

Quality information you can use, presented in a lively, reader-friendly format!

The health care quality field has come of age as today's health care providers face intense scrutiny of the quality and value of the care patients receive.

The Joint Commission Journal on Quality Improvement, a monthly, peer-reviewed journal, brings you authoritative, detailed accounts of how to measure, assess, and improve the quality of care. You'll find case studies, success stories, and interviews with practical advice and suggestions straight from the practitioners and experts in quality measurement and improvement. Articles show you methods, approaches, and programs you can adapt to your own organization.

Subscription Price: $145.00
Canadian Rate: $165.85
International Rate: $155.00

Videos

When Bad Things Happen to Good Health Care Organizations: Responding Appropriately to a Sentinel Event

These two new videos explain the Joint Commission's Sentinel Event Policy and how to develop a methodology for responding appropriately to a sentinel event. In Part One you learn about the legal issues of the Sentinel Event Policy, what constitutes a reportable sentinel event, and how to report a sentinel event. In Part Two you learn how about how to conduct a root cause analysis, effective risk reduction and measurement strategies, and how the Joint Commission processes root cause analysis reports.

Part One: Meeting the Joint Commission Sentinel Event Policy Requirements (V98/03) $195
Part Two: How to Respond to a Sentinel Event (V98/04) $195
Parts One and Two (V98/75) $330

Solving the Mystery...Competence Assessment
Get the straight facts regarding the Joint Commission requirements relating to assessing, measuring, and improving the competence of all employees (clinical and nonclinical) across your organization. Examples from organizations that have been successful in "taking the mystery out" of competence assessment are featured, along with key information that will assist you in understanding and meeting the Joint Commission standards relating to competency.
V97/08 $195

Assessing Age-Specific Competencies: A Case Study Approach
Compare your own approach to assessing age-specific competencies with our case study and learn new, practical approaches to develop, implement, and assess age-specific competencies for all levels of staff throughout your organization.
V97/02 $195

Measuring, Assessing and Improving Competency for Non-Direct Patient Care Providers
Through this video's case studies, you will understand how to identify competencies required for non-clinical staff and assess how well you are meeting the standards, from new employee orientation to ongoing evaluation. This video contains useful information for human resource professionals, department heads, supervisors, and all others who conduct performance appraisals.

V95/50	$195
Order two competency videos	$330
Order all three competency videos (V97/20)	$485

Your Video Guide to the Hospital Survey Process
View key survey process activities prior to your survey! Each 20- to 30-minute video reviews one or more survey activities and answers commonly asked questions.

The video series covers the following survey activities:
- Document Review Session (V-61)
- Medical Staff Activities (V-62)
- Performance Improvement Overview Presentation (V-63)
- Leadership Interview; CEO Strategic Planning; Resource Allocation Interview (V-64)
- Human Resources Interview (V-65)

Order as a set, as a group of three, or individually.

Order the complete set of five videos (V-80)	$650
Order individual tapes (see above order codes)	$160
Order any three topics	$440